Pulmonary Manifestations of Pediatric Diseases

Editor

NELSON L. TURCIOS

PEDIATRIC CLINICS OF NORTH AMERICA

www.pediatric.theclinics.com

Consulting Editor

BONITA F. STANTON

February 2021 • Volume 68 • Number 1

ELSEVIER

1600 John F. Kennedy Boulevard • Suite 1800 • Philadelphia, Pennsylvania, 19103-2899

http://www.theclinics.com

THE PEDIATRIC CLINICS OF NORTH AMERICA Volume 68, Number 1
February 2021 ISSN 0031-3955, ISBN-13: 978-0-323-83614-2

Editor: Kerry Holland
Developmental Editor: Casey Potter

The Pediatric Clinics of North America (ISSN 0031-3955) is published bimonthly by Elsevier Inc., 360 Park Avenue South, New York, NY 10010-1710. Months of issue are February, April, June, August, October, and December. Periodicals postage paid at New York, NY and additional mailing offices. Subscription prices are $250.00 per year (US individuals), $984.00 per year (US institutions), $315.00 per year (Canadian individuals), $1048.00 per year (Canadian institutions), $376.00 per year (international individuals), $1048.00 per year (international institutions), $100.00 per year (US students and residents), $100.00 per year (Canadian students and residents), and $165.00 per year (international residents and students). To receive students/resident rare, orders must be accompanied by name of affiliated institution, date of term, and the signature of program/residency coordinator on institution letterhead. Orders will be billed at individual rate until proof of status is received. Foreign air speed delivery is included in all *Clinics* subscription prices. All prices are subject to change without notice. **POSTMASTER:** Send address changes to *The Pediatric Clinics of North America*, Elsevier Health Sciences Division, Subscription Customer Service, 3251 Riverport Lane, Maryland Heights, MO 63043. **Customer Service: 1-800-654-2452 (US and Canada). From outside of the US and Canada: 1-314-447-8871. Fax: 1-314-447-8029. For print support, E-mail: JournalsCustomerService-usa@elsevier.com. For online support, E-mail: JournalsOnlineSupport-usa@elsevier.com.**

Reprints. For copies of 100 or more, of articles in this publication, please contact the Commercial Reprints Department, Elsevier Inc., 360 Park Avenue South, New York, NY 10010-1710. Tel.: 212-633-3874; Fax: 212-633-3820; E-mail: reprints@elsevier.com.

The Pediatric Clinics of North America is also published in Spanish by McGraw-Hill Inter-americana Editores S.A., Mexico City, Mexico; in Portuguese by Riechmann and Affonso Editores, Rua Comandante Coelho 1085, CEP 21250, Rio de Janeiro, Brazil; and in Greek by Althayia SA, Athens, Greece.

The Pediatric Clinics of North America is covered in *MEDLINE/PubMed (Index Medicus), Excerpta Medica, Current Contents, Current Contents/Clinical Medicine, Science Citation Index, ASCA, ISI/BIOMED*, and *BIOSIS*.

PROGRAM OBJECTIVE

The goal of the *Pediatric Clinics of North America* is to keep practicing physicians and residents up to date with current clinical practice in pediatrics by providing timely articles reviewing the state-of-the-art in patient care.

TARGET AUDIENCE

All practicing pediatricians, physicians and healthcare professionals who provide patient care to pediatric patients.

LEARNING OBJECTIVES

Upon completion of this activity, participants will be able to:

1. Review pathophysiologic issues, common congenital myopathies, and interventions that may help prevent respiratory complications and improve quality of life.
2. Discuss the impact various medical conditions, not primarily associated with the lung, have on pulmonary structure and function.
3. Recognize the importance of addressing air pollution and climate change, and the role they play in childhood lung disease as well as the adverse impact on human health overall.

ACCREDITATIONS

Physician Credit

The Elsevier Office of Continuing Medical Education (EOCME) is accredited by the Accreditation Council for Continuing Medical Education (ACCME) to provide continuing medical education for physicians.

The EOCME designates this journal-based activity for a maximum of 18 *AMA PRA Category 1 Credit*(s)™. Physicians should claim only the credit commensurate with the extent of their participation in the activity.

All other healthcare professionals requesting continuing education credit for this this journal-based activity will be issued a certificate of participation.

ABP Maintenance of Certification Credit

Successful completion of this CME activity, which includes participation in the activity and individual assessment of and feedback to the learner, enables the learner to earn up to 18 MOC points in the American Board of Pediatrics' (ABP) Maintenance of Certification (MOC) program. It is the CME activity provider's responsibility to submit learner completion information to ACCME for the purpose of granting ABP MOC credit.

DISCLOSURE OF CONFLICTS OF INTEREST

The EOCME assesses conflict of interest with its instructors, faculty, planners, and other individuals who are in a position to control the content of CME activities. All relevant conflicts of interest that are identified are thoroughly vetted by EOCME for fair balance, scientific objectivity, and patient care recommendations. EOCME is committed to providing its learners with CME activities that promote improvements or quality in healthcare and not a specific proprietary business or a commercial interest.

The planning committee, staff, authors and editors listed below have identified no financial relationships or relationships to products or devices they or their spouse/life partner have with commercial interest related to the content of this CME activity:

Adriana Asturizaga, MD, MSc; John R. Bach, MD; Alexander A. Broomfield, MBBS; Mary M. Buckley, MD; Paulo Augusto Moreira Camargos, MD, PhD; Regina Chavous-Gibson, MSN, RN; Bernard A. Cohen, MD; Lama Elbahlawan, MD; Julie L. Fierro, MD; Dominic A. Fitzgerald, MBBS, PhD; Antonio Moreno Galdo, MD; Leah Githinji, MD, PhD; Robert Giusti, MD; John Grayhack, MD, MS; Alexandra Heath-Freudenthal, MD, MSc; Kerry Holland; Manju Hurvitz, MD; Brandy N. Johnson, MD; Muserref Kasap Cuceoglu, MD; Emily R. Le Fevre, MBBS; Nair Lovaton, MD; Laura Malaga-Dieguez, MD, PhD; Rajkumar Mayakrishnann; Kathleen H. McGrath, FRACP, MBBS, BSc(Med); Theresa J. Ochoa, MD, PhD; Seza Ozen, MD; Susan E. Pacheco, MD; Raja Padidela, MD; Howard B. Panitch, MD; Beth A. Pletcher, MD; C. Egla Rabinovich, MD, MPH; Raul C. Ribeiro, MD; Jose Serpa, MD, MS; Diane Dudas Sheehan, ND, APN, FNP-BC; Peter D. Sly, MBBS, MD, DSc; James M. Stark, MD, PhD; Howard Trachtman, MD; Nelson L. Turcios, MD; Nelson Villca, MD, MPH; Liping Wang, MD; Kimberly Danieli Watts, MD, MS; Miles Weinberger, MD; Stuart Wilkinson, MBchB; Teena Huan Xu, MD; Heather J. Zar, MD, PhD; Gustavo Zubieta-Calleja, MD; Natalia Zubieta-DeUrioste, MD

UNAPPROVED/OFF-LABEL USE DISCLOSURE

The EOCME requires CME faculty to disclose to the participants:

- When products or procedures being discussed are off-label, unlabelled, experimental, and/or investigational (not US Food and Drug Administration [FDA] approved); and
- Any limitations on the information presented, such as data that are preliminary or that represent ongoing research, interim analyses, and/or unsupported opinions. Faculty may discuss information about pharmaceutical agents that is outside of FDA-approved labelling. This information is intended solely for CME and is not intended to promote off-label use of these medications. If you have any questions, contact the medical affairs department of the manufacturer for the most recent prescribing information.

TO ENROLL

To enroll in the *Pediatric Clinics of North America* Continuing Medical Education program, call customer service at 1-800-654-2452 or sign up online at http://www.theclinics.com/home/cme. The CME program is available to subscribers for an additional annual fee of USD 324.00.

METHOD OF PARTICIPATION

In order to claim credit, participants must complete the following:

- Complete enrolment as indicated above.
- Read the activity.
- Complete the CME Test and Evaluation. Participants must achieve a score of 70% on the test. All CME Tests and Evaluations must be completed online.

In order to claim MOC points, participants must complete the following:

- Complete steps listed above for claiming CME credit
- Provide your specialty board ID#, birth date (MM/DD), and attestation.
- Online MOC submission is only available for the American Board of pediatrics' (ABP) Maintenance of Certification (MOC) program

CME INQUIRIES/SPECIAL NEEDS

For all CME inquiries or special needs, please contact elsevierCME@elsevier.com.

Contributors

CONSULTING EDITOR

BONITA F. STANTON, MD
Founding Dean, and Robert C. and Laura C. Garrett Endowed Chair, Hackensack Meridian School of Medicine, President, Academic Enterprise, Hackensack Meridian Health, Nutley, New Jersey, USA

EDITOR

NELSON L. TURCIOS, MD
Professor of Pediatrics, Hackensack Meridian School of Medicine, Nutley, New Jersey, USA

AUTHORS

ADRIANA ASTURIZAGA, MD
Pediatric Pulmonology Consultant, Hospital de la Banca Privada, La Paz, Bolivia

JOHN R. BACH, MD
Professor of Physical Medicine and Rehabilitation and Neurology, Department of Physical Medicine and Rehabilitation, Rutgers University, New Jersey Medical School, Newark, New Jersey, USA

ALEXANDER A. BROOMFIELD, MBBS
Willink Biochemical Genetics Unit, Manchester Centre for Genomic Medicine, St. Mary's Hospital, Manchester University NHS Foundation Trust, Manchester, United Kingdom

MARY M. BUCKLEY, MD
Fellow, Department of Pediatrics, Division of Rheumatology, Duke University Medical Center, Durham, North Carolina, USA

PAULO CAMARGOS, MD, PhD
Professor, Department of Pediatrics, Medical School, Pediatric Pulmonology Unit, University Hospital, Federal University of Minas Gerais, Belo Horizonte, Brazil

BERNARD A. COHEN, MD
Professor of Pediatrics and Dermatology, Division of Pediatric Dermatology, Johns Hopkins Children's Center, Baltimore, Maryland, USA

MUSERREF KASAP CUCEOGLU, MD
Fellow, Department of Pediatric Rheumatology, Hacettepe University, Ankara, Turkey

LAMA ELBAHLAWAN, MD
Division of Critical Care, Department of Pediatrics, St. Jude Children's Research Hospital, Memphis, Tennessee, USA

JULIE L. FIERRO, MD
Attending Physician, Division of Pulmonary Medicine, Assistant Professor of Clinical Pediatrics, The Perelman School of Medicine at the University of Pennsylvania, Children's Hospital of Philadelphia, Philadelphia, Pennsylvania, USA

DOMINIC A. FITZGERALD, MBBS, PhD, FRACP
Paediatric Respiratory and Sleep Physician, Department of Respiratory Medicine, The Children's Hospital at Westmead, Westmead, New South Wales, Australia; Clinical Professor of Paediatric Respiratory and Sleep Medicine, Faculty Health Sciences, University of Sydney, Sydney, New South Wales, Australia

ANTONIO MORENO GALDO, MD
Pediatric Pulmonology Section, Hospital Vall d2b9Hebron, Universitat Autònoma de Barcelona, Barcelona, Spain

LEAH GITHINJI, MD, PhD
Department of Paediatrics and Child Health, South Africa MRC Unit on Child and Adolescent Health, University of Cape Town, Red Cross War Memorial Children's Hospital, Rondebosch, South Africa

ROBERT GIUSTI, MD
Division of Pediatric Pulmonology, Department of Pediatrics, NYU School of Medicine, Hassenfeld Children's Hospital at NYU Langone, New York, New York, USA

JOHN GRAYHACK, MD, MS
Orthopaedic Surgeon, Division of Orthopaedic Surgery and Sports Medicine, Ann and Robert H. Lurie Children's Hospital of Chicago, Professor, Department of Orthopaedic Surgery, Feinberg School of Medicine of Northwestern University, Chicago, Illinois, USA

ALEXANDRA HEATH-FREUDENTHAL, MD, PhD
Pediatric Cardiology Consultant, Kardiozentrum, La Paz, Bolivia

MANJU HURVITZ, MD
Senior Fellow in Pediatric Pulmonology, Rady Children's Hospital, University of California San Diego, San Diego, California, USA

BRANDY N. JOHNSON, MD
Fellow, Pediatric Pulmonology, Division of Pulmonary Medicine, Children's Hospital of Philadelphia, Philadelphia, Pennsylvania, USA

CHRYSOULA KOSMERI, MD, PhD
Department of Pediatrics, University Hospital of Ioannina, Ioannina, Greece

EMILY R. LE FEVRE, MBBS
Paediatric Registrar, Department of Respiratory Medicine, The Children's Hospital at Westmead, Westmead, New South Wales, Australia

NAIR LOVATON, MD
Assistant Professor, Department of Pediatrics, Faculty of Medicine, Universidad Peruana Cayetano Heredia, Lima, Peru

ALEXANDROS MAKIS, MD, PhD
Associate Professor in Pediatrics/Pediatric Hematology, Department of Pediatrics, Faculty of Medicine, University of Ioannina, Ioannina, Greece

LAURA MALAGA-DIEGUEZ, MD, PhD
Division of Pediatric Nephrology, Department of Pediatrics, NYU School of Medicine, Hassenfeld Children's Hospital at NYU Langone, New York, New York, USA

KATHLEEN H. McGRATH, MBBS, BSc(Med), FRACP
Paediatric Gastroenterologist, Department of Gastroenterology and Clinical Nutrition, The Royal Children's Hospital, Parkville, Victoria, Australia; Clinical Fellow, Department of Paediatrics, The University of Melbourne, Melbourne, Victoria, Australia

THERESA J. OCHOA, MD, PhD
Associate Professor, Department of Pediatrics, Faculty of Medicine, Instituto de Medicina Tropical Alexander von Humboldt, Universidad Peruana Cayetano Heredia, Lima, Peru

SEZA OZEN, MD
Professor of Pediatrics, Department of Pediatric Rheumatology, Hacettepe University, Ankara, Turkey

SUSAN E. PACHECO, MD
Professor, Department of Pediatrics, Division of Pulmonary Medicine, Allergy-Immunology, and Sleep, McGovern Medical School at UTHealth, Houston, Texas, USA

RAJA PADIDELA, MD
Department of Paediatric Endocrinology, Royal Manchester Children's Hospital, Faculty of Biology, Medicine and Health, University of Manchester, Manchester, United Kingdom

HOWARD B. PANITCH, MD
Director, Technology Dependence Center, Division of Pulmonary Medicine, Professor of Pediatrics, The Perelman School of Medicine at the University of Pennsylvania, Children's Hospital of Philadelphia, Philadelphia, Pennsylvania, USA

BETH A. PLETCHER, MD, FAAP, FACMG
Associate Professor, Departments of Pediatrics and Medicine, Rutgers New Jersey Medical School, Newark, New Jersey, USA

C. EGLA RABINOVICH, MD, MPH
Professor, Department of Pediatrics, Division of Rheumatology, Duke University Medical Center, Durham, North Carolina, USA

RAUL C. RIBEIRO, MD
Director, Leukemia/Lymphoma Division, Director, International Outreach Program, Department of Oncology, St. Jude Children's Research Hospital, Memphis, Tennessee, USA

JOSE SERPA, MD, MS
Associate Professor, Section of Infectious Diseases, Department of Medicine, Baylor College of Medicine, Houston, Texas, USA

DIANE DUDAS SHEEHAN, ND, APRN, FNP-BC
Advanced Practice Registered Nurse, Division of Orthopaedic Surgery and Sports Medicine, Ann and Robert H. Lurie Children's Hospital of Chicago, Assistant Professor, Department of Physical Medicine and Rehabilitation, Feinberg School of Medicine of Northwestern University, Chicago, Illinois, USA

EKATERINI SIOMOU, MD, PhD
Associate Professor of Pediatrics/Pediatric Nephrology, Department of Pediatrics, Faculty of Medicine, University of Ioannina, Ioannina, Greece

PETER D. SLY, AO, MBBS, MD, DSc
Director, Children's Health and Environment Program, Child Health Research Centre, The University of Queensland, South Brisbane, Queensland, Australia

JAMES M. STARK, MD, PhD
Professor, Department of Pediatrics, Division of Pulmonary Medicine, Allergy-Immunology, and Sleep, McGovern Medical School at UTHealth, Houston, Texas, USA

HOWARD TRACHTMAN, MD
Division of Pediatric Nephrology, Department of Pediatrics, NYU School of Medicine, Hassenfeld Children's Hospital at NYU Langone, New York, New York, USA

SOPHIA TSABOURI, MD, PhD
Associate Professor of Pediatrics and Pediatric Allergy, Department of Pediatrics, Faculty of Medicine, University of Ioannina, Ioannina, Greece

NELSON L. TURCIOS, MD
Professor of Pediatrics, Hackensack Meridian School of Medicine, Nutley, New Jersey, USA

NELSON VILLCA, MD, MPH
Pediatric Pulmonology Consultant, Hospital Materno Infantil, La Paz, Bolivia

LIPING WANG, MD
Department of Neurology, Peking University Third Hospital, Beijing, China

KIMBERLY DANIELI WATTS, MD, MS
Division of Pediatric Pulmonary Medicine, Advocate Children's Hospital, Park Ridge, Illinois, USA; Assistant Professor of Clinical Pediatrics, Rosalind Franklin University of Medicine and Science, North Chicago, Illinois, USA

MILES WEINBERGER, MD
Professor Emeritus, University of Iowa, Iowa City, Iowa, USA; Visiting Professor of Pediatrics, University of California San Diego, San Diego, Rady Children's Hospital, San Diego, California, USA

STUART WILKINSON, MBChB
Respiratory Department Royal Manchester Children's Hospital, Manchester University, NHS Foundation Trust, Manchester Academic Health Science Centre, Manchester, United Kingdom

TEENA HUAN XU, MD
Infectious Diseases Fellow, Section of Infectious Diseases, Department of Medicine, Baylor College of Medicine, Houston, Texas, USA

HEATHER J. ZAR, MD, PhD
Department of Paediatrics and Child Health, South Africa MRC Unit on Child & Adolescent Health, University of Cape Town, Red Cross War Memorial Children's Hospital, Rondebosch, South Africa

Contents

Foreword: Pediatric Pulmonary Disorders: A Combination of Breakthroughs and New Disorders xvii

Bonita F. Stanton

Preface: Lung Involvement in Pediatric Disorders xix

Nelson L. Turcios

Pulmonary Manifestations of Genetic Disorders in Children 1

Beth A. Pletcher and Nelson L. Turcios

Congenital bronchopulmonary malformations are relatively common and arise during various periods of morphogenesis. Although some are isolated or sporadic occurrences, others may result from single gene mutations or cytogenetic imbalances. Single gene mutations have been identified, which are etiologically related to primary pulmonary hypoplasia, lung segmentation defects as well as pulmonary vascular and lymphatic lesions. Functional defects in cystic fibrosis, primary ciliary dyskinesias, alpha-1-antitrypsin deficiency, and surfactant proteins caused by gene mutations may result in progressive pulmonary disease. This article provides an overview of pediatric pulmonary disease from a genetic perspective.

Pulmonary Manifestations of Congenital Heart Disease in Children 25

Brandy N. Johnson, Julie L. Fierro, and Howard B. Panitch

This review addresses how anomalous cardiovascular anatomy imparts consequences to the airway, respiratory system mechanics, pulmonary vascular system, and lymphatic system. Abnormal formation or enlargement of great vessels can compress airways and cause large and small airway obstructions. Alterations in pulmonary blood flow associated with congenital heart disease (CHD) can cause abnormalities in pulmonary mechanics and limitation of exercise. CHD can lead to pulmonary arterial hypertension. Lymphatic abnormalities associated with CHD can cause pulmonary edema, chylothorax, or plastic bronchitis. Understanding how the cardiovascular system has an impact on pulmonary growth and function can help determine options and timing of intervention.

Pulmonary Manifestations of Gastrointestinal, Pancreatic, and Liver Diseases in Children 41

Emily R. Le Fevre, Kathleen H. McGrath, and Dominic A. Fitzgerald

Pulmonary manifestations of gastrointestinal (GI) diseases are often subtle, and underlying disease may precede overt symptoms. A high index of suspicion and a low threshold for consultation with a pediatric pulmonologist is warranted in common GI conditions. This article outlines the pulmonary manifestations of different GI, pancreatic, and liver diseases

in incidence with early diagnosis and use of antiretroviral therapy (ART) but is widespread in areas with limited access to ART. HIV-exposed uninfected infants have a higher risk of LRTI early in life than unexposed infants. Pulmonary tuberculosis (PTB) presenting as acute or chronic disease is common in highly TB endemic areas. Chronic lung disease is common; preceding LRTI, PTB or late initiation of ART are risk factors.

Pulmonary Manifestations of Rheumatic Diseases in Children **147**

Mary M. Buckley and C. Egla Rabinovich

Children with rheumatic disease have rare pulmonary manifestations that may cause significant morbidity and mortality. These children are often clinically asymptomatic until disease has significantly progressed, so they should be screened for pulmonary involvement. There has been recent recognition of a high mortality-related lung disease in systemic-onset juvenile idiopathic arthritis; risk factors include onset of juvenile idiopathic arthritis less than 2 years of age, history of macrophage activation syndrome, presence of trisomy 21, and history of anaphylactic reaction to biologic therapy. Early recognition and treatment of lung disease in children with rheumatic diseases may improve outcomes.

Pulmonary Manifestations of Systemic Vasculitis in Children **167**

Muserref Kasap Cuceoglu and Seza Ozen

Vasculitides are defined according to the vessel size involved, and they tend to affect certain organ systems. Pulmonary involvement is rare in the common childhood vasculitides, such as Kawasaki disease, IgA vasculitis (Henoch Schonlein purpura). On the other hand, lung involvement is common in a rare pediatric vasculitis, granulomatosis with polyangiitis (GPA) (Wegener granulomatosis), where respiratory system findings are common. A criterion in the Ankara 2008 classification criteria for GPA is the presence of nodules, cavities, or fixed infiltrates. The adult data suggest that rituximab may be an alternative to cyclophosphamide in induction treatment.

Respiratory Complications of Pediatric Neuromuscular Diseases **177**

John R. Bach, Nelson L. Turcios, and Liping Wang

Respiration is an event of oxygen consumption and carbon dioxide production. Respiratory failure is common in pediatric neuromuscular diseases and the main cause of morbidity and mortality. It is a consequence of lung failure, ventilatory pump failure, or their combination. Lung failure often is due to chronic aspiration either from above or from below. It may lead to end-stage lung disease. Ventilatory pump failure is caused by increased respiratory load and progressive respiratory muscles weakness. This article reviews the normal function of the respiratory pump, general pathophysiology issues, abnormalities in the more common neuromuscular conditions and noninvasive interventions.

Pulmonary Manifestations of Skin Disorders in Children **261**

Bernard A. Cohen and Nelson L. Turcios

Systemic diseases often manifest with cutaneous findings. Many pediatric conditions with prominent skin findings also have significant pulmonary manifestations. These conditions include both inherited multisystem genetic disorders such as yellow-nail syndrome, neurofibromatosis type 1, tuberous sclerosis complex, hereditary hemorrhagic telangiectasia, Klippel–Trénaunay–Weber syndrome, cutis laxa, Ehlers–Danlos syndrome, dyskeratosis congenita, reactive processes such as mastocytosis, and aquagenic wrinkling of the palms. This overview discusses the pulmonary manifestations of skin disorders.

Adverse Environmental Exposure and Respiratory Health in Children **277**

Peter D. Sly

The burden imposed by pollution falls more on those living in low-income and middle-income countries, affecting children more than adults. Most air pollution results from incomplete combustion and contains a mixture of particulate matter and gases. Air pollution exposure has negative impacts on respiratory health. This article concentrates on air pollution in 2 settings, the child's home and the ambient environment. There is an inextricable 2-way link between air pollution and climate change, and the effects of climate change on childhood respiratory health also are discussed.

Inequalities and Inequities in Pediatric Respiratory Diseases **293**

Paulo Camargos and Kimberly Danieli Watts

Social inequality refers to disparities in society that have the effect of limiting a group's socioeconomic, educational, and intellectual potential. Inequity in health means any limitation to access comprehensive health services that also hinders the achievement of well-being and favorable health outcomes. Strategies for more equitable growth to eradicate global poverty would contribute to reducing health inequities and improve health care outcomes. Coordinated efforts between governments, private sector, families, and interested stakeholders are needed. This article discusses inequality and inequity in pediatric respiratory diseases, the challenges confronted, and the strategies needed to mitigate these disparities.

High-altitude Illnesses and Air Travel: Pediatric Considerations **305**

Nelson Villca, Adriana Asturizaga, Alexandra Heath-Freudenthal

Healthy children may present acute mountain sickness (AMS) within a few hours after arrival at high altitudes. In few cases, serious complications may occur, including high-altitude pulmonary edema and rarely high-altitude cerebral edema. Those with preexisting conditions especially involving hypoxia and pulmonary hypertension shall not risk travelling to high altitudes. Newborn from low altitude mothers may have prolonged time to complete postnatal adaptation. The number of children and adolescents traveling on commercial aircrafts is growing, and this poses a need for their treating physicians to be aware of the potential risks of hypoxia while air traveling.

Risk Factors for Severity in Children with Coronavirus Disease 2019: A Comprehensive Literature Review 321

Sophia Tsabouri, Alexandros Makis, Chrysoula Kosmeri, and Ekaterini Siomou

The coronavirus disease 2019 (COVID-19) pandemic has affected hundreds of thousands of people. The authors performed a comprehensive literature review to identify the underlying mechanisms and risk factors for severe COVID-19 in children. Children have accounted for 1.7% to 2% of the diagnosed cases of COVID-19. They often have milder disease than adults, and child deaths have been rare. The documented risk factors for severe disease in children are young age and underlying comorbidities. It is unclear whether male gender and certain laboratory and imaging findings are also risk factors. Reports on other potential factors have not been published.

PEDIATRIC CLINICS OF NORTH AMERICA

FORTHCOMING ISSUES

April 2021
Ending the War against Children: The Rights of Children to Live Free of Violence
Bonita Stanton and Danielle Laraque-Arena, *Editor*

June 2021
Integrated Behavioral Health in Pediatric Practice
Roger W. Apple, *Editor*

August 2021
Pediatric Neurosurgery in Primary Care
Jonathan Martin, *Editor*

RECENT ISSUES

December 2020
Max J Coppes and Leontine C.M. Kremer, *Editors*
Challenges After Treatment for Childhood Cancer

October 2020
Pediatric Cardiology
Pei-Ni Jone, D. Dunbar Ivy, Stephen R. Daniels, *Editors*

August 2020
Telehealth for Pediatricians
C. Jason Wang, Josip Car, and Barry S. Zuckerman, *Editors*

Foreword

Pediatric Pulmonary Disorders: A Combination of Breakthroughs and New Disorders

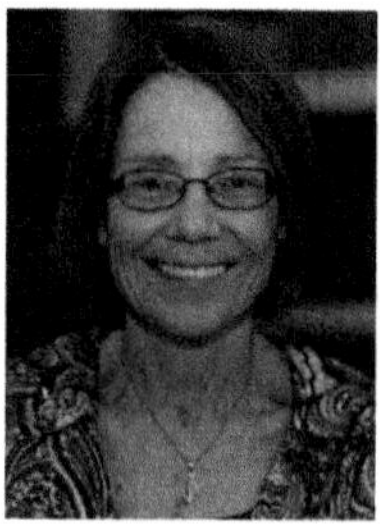

Bonita F. Stanton, MD
Consulting Editor

This issue of *Pediatric Clinics of North America* updates and summarizes our current understanding of the vast array of conditions leading to difficulties with the pulmonary system in children. The wide range of disorders that are not pulmonary in origin but are, or can be, associated with pulmonary manifestations is substantial and appears to be growing. The authors describe many common disorders associated with pulmonary compromise, including genetic, cardiac, gastrointestinal, rheumatologic, pancreatic, hepatic, endocrinologic, renal, dermatologic, and neuromuscular disorders. New information regarding the pulmonary manifestations of these disorders reflects advances in diagnosis and treatment as well as the emergence of some new disease entities, symptoms, and manifestations. Encouragingly, some of the newly identified pulmonary manifestations, such as some of the pulmonary complications of the human immunodeficiency disorders, reflects greater overall longevity of persons infected with the disease.

Appropriately, this issue also addresses emerging pulmonary issues resulting from global warming and its associated environmental challenges: increased air pollution and water pollution. Predicted in 1979,[1] global warming is now well described in the literature and well recognized as an international crisis.[2,3] "Climate change" includes global warming and associated conditions of increasing air pollution, water pollution, and ground-level ozone.[4,5] Although few of the myriad pulmonary disorders recognized are directly "caused" by global warming/climate change, the increases in global temperature and in the incidence and severity of wildfires appear to be contributing to the severity and incidence of pediatric pulmonary disease. Global warming directly triggers or aggravates preexisting respiratory diseases and increases exposure to risk factors (such as the increasing levels of ground-level ozone) for respiratory

Pediatr Clin N Am 68 (2021) xvii–xviii
https://doi.org/10.1016/j.pcl.2020.10.002 pediatric.theclinics.com
0031-3955/21/© 2020 Published by Elsevier Inc.

disorders. Ground-level ozone, a major component of "urban smog," results from a sun-induced chemical reaction between nitrogen oxide and organic compounds contained in emissions. It appears to be particularly harmful to children with asthma, causing airway inflammation and lung tissue damage.[4]

This update on pediatric pulmonary disorders is especially important, as it represents a broad look at the advances in the field combating known disorders and also alerts pediatricians and other child health providers to the growing reality of pulmonary health consequences for children resulting from the accelerated global warming.

Bonita F. Stanton, MD
Hackensack Meridian School of Medicine
340 Kingsland Street, Building 123
Nutley, NJ 07110, USA

E-mail address:
Bonita.Stanton@hackensackmeridian.org

REFERENCES

1. National Academy of Sciences: Ad hoc study group on carbon dioxide and climate: a scientific assessment. Washington, DC: National Academy of Sciences; 1979.
2. Asthma and Allergy Foundation Association of America. Climate and Health. Available at: https://www.aafa.org/climate-and-health/#:~:text=Climate%20change%20increases%20water%20and,respiratory%20disease%2C%20such%20as%20asthma.&text=Increased%20temperatures%20due%20to%20climate,inflammation%20and%20damages%20lung%20tissue. Accessed September 19, 2020.
3. Amato G, Cecchi L, Amato M, et al. Climate change and respiratory diseases. Eur Respir Rev 2014;23(132):161–9. Available at: http://err.ersjournals.com/content/23/132/161.full.
4. Amato G, Cagani CA, Cecchi L, et al. Climate change, air pollution, and extreme events leading to increasing prevalence of allergic respiratory diseases. Multidiscip Respir Med 2013;8(1):12. Available at: http://www.ncbi.nlm.nih.gov/pmc/articles/PMC3598823/pdf/2049-6958-8-12.pdf.
5. Environmental Protection Agency (EPA). Ground level ozone. Available at: http://www.epa.gov/groundlevelozone/index.html. Accessed September 19, 2020.

Preface

Lung Involvement in Pediatric Disorders

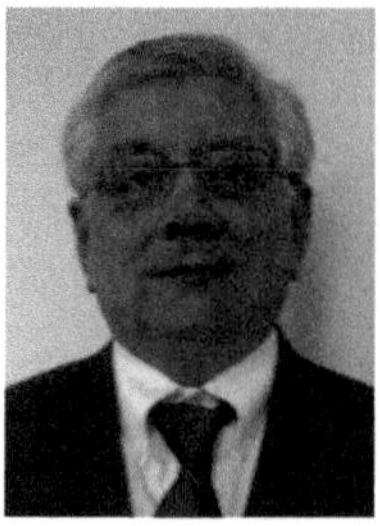

Nelson L. Turcios, MD
Editor

From its humble beginnings in the 1970s, pediatric pulmonology now has a considerable presence at all major children's hospitals worldwide. As the body of medical information grows and the field of pediatric pulmonology continues to expand, it has become increasingly evident that even those conditions not primarily associated with the lung will often have significant ramifications on lung structure and function.

It is upon these interactions and effects that this special issue of *Pediatric Clinics of North America* is focused. As such, we have attempted to compile in a series of articles many of the more intriguing pulmonary manifestations of many pediatric diseases. Genetic disorders discussed herein may help health practitioners recognize the underlying genetic cause for an apparently isolated pulmonary abnormality to better manage the patient, while providing the patients and their families with long-term prognostic and future reproductive information. In addition, this special issue spotlights the variety of ways in which congenital heart disease impacts the lung anatomically and pathophysiologically as well as the effects that cardiac surgery may have on pulmonary structure and function.

Pulmonary manifestations of different gastrointestinal, pancreatic, and liver diseases in children and adolescents are also reviewed. Respiratory complications are commonplace in pediatric hematologic and oncologic disorders, and these frequently present as pulmonary manifestations.

The section on the fields of both endocrinology and inborn errors of metabolism updates clinicians on lung involvement in these disorders. The respiratory complications in children and adolescents infected with the human immunodeficiency virus as well as those of other immunodeficiency and immunosuppressive disorders are also considered in depth.

The articles on rheumatic disease and systemic vasculitis examine the pulmonary manifestations in each subtype of pediatric rheumatic disease and the different forms

Pediatr Clin N Am 68 (2021) xix–xxi
https://doi.org/10.1016/j.pcl.2020.10.003
0031-3955/21/© 2020 Published by Elsevier Inc.

of small vessel vasculitis that affect the lung. The section on respiratory complications of neuromuscular disorders reviews pathophysiologic issues, common congenital myopathies, and interventions, including novel medications that may help prevent respiratory complications and improve quality of life.

The large spectrum of parasitic infestations linked to respiratory illnesses is illustrated in the related section. Pulmonary complications of renal diseases provide an understanding of the relationship between the kidney on fetal lung growth and how renal disease may disrupt pulmonary function. Many pediatric conditions with prominent dermatologic findings also have significant pulmonary manifestations, as described on pulmonary involvement of skin disorders.

The article on adverse environmental exposure and respiratory health in children highlights the vital importance of addressing air pollution in decreasing childhood lung disease and improving long-term lung health outcomes and climate change and the adverse impacts on human health as well.

Functional respiratory disorders characterized by persistent respiratory symptoms lacking an identifiable organic basis are examined, followed by a discussion of health care inequality and inequity on pediatric respiratory diseases, the challenges confronted, and the strategies needed, including redesigning medical education to mitigate these disparities.

The section on the pulmonary implications of primary structural spinal deformities describes the impact of developing surgical devices and procedures on respiratory function in affected pediatric patients. The writing on high-altitude illnesses and air travel reviews the expected physiological responses and the most relevant acute high-altitude illnesses, their prevention, and treatment and presents an overview of the most up-to-date recommendations to ensure the safety of children during air travel.

This special issue concludes with a timely comprehensive review that offers the clinician a balanced analysis of the literature on what is known from the cases reported to date on the risk factors for the progression and severity of coronavirus infection in infants and children. It also discusses the possible mechanisms underlying the unusual clinical features of coronavirus infection in children.

Although these outstanding clinical reviews have been contributed by some of the most prominent physicians from many of the world's most eminent institutions of higher learning, this special issue is notable in that many of these authors are not, in fact, pediatric pulmonologists. Thus, both pulmonologists and other health care practitioners whose patients have nonpulmonary diagnoses but also exhibit acute or chronic respiratory symptoms might welcome these contributors' perspectives.

Pulmonary manifestations of pediatric diseases are common but often undiagnosed or misdiagnosed. As such, the authors hope that their efforts lead to early recognition and prompt treatment of this very variable, but important, group of respiratory manifestations.

We hope that this special issue will become an invaluable source of information for medical students, pediatric residents, fellows, pediatricians, family practitioners, pediatric subspecialists, and other health professionals—to not only educate but also improve patient care, for this is and has always been our most important endeavor.

Nelson L. Turcios, MD
Hackensack Meridian School of Medicine
Nutley, NJ 07110, USA

E-mail address:
nelson.turcios@shu.edu

Pulmonary Manifestations of Genetic Disorders in Children

Beth A. Pletcher, MD[a,*], Nelson L. Turcios, MD[b]

KEYWORDS

- Pulmonary genetics • Congenital lung malformations
- Pediatric pulmonary disorders

KEY POINTS

- Congenital anomalies of the lung are relatively common and arise during various periods of morphogenesis. Although some are isolated or sporadic occurrences, others may result from single gene mutations or cytogenetic imbalances.
- Single gene mutations have been identified, which are etiologically related to primary pulmonary hypoplasia, lung segmentation defects as well as pulmonary vascular and lymphatic lesions.
- Functional defects in cystic fibrosis, primary ciliary dyskinesias, alpha-1-antitrypsin deficiency, and surfactant proteins caused by genetic mutations may result in progressive pulmonary disease.
- Some inborn errors of metabolism and connective tissue disorders are also associated with a host of pulmonary symptoms.
- Identification of a specific cause for pulmonary symptoms enables a provider to better manage the patient, while providing patients and families with important prognostic and future reproductive information.

INTRODUCTION

Congenital bronchopulmonary malformations (BPM) may occur as isolated anomalies resulting from disruptions of normal lung development as well as part of multiple anomaly syndromes. Myriad pulmonary findings are associated with certain cytogenetic conditions and many single gene disorders. This writing includes a discussion about prenatal lung development and various congenital bronchopulmonary anomalies. Genetic underpinnings for various pulmonary disorders are also reviewed and

[a] Department of Pediatrics, Rutgers New Jersey Medical School, Newark, NJ, USA; [b] Hackensack Meridian School of Medicine, Nutley, NJ 07110, USA
* Corresponding author. Doctor's Office Center, 90 Bergen Street, Suite 5400, Newark, NJ 07103.
E-mail address: pletchba@njms.rutgers.edu

Pediatr Clin N Am 68 (2021) 1–24
https://doi.org/10.1016/j.pcl.2020.09.010
pediatric.theclinics.com

outlined in detailed tables. Recognizing the underlying genetic cause for specific pulmonary disorders provides a foundation for making therapeutic decisions and counseling the patients and families about the long-term prognosis for the condition as well as reproductive risks for future children. In many cases, molecular genetic testing may confirm a suspected diagnosis, guide medical management, and augment decision making over time.

Congenital Bronchopulmonary Malformations

Embryologic development of the human lung transitions through distinct periods to form the tracheobronchial tree, as outlined in **Table 1**. It is hypothesized that developmental disruption of airway embryogenesis may result in a variety of anomalies, with type and histopathology both related to the timing of the embryonic insult.[1] Prenatal ultrasound (US) and ultrafast MRI have allowed a better definition of these lesions.

Most newborns with congenital BPM are asymptomatic. However, for some, the clinical presentation is variable: respiratory distress, stridor, bubbly oral secretions, failure to pass nasogastric tube, cyanosis, heart failure, or poor respiratory effort.

In later childhood/adolescence, presentations may be related to undetected or untreated congenital BPM: recurrent pneumonia in the same location, hemoptysis, heart failure, cyanosis, malignant changes, or unexpected chest radiograph finding. In this group, important considerations of congenital lung disease are the "steroid-resistant asthma" or "recurrent croup." Large airway narrowing (eg, tracheomalacia, vascular

Table 1
Morphogenic periods of human lung development

Period	Gestational Age (wk)	Developmental Processes	Typical Defects
Embryonic	3–6	Lung buds, trachea, main stem, lobar, and segmental bronchi	Tracheal, laryngeal and esophageal atresia, tracheal stenosis, TEFs, and bronchial malformations
Pseudoglandular	6–16	Subsegmental bronchi, terminal bronchioles, acinar tubules, mucous glands, cartilage, smooth muscle	Tracheobronchomalacia, cystic adenomatoid malformation, ectopic lobes, cyst formation, and pulmonary lymphangiectasia
Canicular	16–26	Respiratory bronchioles, acinus formation and vascularization, type I and type II cell differentiation	Pulmonary hypoplasia secondary to extrinsic compression or oligohydramnios
Saccular	26–36	Dilation and subdivision of alveolar saccules, increase of gas-exchange surface area	Pulmonary hypoplasia or CSL
Alveolar	36 to maturity	Further growth and alveolarization, maturation of alveolar-capillary network	Pulmonary hypoplasia or CSL

ring, or pulmonary artery sling) enters the differential diagnosis, and a physiologic clue comes from the flow-volume curve.

Lung agenesis and hypoplasia

Tracheal atresia accompanied by bilateral lung agenesis is most likely to arise as an isolated defect, possibly secondary to a vascular event occurring very early in the embryonic period. However, variable degrees of lung agenesis have been reported in several sibships, with and without consanguinity.[2] Developmental anomalies of the lungs have also been described in association with other birth defects, as part of a single gene disorder,[3] and as an occasional finding in a microdeletion syndrome (**Table 2**).

Primary pulmonary hypoplasia (PH), also known as congenital small lung (CSL), is occasionally reported as an isolated finding, yet it has been described in several sibships, suggesting autosomal recessive inheritance in at least some cases.[4] This means for some families who have given birth to 1 child with PH, recurrence may be as high as 25% in subsequent pregnancies.

At birth, PH may present with severe respiratory distress secondary to another disorder. Primary problems may be divided into 3 broad categories: (a) renal problems leading to oligohydramnios, (b) skeletal dysplasia resulting in thoracic cage limitation and pulmonary insufficiency, and (c) neuromuscular disorders leading to PH secondary to insufficient respiratory efforts in utero.

Any renal abnormality, developmental or obstructive, leading to decreased urine output in utero with concomitant oligohydramnios has the potential to cause PH. The degree of oligohydramnios and length of time the fetus is exposed to limitation of movement will likely determine the severity of PH and potential for long-term survival. Most instances of oligohydramnios are not genetically determined, but instead

Table 2
Genetic conditions associated with primary pulmonary hypoplasia

Syndrome	Clinical Features	Inheritance
Lethal pulmonary hypoplasia	Primary PH	AD (multigene or epistatic)
Total anomalous pulmonary venous return (TAPVR) (Scimitar syndrome)	Right lung hypoplasia Pulmonary hypertension TAPVR Dextrocardia	AD, incompletė penetrance
Matthew-Wood syndrome	PH (with or without diaphragmatic hernia) Anophthalmia	AR
PH with posterior amelia syndrome	PH with segmentation defects Fetal akinesia Sacral/pelvic hypoplasia	AR
McKusick-Kaufman syndrome	PH Hydrometrocolpos in female patients Cardiac, genitourinary (GU), and renal malformations	AR

Abbreviations: AD, autosomal dominant; AR, autosomal recessive.

Adapted from Pletcher, BA. Pulmonary Manifestations of Genetic Diseases in Turcios and Fink, editors. Pulmonary Manifestations of Pediatric Diseases. Philadelphia, PA Elsevier (2009). p 295-338; with permission.

are secondary to prelabor rupture of membranes. However, late loss of amniotic fluid is less likely to cause significant respiratory compromise. Conversely, prolonged, severe oligohydramnios secondary to renal agenesis or sirenomelia results in the so-called Potter sequence, with severe PH and neonatal death. See Laura Malaga-Dieguez and colleagues' article, "Pulmonary Manifestations of Renal Disorders in Children," in this issue.

A relatively common isolated birth defect in male fetuses, posterior urethral valves, may result in oligohydramnios, bladder distension, hydronephrosis, and ultimately, renal damage. In severe cases, the bladder distension leads to anterior abdominal wall musculature hypoplasia and renal failure (prune belly syndrome). These boys may also have respiratory compromise that correlates with the duration and severity of the oligohydramnios. See Laura Malaga-Dieguez and colleagues' article, "Pulmonary Manifestations of Renal Disorders in Children," in this issue.

Suboptimal urine output associated with several genetic conditions may be seen with varying degrees of PH at birth. A list of some of these syndromes is included in **Table 3**. It should be noted, however, that bilateral or unilateral renal agenesis may occur as an isolated (nonhereditary) defect during early fetal development.

Skeletal dysplasias with associated thoracic anomalies may in some instances result in secondary PH. In addition to severe and universally fatal skeletal dysplasias, such as achondrogenesis, osteogenesis imperfecta type 2, a few short-rib polydactyly syndromes, and thanatophoric dysplasia, there are several less severe skeletal dysplasias that may result in pulmonary compromise and respiratory difficulties at or shortly after birth. The long-term prognosis for each depends on the extent of the PH and ability for the lungs to grow within the confines of the thoracic cage over time. **Table 4** includes some of the skeletal dysplasias associated with respiratory difficulties at birth, but with the possibility of long-term survival.

Table 3
Genetic conditions associated with renal problems and secondary pulmonary hypoplasia

Syndrome	Clinical Features	Inheritance
Renal hypoplasia/aplasia	Renal agenesis Other GU anomalies Potters facies	AR AD
Polycystic kidney disease	Enlarged cystic kidneys with interstitial fibrosis Hepatic and pancreatic cysts Potters facies	AR
Meckel syndrome	Polycystic kidneys ± renal agenesis Occipital encephalocele Postaxial polydactyly	AR
Nephronophthisis 2	Hyperechogenic kidneys with cortical microcysts and tubulo-interstitial nephritis	AR
Genitopatellar syndrome	Polyhydramnios Multicystic kidneys Hydronephrosis Cardiac septal defects Joint flexion deformities	AR

Adapted from Pletcher, BA. Pulmonary Manifestations of Genetic Diseases in Turcios and Fink, editors. Pulmonary Manifestations of Pediatric Diseases. Philadelphia, PA Elsevier (2009). p 295-338; with permission.

Table 4
Nonlethal skeletal dysplasias associated with pulmonary hypoplasia

Syndrome	Clinical Features	Inheritance
Campomelic dysplasia	Small thorax Acromelia Cystic hygroma, lymphedema	AD
Asphyxiating thoracic dystrophy (Jeune syndrome)	Pulmonary insufficiency Narrow thorax Rib & clavicular anomalies	AR
Spondylocostal dysostosis (Jarcho-Levin dysplasia)	Pulmonary insufficiency Vertebral and rib anomalies Crablike chest Short neck with normal limbs	AD
Spondyloepiphyseal dysplasia congenita	Pulmonary insufficiency Barrel chest with platyspondyly Scoliosis, kyphosis, lordosis Pectus carinatum	AD
Rhizomelic chondrodysplasia punctata, type 1	Pulmonary insufficiency Rhizomelic limb shortening with epiphyseal calcifications Coronal vertebral clefts and kyphoscoliosis	AR

Adapted from Pletcher, BA. Pulmonary Manifestations of Genetic Diseases in Turcios and Fink, editors. Pulmonary Manifestations of Pediatric Diseases. Philadelphia, PA Elsevier (2009). p 295-338; with permission.

Severe neuromuscular disorders associated with lack of fetal movement (fetal akinesia) may cause a host of problems in addition to PH. Prenatal history is often significant for polyhydramnios (thought to be secondary to failure of normal fetal swallowing), joint contractures, and clubfeet. Whether the fetal akinesia is secondary to an inherent muscle or peripheral nerve problem, or instead a central nervous system (CNS) problem, the clinical presentations are quite similar. Severe, congenital forms of inborn errors of metabolism (IEM), myopathies, or neuropathies may be clinically indistinguishable unless specific diagnostic tests are performed. **Table 5** outlines genetic conditions with neuromuscular underpinnings that may result in secondary PH.

Congenital diaphragmatic hernia

Congenital diaphragmatic hernia (CDH) is relatively common with an incidence of about 1 in 2000 liveborn. Eighty percent of CDHs are left sided and result in abdominal contents sliding up into the chest, inhibiting normal lung development and resulting in PH.[5] CDH occurs as an isolated event as well as in association with more than 15 genetic syndromes (**Table 6**). Up to 15% of infants with CDH have a structural or numeric cytogenetic abnormality. It is associated with cardiac defects and midline anomalies (cleft lip and cleft palate). Therefore, prenatal or postnatal detection of a CDH should include a thorough search for additional birth defects that may be diagnostic of a specific syndrome.

Postnatal survival varies between 39% and 95% after repair of CDH. This large variation in mortality depends on the severity of the resulting PH and abnormal pulmonary vasculature. If extracorporeal membrane oxygenation is required, the prognosis is not favorable. The overall outcome of CDH is worse when it is associated with certain

Table 5
Neuromuscular conditions associated with pulmonary hypoplasia

Syndrome	Clinical Features	Inheritance
Fetal akinesia deformation sequence (Pena-Shokeir syndrome)	Small thorax and thin ribs Generalized joint contractures with clubfeet Polyhydramnios	AR (~50% of cases) Recurrence 10%–15%
Multiple pterygium syndrome (Escobar variant)	Eventration of the diaphragm Joint contractures with pterygia (webbing) neck Reduced muscle mass	AR
Stuve-Wiedemann syndrome	Pulmonary hypertension Short neck; thin ribs Progressive scoliosis	AR
Marden-Walker syndrome	Prenatal and postnatal growth retardation Microcephaly with CNS malformations Hypotonia and decreased muscle mass Kyphoscoliosis	AR
Spinal muscular atrophy (SMA type 1)	Pulmonary hypoplasia (one-fourth of SMA type 1) Prenatal onset of hypotonia Joint contractures	AR
Gaucher disease	Small thorax Severe fetal hydrops (30% stillborn) Polyhydramnios Fetal akinesia	AR

Adapted from Pletcher, BA. Pulmonary Manifestations of Genetic Diseases in Turcios and Fink, editors. Pulmonary Manifestations of Pediatric Diseases. Philadelphia, PA Elsevier (2009). p 295-338; with permission.

syndromes, such as Fryns.[6] Recurrence risks for siblings of a child with an isolated CDH, based on empiric data, is approximately 2%.[7]

Isolated CDH is generally thought to be a sporadic occurrence, although both autosomal dominant and autosomal recessive pedigrees have been described. Several loci and putative predisposition genes have been found in cases of CDH with cytogenetic deletions, duplications, and translocations often uncovering a CDH locus.[8]

Lung segmentation and laterality defects

During the embryologic stage, the right and left bronchial buds begin to grow, subsequently dividing into secondary bronchi. Normally, the right lung bud divides into 3 segments (lobes) and the left lung bud divides into 2 segments (lobes). On rare occasions, segmentation or lobulation anomalies occur, which may or may not be associated with heterotaxy.

Heterotaxy (defect of laterality), also called “situs ambiguous” (discordance of right and left patterns of ordinarily asymmetric structures), is different from situs inversus and is often grouped clinically as *asplenia* (bilateral right-sidedness, or right isomerism) or *polysplenia* or multiple small spleens (bilateral left-sidedness, or left isomerism).[9]

Table 6
Genetic conditions associated with congenital diaphragmatic hernia

Syndrome	Clinical Features	Inheritance
CDH	Diaphragmatic hernia alone	AD AR
Anterior diaphragmatic hernia	Anterior diaphragmatic hernia	X-linked or Multifactorial M > F
Cornelia de Lange syndrome	Abnormal cry at birth Classic facial dysmorphism Microcephaly and congenital heart defects	AD
Fryns syndrome	Pulmonary lobulation defect Small thorax Large for gestational age	AR Three recognized microdeletions
Meacham syndrome	Pulmonary rhabdomyomatous dysplasia Congenital heart defects Boys: ambiguous genitalia or sex reversal	AD (de novo)
Simpson-Golabi-Behmel syndrome	Lung segmentation defects Accessory nipples; 13 rib pairs Cardiac and GI defects Large, cystic kidneys	X-linked recessive
Goltz syndrome	Ocular, dental, GI, and GU defects Papillomas ± telangiectasias Absent or hypoplastic nails	X-linked dominant (lethal in boys)
Autosomal recessive cutis laxa, type 1C	Emphysema and lung hypoplasia Cutis laxa Joint laxity	AR
Epidermolysis bullosa with diaphragmatic hernia	Epidermolysis bullosa Infants die shortly after birth	AR
MIDAS syndrome	Unilateral or bilateral microphthalmia Sclerocornea Linear skin defects on face and neck Cardiac defects Genital ± anal anomalies	X-linked dominant (lethal in boys)
Syndromic microphthalmia	Pulmonary dysplasia even in absence of diaphragmatic defect	AR
Thoracoabdominal syndrome (X-linked midline defects, including pentalogy of Cantrell)	Diaphragmatic hernia Cleft lip ± palate Cardiac defects Omphalocele; ventral hernias Hydrocephaly; anencephaly Renal agenesis; hypospadias	X-linked recessive or X-linked dominant
Donnai-Barrow syndrome	Ventral abdominal wall defects Agenesis of the corpus callosum	AR

(continued on next page)

Table 6
(continued)

Syndrome	Clinical Features	Inheritance
Gershon-Baruch syndrome	Omphalocele Single umbilical artery Scoliosis	Probable AR
Froster syndrome	Omphalocele Limb deficiencies with syndactyly Cranial ossification defects	AR
Denys-Drash syndrome (Wilms tumor and pseudo or true hermaphroditism)	Ambiguous genitalia (M or F) Gonadal dysgenesis (M or F) Wilms tumor	AD (de novo)
PAGOD syndrome	PH even without diaphragmatic defect Omphalocele Dextrocardia and cardiac defects	AR
Perlman syndrome	Polyhydramnios Renal hamartomas Nephroblastomatosis Wilms tumor	AR
Pallister-Killian syndrome (Mosaic tetrasomy 12p)	Short, webbed neck Cardiac and GU defects Ventral wall defects	Cytogenetic
Emanuel syndrome (supernumerary derivative 22 chromosome)	Prenatal growth retardation Microcephaly Cleft palate Cardiac, GU, and anal defects	Cytogenetic (3:1 segregation from parent balanced carrier of 11q23; 22q11 translocation)
Deletion 1q32.3-q42.3	Postnatal growth retardation Microcephaly Coarse facies	Cytogenetic

Adapted from Pletcher, BA. Pulmonary Manifestations of Genetic Diseases in Turcios and Fink, editors. Pulmonary Manifestations of Pediatric Diseases. Philadelphia, PA Elsevier (2009). p 295-338; with permission.

Pulmonary isomerism may be right isomerism (bilateral right lung) with bilateral eparterial bronchi. Eighty percent of children with right isomerism lack a spleen (asplenia), leading to a risk of overwhelming pneumococcal sepsis. Pulmonary left isomerism (bilateral left lung) is associated with polysplenia, a midline liver, malrotation of the gut, and cardiovascular defects.[9] Although nonfamilial, Ivemark syndrome, which consists of right isomerism, is confined to males, whereas the other isomerism syndromes may affect either sex. A few genetic syndromes have been associated with these types of defects (**Table 7**). Mirror-image arrangement and other laterality disorders may be a feature of primary ciliary dyskinesia (PCD; discussed later).

Congenital bronchobiliary fistula (CBBF), a rare anomaly, represents a direct, abnormal connection between the trachea or bronchus and biliary tract. CBBF often presents in neonates with respiratory distress, cyanosis, and a large amount of bilelike (green-colored) respiratory secretions. CBBFs are isolated occurrences with no recognized genetic associations.

Table 7
Genetic conditions associated with lung segmentation defects with or without heterotaxy

Syndrome	Clinical Features	Inheritance
Smith-Lemli-Opitz syndrome (RSH syndrome)	Incomplete lung lobulation ± lung hypoplasia Microcephaly; epicanthal folds Cardiac defects	AR
Pallister-Hall syndrome	Abnormal lung lobulation Cardiac & GU defects Hypopituitarism	AD Most cases sporadic
Simpson-Golabi-Behmel syndrome	See **Table 5**	See **Table 5**
Right isomerism (Ivemark syndrome)	Right isomerism (bilateral right lung) Asplenia Severe cardiac defects Midline liver, malrotation of the gut	AR

Adapted from Pletcher, BA. Pulmonary Manifestations of Genetic Diseases in Turcios and Fink, editors. Pulmonary Manifestations of Pediatric Diseases. Philadelphia, PA Elsevier (2009). p 295-338; with permission.

Congenital pulmonary airway malformations

Congenital pulmonary airway malformations (CPAM), formerly congenital cystic adenomatoid malformations (CCAMs), are the most commonly diagnosed BPM. It is thought that these malformations are related to insults to the pulmonary airways at different developmental levels. A pathologic classification of these abnormalities in 5 types (0–4) has been proposed: 0, bronchial; 1, bronchial/bronchiolar; 2, bronchiolar; 3, bronchiolar/alveolar, and 4, peripheral. Based on prenatal US, they may be classified as macrocystic (>5.0 mm in diameter) and microcystic, presenting as a solid echogenic mass. Macrocystic lesions may resemble CDH and may compress adjacent lung tissue and cause PH with a mediastinal shift.[10]

Depending on the degree of pulmonary compromise, infants may or may not be symptomatic at birth. A small percentage may be asymptomatic until later in childhood and often present with recurrent pneumonia. Increased risks for malignancy have been a rationale for the early surgical resection of these lesions even when there are no clinical symptoms, particularly for those with a close relative with childhood malignancy.[11] Most CPAM are isolated occurrences; although associated pulmonary sequestration (PS) and CDH have been reported, CPAM are not thought to be genetically determined.

Bronchogenic cysts and other cystic lesions

Foregut cysts are closed epithelium-lined sacs developing abnormally from the primitive respiratory tract and developing upper gut.[11,12] When these structures differentiate toward airway and contain cartilage in the wall, they are called *bronchogenic cysts*, whereas those developing toward the gut are termed *enterogenous (or enteric) cysts*. Bronchogenic cysts are the most common thoracic cysts in infancy, although many do not present until older age. Most are situated in the mediastinum close to the carina, but do not communicate with the trachea or bronchi. Less frequently, they are adjacent to the esophagus. They are usually single, unilocular, and more common on the right.[2] Because of inadequate drainage, such cysts may be associated with recurrent infections and may appear as a consolidation or area of atelectasis on chest radiograph. Preexisting bronchogenic cyst has been associated pulmonary pleuroblastoma and bronchioloalveolar carcinoma in children and adults and, with the development of pulmonary adenocarcinoma, in adulthood.[12] Rarely, congenital lung cysts are seen in conjunction with genetic syndromes (**Table 8**).

Pulmonary sequestration

PS consists of a nonfunctioning mass of lung tissue that receives its arterial blood supply from the thoracic or abdominal aorta rather than from the pulmonary circulation and lacks communication with the bronchial tree.[13] Rarely symptomatic at birth, PS may appear as a cystic or solid infiltrate on US and chest radiograph. *Extralobar PS*, which has its own pleural lining, is usually situated below the left lower lobe (subdiaphragmatic) and is less common than *intralobar PS*, which is mainly located within normal parenchyma of the left lower lobe.[10]

Unless an intralobar PS becomes infected, most cases are diagnosed in adolescence. Extralobar PS is usually detected in infancy because of associated malformations, and it affects boys more than girls (4:1). There are no strong genetic factors predisposing to the development of PS.

Congenital lobar emphysema

Congenital lobar emphysema (CLE) is a misnomer, because it implies lung destruction, whereas in some cases, there may be too many alveoli (polyalveolar lobe). The term congenital large hyperlucent lobe is more appropriate, a developmental anomaly characterized by hyperinflation of one or more pulmonary lobes. CLE most commonly affects the left upper or right middle lobes. Mechanisms proposed to explain the obstruction of the developing airway include dysplastic or deficient bronchial cartilage, excessive mucosal proliferation, bronchial torsion, and bronchial compression by cardiopulmonary vessels.[13] The airway obstruction leads to a "ball-valve" effect whereby a greater volume of air enters the affected lobe during inspiration than leaves during expiration, producing air trapping. The hyperinflation of the affected lung has been associated with compression of adjacent lung tissue and respiratory distress. Most cases of CLE are isolated occurrences.

Tracheoesophageal fistula and tracheal agenesis

Tracheoesophageal fistula (TEF), the most common congenital tracheal abnormality, with an incidence of about 1 in 3500 live births, typically occurs with esophageal atresia (EA). TEF results from failure of the tracheoesophageal ridges to fully fuse

Table 8
Genetic conditions associated with pulmonary cysts

Syndrome	Clinical Features	Inheritance
Cystic disease of the lung	Recurrent lung infections Spontaneous pneumothorax in neonates	AR (Common in Yemenite, & non-Ashkenazi Jews)
Proteus syndrome	Macrocephaly Hemihypertrophy with localized overgrowth Lymphangiomas, epidermal nevi, hemangiomas Kyphoscoliosis	Somatic mutations

Adapted from Pletcher, BA. Pulmonary Manifestations of Genetic Diseases in Turcios and Fink, editors. Pulmonary Manifestations of Pediatric Diseases. Philadelphia, PA Elsevier (2009). p 295-338; with permission.

during early embryologic life, with incomplete separation of the esophagus from the trachea.[13] EA and TEF are classified according to their anatomic configuration. Type A, which consists of a proximal esophageal pouch and distal TEF, accounts for 85% of cases. Up to one-third of infants born with a TEF have additional birth defects and may be seen as part of multiple anomaly associations as well as in several mendelian disorders (**Table 9**).

The clinical presentation of TEF depends on the presence or absence of EA. In cases with EA, polyhydramnios occurs in approximately two-thirds of pregnancies.

Table 9
Genetic conditions associated with tracheoesophageal fistula

Syndrome	Clinical Features	Inheritance
TEF with or without EA	TEF EA	Multifactorial
X-linked VACTERL	TEF Hydrocephalus Vertebral malformations Anal atresia Cardiac and GU defects	X-linked recessive
VATER association	Tracheal agenesis (occasional) TEF Single umbilical artery Vertebral defects Cardiac and renal defects Radial dysplasia and thumb anomalies	Isolated cases (similar defects with Fanconi anemia, which is AR)
Goldenhar syndrome	TEF (5%) Hemifacial facial microsomia Cardiac, vertebral, and renal defects	Isolated cases AD (rare)
CHARGE syndrome	TEF Choanal atresia Anal atresia or stenosis Cardiac, renal, and genital anomalies Ocular colobomas	AD
Opitz-Frias syndrome, type 2	TEF Pulmonary hypoplasia Cardiac and renal defects	AD
Feingold syndrome	TEF Asplenia or polysplenia Polyhydramnios	AD
Syndromic microphthalmia 3	EA Microphthalmia; anophthalmia Cardiac, vertebral, GU, and CNS defects	AD
Martinez-Frias syndrome	TEF Duodenal atresia Hypoplasia pancreas, gallbladder, biliary ducts, and intestines	AR

Adapted from Pletcher, BA. Pulmonary Manifestations of Genetic Diseases in Turcios and Fink, editors. Pulmonary Manifestations of Pediatric Diseases. Philadelphia, PA Elsevier (2009). p 295-338; with permission.

Infants with EA are symptomatic immediately after birth with excessive secretions resulting in drooling, choking, respiratory distress, and inability to feed. A fistula between the trachea and distal esophagus often leads to gastric distention and reflux of gastric contents through the TEF, resulting in aspiration pneumonia.[14] A TEF type H may present with a history of recurrent bouts of coughing after drinking.

Respiratory and gastrointestinal (GI) complications are common in patients with all types of TEF, even after repair. These complications include recurrent pneumonia, impaired esophageal peristalsis, gastroesophageal reflux disease, recurrent TEF, tracheomalacia, esophageal stenosis, anastomosis leak, and tracheal diverticulum.[15] Because chronic aspiration may lead to recurrent pneumonia and impaired pulmonary function, it is important that, in patients with a history of TEF/EA, these recognized complications be excluded before respiratory symptoms are attributed to "asthma."[16]

Congenital pulmonary lymphangiectasis

Congenital pulmonary lymphangiectasis (CPL) is a rare vascular malformation characterized by dilated lymphatic vessels and disturbed drainage of lymph fluid in multiple areas of the lungs, including subpleural, interlobar, perivascular, and peribronchial regions.[17] CPL is classified as *primary* or *secondary* CPL.[18] Primary CPL fits into a development disorder persisting beyond the neonatal period or manifesting at any age that includes hydrops fetalis, chylous ascites, intestinal lymphangiectasis, pleural and pericardial effusions, and pulmonary lymphangiectasis. Secondary PL are heterogeneous conditions associated with severe congenital heart disease and thoracic duct anomalies, all causing obstruction and extravasation.[18]

Although most CPL are isolated occurrences, primary CPLs have been reported to be generalized, or as part of known or unknown genetic syndromes included in **Table 10**. Primary CPL limited to the lung often presents with severe respiratory distress because of unilateral or bilateral pleural effusions, PH, and surfactant deficiency of prematurity. Patients with generalized lymphangiectasis usually have less pulmonary involvement, but develop more subcutaneous edema and visceral effusions, as described in some congenital genetic lymphedema syndromes.

Table 10
Genetic conditions associated with congenital pulmonary lymphangiectasia

Syndrome	Clinical Features	Inheritance
CPL	Pulmonary lymphangiectasia Polyhydramnios Hydrothorax, chylothorax Recurrent respiratory infections	AR
Urioste syndrome	Polyhydramnios Narrow thorax Boys with persistent Mullerian ducts (uterus & fallopian tubes) Intestinal lymphangiectasia	AR
Lymphedema-hypoparathyroidism syndrome	Pulmonary lymphangiectasia Hypoparathyroidism Mitral valve prolapse	AR vs X-linked recessive
Hennekam lymphangiectasia-lymphedema syndrome	Lymphangiectasia Lymphedema (pleural, renal pericardial, intestinal, thyroid) Cardiac, renal, & CNS defects	AR

Adapted from Pletcher, BA. Pulmonary Manifestations of Genetic Diseases in Turcios and Fink, editors. Pulmonary Manifestations of Pediatric Diseases. Philadelphia, PA Elsevier (2009). p 295-338; with permission.

Pulmonary arteriovenous malformations and hemangiomas

Vascular anomalies are classified into 2 groups: vascular malformations (arterial, venous, capillary, lymphatic, or combined) and vascular tumors. Pulmonary arteriovenous malformation (PAVM) affects blood flow between the heart and the lungs. Affected people have a direct connection, without intervening capillary networks, between the pulmonary vein (carries blood from the lungs to the heart) and pulmonary artery (carries blood from the heart to the lungs). As a result, blood may not be properly oxygenated by the lungs. PAVM may present at birth or may occasionally develop postnatally. Some affected people may be asymptomatic. When present, symptoms may include epistaxis, dyspnea, and cyanosis. Most individuals with PAVM have an inherited condition called hereditary hemorrhagic telangiectasia (HHT) or (Osler-Weber-Rendu syndrome), an autosomal dominant disorder leading to vascular malformations[19] (**Table 11**). See Bernard A. Cohen and Nelson L. Turcios' article, "Pulmonary Manifestations of Skin Disorders in Children", in this issue.

Mucoobstructive Lung Diseases

Cystic fibrosis

Cystic fibrosis (CF), an autosomal recessive disease, is caused by a mutation (chemical change) in the CF gene named the *CFTR* (cystic fibrosis transmembrane conductance regulator) protein.[20] CF occurs wherever Europeans have settled. However, CF has been reported among all ethnicities and nationalities. Therefore, CF should *not* be excluded in a patient with suggestive clinical findings solely because of that patient's ethnicity[21] (**Box 1**).

The earliest manifestations of CF are GI and nutritional disorders. Approximately 15% of infants with CF present with *meconium ileus* at birth[22] (**Table 12**). Respiratory manifestations are uncommon in newborns, but older infants may present with persistent coughing, recurrent wheezing, and frequent lung infections. In some countries, where neonatal screening for CF is not available, these respiratory symptoms are often misdiagnosed as asthma or "recurrent bronchitis," and, as a result, appropriate therapy is frequently delayed. Consensus guidelines from the Cystic Fibrosis Foundation review the diagnostic approach to CF[23] (**Fig. 1**).

The consequences of the *CFTR* mutations may be grouped into classes that represent alterations of normal protein production, trafficking, and function at the epithelial cell membrane, or a combination of these abnormalities. These classes of mutations give rise to a range of phenotypes extending from classic CF to single-organ

Table 11
Genetic conditions associated with pulmonary arteriovenous malformations

Syndrome	Clinical Features	Inheritance
(HHT, types 1–5 (Osler-Weber-Rendu)	PAVM Recurrent epistaxis (common) Telangiectasias (mucocutaneous) Visceral AVMs Heart failure (high output)	AD
Juvenile polyposis HHT syndrome	PAVM Other features of HHT Juvenile GI polyps with rectal bleeding	AD

Adapted from Pletcher, BA. Pulmonary Manifestations of Genetic Diseases in Turcios and Fink, editors. Pulmonary Manifestations of Pediatric Diseases. Philadelphia, PA Elsevier (2009). p 295-338; with permission.

Box 1
Cystic fibrosis estimated birth prevalence

Whites 1:2500

Hispanics 1:3500

African Americans 1:15,100

Asians, native Hawaiians, and Pacific Islanders 1:31,000 to 1:100,000.

involvement. For more information on *CFTR* mutation databases, visit www.genet.sickkids.on.ca/cftr/ and https://www.cftr2.org (**Fig. 2**).

Primary ciliary dyskinesia

Kartagener described a combination of situs inversus, chronic sinusitis, and bronchiectasis, which became known as Kartagener triad. The term Kartagener syndrome (KS) was later adopted when additional features of rhinitis, nasal polyps, chronic otitis media, and reduced fertility were recognized. It was later found that individuals with this syndrome have ultrastructural defects in the motor cilia.[24] The now commonly used name of "primary ciliary dyskinesia" appropriately describes the spectrum of ciliary abnormalities and distinguishes genetic ciliary defects from "secondary" or acquired defects associated with epithelial injury.

PCD is a heterogenous, autosomal recessive disorder associated with abnormal ciliary ultrastructure and function that result in retention of mucus and bacteria in the respiratory tract leading to chronic otosinopulmonary disease and abnormal flagellar structure resulting in abnormal sperm motility.[25] **Box 2** highlights the major clinical features of PCD in childhood.[26]

Virtually all men are infertile because of abnormal sperm motility. Some women have normal fertility; others have impaired fertility and are at increased risk for ectopic pregnancy because of ciliary dysfunction in the Fallopian tubes.[25] Situs inversus totalis (mirror-image reversal of all visceral organs with no apparent functional consequences) is observed in 40% to 50% of individuals with PCD.

Heterotaxy ("situs ambiguous") is present in ~12% of individuals with PCD.[25]

In addition to the major clinical features, the diagnosis of PCD in childhood includes genetic testing, which may confirm the diagnosis. To date, mutations in 45 genes are

Table 12
Clinical manifestations of cystic fibrosis

Meconium ileus, meconium peritonitis	Gallstones
Prolonged obstructive jaundice	CBAVD/azoospermia
Hyponatremic or hypochloremic dehydration	Staphylococcal pneumonia
Chronic metabolic alkalosis	Recurrent or persistent pneumonia
Heat prostration	Unexplained cirrhosis
Failure to thrive	Bronchiectasis
Hypoproteinemia with or without edema	Mucoid *pseudomonas* in lung
Fat-soluble vitamin deficiency	Recurrent pancreatitis
Rectal prolapse	Pansinusitis
Nasal polyposis	Family history (sibling, first cousin)

Abbreviation: CBAVD, Congenital bilateral absence of the vas deferens.

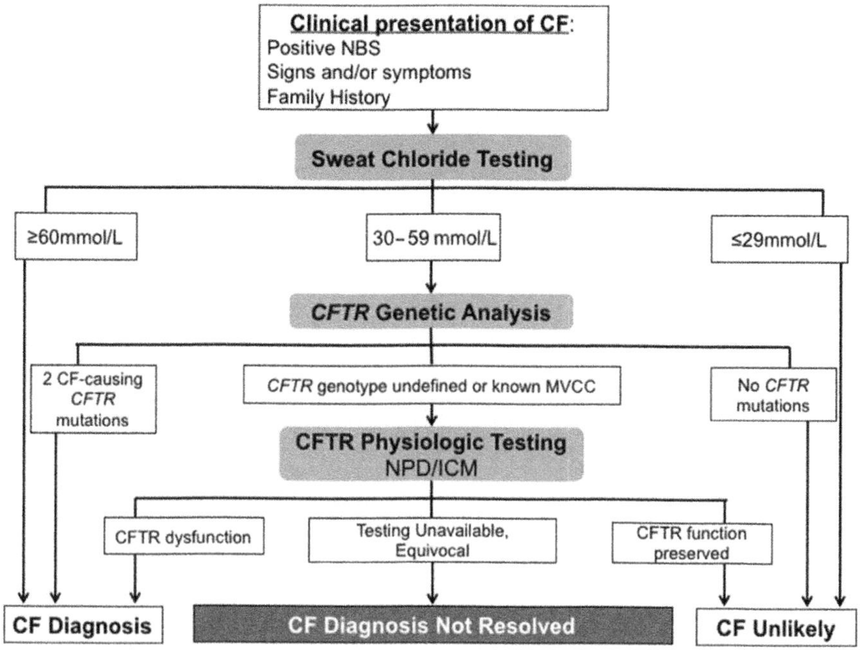

Fig. 1. How consensus should be applied to individuals suspected of having CF. ICM, intestinal current measurement; MVCC, mutation of varying clinical consequence; NBS, newborn screening; NPD, nasal potential difference. (*From* Farrell PM, White TB, Ren CL, Hempstead SE, Accurso F, Derichs N, et al: Diagnosis of cystic fibrosis: consensus guidelines from the Cystic Fibrosis Foundation. J Pediatr 2017;181(Suppl 4):S4-S15; with permission.)

known to cause PCD. Genetic testing now is good for diagnostic confirmation in the majority (about 70%) of cases of PCD. However, 20% to 30% of individuals with well-characterized PCD do *not* have identifiable mutations in any of associated genes. Transmission electron microscopy (EM) analysis of ciliary biopsy may also be performed; however, an estimated 30% of individuals do *not* have ciliary ultrastructural abnormalities. Nasal nitric oxide measurement may be obtained in children older than 5 years of age for additional diagnostic support.[25] However, the most common diagnostic problem is in fact usually failure to consider the diagnosis.

Genetic abnormalities in cilia shaft proteins, cilia beat frequency, and defective mucociliary clearance have been considered the underlying pathogenesis of PCD. However, the sputum is also abnormally hyperconcentrated, suggesting that it may also contribute to its pathogenesis[27] (**Fig. 3**).

Table 13 describes the most prevalent ultrastructural ciliary defects in PCD.

Bronchiectasis is the pathologic term for bronchial destruction and dilatation with accumulation of infected secretions, which occurs most often in the setting of chronic lung infections.[28] Several genetic syndromes with bronchiectasis as a major feature have been described[25] (**Table 14**).

Alpha-1-Antitrypsin Deficiency

Alpha$_1$-antitrypsin deficiency (AATD), an autosomal recessive condition, affects about 1 in 1500 to 3500 individuals with European ancestry.[29] Most persons carry 2 copies of the wild-type M allele of *SERPINA1*, which encodes AAT, and have normal circulating

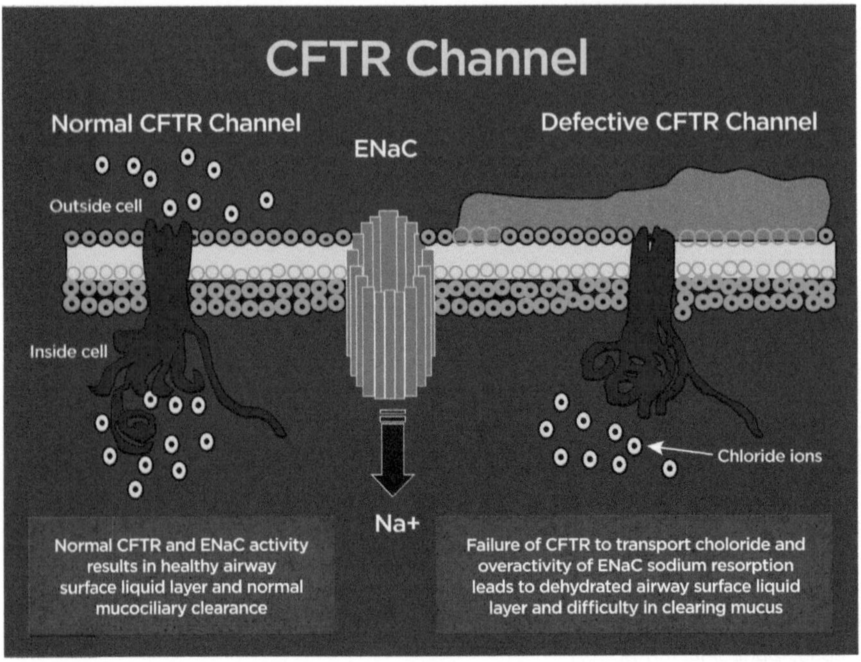

Fig. 2. Pathogenesis of CF lung disease. In healthy people (*left*), balanced epithelial sodium (Na^+) absorption and secretion of chloride anions hydrate airway surfaces and promote efficient mucociliary transport. In the CF airway (*right*), the defective CFTR channel and increased activity of the epithelial sodium channel (ENaC) lead to dehydrated mucus and failed mucus clearance. The abnormal concentration of mucus reflects a primary abnormality of airway epithelial ion transport. Mucus hyperconcentration is a feature of CF. (*Courtesy of* ABcomm.Inc, Champaign, IL; with permission.)

levels of the protein. Alpha-1-antitrypsin (AAT) is a serine protease inhibitor (SERPIN) and functions inhibiting the activity of proteolytic enzymes with a serine residue. AAT inhibits neutrophil elastase, which, when unopposed, may cleave several structural proteins of the lung as well as innate immune proteins.

The clinical manifestations of lung disease associated with AATD are mainly indistinguishable from those of nonhereditary emphysema.[29] The classic clinical

Box 2
Key clinical features of primary ciliary dyskinesia in childhood

Unexplained neonatal respiratory distress (at term birth)

Any organ laterality defect: situs inversus totalis or situs ambiguous (heterotaxy)

Daily, year-round wet cough starting in first year of life or bronchiectasis on chest computed tomographic (CT) scan

Daily, year-round nasal congestion starting in first year of life or pansinusitis on sinus CT scan

The diagnosis of PCD is highly likely if 2 or more of these key clinical features are present.

Data from Leigh MW, Ferkol TW, Davis SD, et al: Clinical features and associated likelihood of primary ciliary dyskinesia in children and adolescents. Ann Am Thoracic Soc 2016;13: 1305-1313.

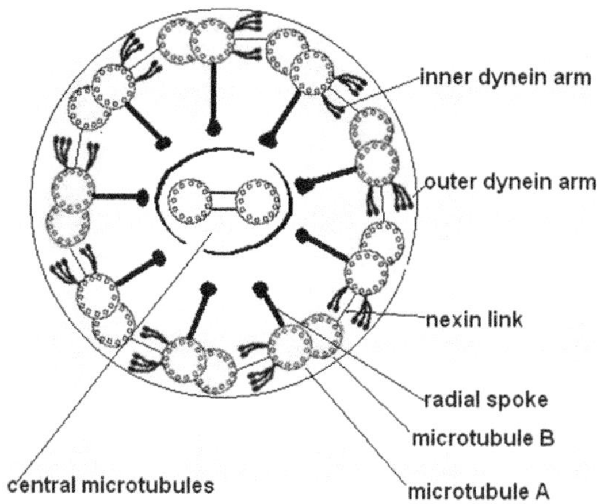

Fig. 3. A cross-section of a cilium revealing "9 + 2" pattern of 9 peripheral microtubule doublets surrounding a central microtubule pair. Shortening and/or absence of outer dynein arms alone (40%) and shortening or absence of both outer and inner dynein arms (10%) are the most prevalent ultrastructural defects in PCD.

description of lung disease associated with AATD is of early-onset obstructive lung disease, panacinar emphysema, affecting mainly the lower lobes.[29] Emphysema is rare in childhood. About 10% of infants with AATD develop neonatal cholestatic jaundice and elevated liver function tests. If the AAT plasma concentration is less than 50% of normal, protease inhibitor analysis should be obtained to confirm the diagnosis. Most affected individuals are homozygous for the "Z" allele.[29] See Emily R.

Table 13
Most prevalent ultrastructural ciliary defects in primary ciliary dyskinesia

	Clinical Features	Inheritance
Shortening or absence of outer dynein arms (~38.5%) Shortening or absence of both outer and inner dynein arms (~10.5%)	Abnormal cilia structure & function Chronic otosinopulmonary disease Bronchiectasis Male infertility (virtually all) Female normal/impaired fertility Situs inversus (~50%) Situs ambiguous (heterotaxy) ~12% EM: absent or abnormal dynein arms of cilia and sperm	AR[a]
Microtubular disruption and absence of inner dynein arm (~14%)	Chronic sinopulmonary infections EM: microtubular disorganization and absent inner dynein arm	AR
Absence/disruption of central microtubules and/or radial spokes (~7%)	Chronic sinopulmonary infections Abnormal sperm motility EM: absent ciliary axoneme and/or radial spokes	AR

[a] Exceptions: FOXJI-PCD (AD) and PIHID3-PCD & OFDI-PCD (X-linked).

Data from Zariwala MA, Knowles, MR and Leigh MW. Primary Ciliary Dyskinesia GeneReviews (internet) Dec 5, 2019; with permission.

Table 14
Genetic conditions associated with bronchiectasis

Syndrome	Clinical Features	Inheritance
Ataxia-telangiectasia	Cerebellar ataxia Telangiectasias Sinopulmonary infections Immune defects with thymus hypoplasia, decreased T cells, defective B-cell differentiation Decreased immunoglobulin A (IgA), IgE, and IgG_2	AR Heterozygotes at risk for certain neoplasias
Bloom syndrome	Telangiectasia Altered pigmented skin Recurrent severe infections IgA, IgG, and IgM deficiency	AR ~1/3 cases are Ashkenazi Jews
Impaired immune function (incomplete list)	Severe combined immunodeficiency Common variable immunodeficiency Natural killer cell deficiency Bare lymphocyte syndrome X-linked lymphoproliferative disease T-cell deficiency Ectodermal dysplasia Cartilage-hair hypoplasia	
Young syndrome	Azoospermia due to obstructed vas deferens Sinopulmonary infections EM: Normal cilia structure	AR Differentiate from congenital bilateral absence of vas deferens due to CFTR mutation
Yellow nail syndrome	Bronchiectasis Nail discoloration, lymphedema	Familial (unknown genetics)
Marfan syndrome	Bronchiectasis Tall, thin habitus Arachnodactyly Ectopia lens Aortic root dilatation	AD
Congenital Tracheobronchomegaly (Mounier-Kuhn syndrome)	Tracheomalacia Bronchiectasis Recurrent lung infections	AR? >Men age 30–50 y
Williams-Campbell syndrome	Bronchiectasis (fourth to sixth bronchial order) Bronchial isomerism Polysplenia	AR
Ehlers-Danlos syndrome	Bronchiectasis Joint hyperextensibility Poor scar formation	AR

Adapted from Pletcher, BA. Pulmonary Manifestations of Genetic Diseases in Turcios and Fink, editors. Pulmonary Manifestations of Pediatric Diseases. Philadelphia, PA Elsevier (2009). p 295-338; with permission.

Le Fevre and colleagues' article, "Pulmonary Manifestations of Gastrointestinal, Pancreatic and Liver Diseases in Children," in this issue.

Spontaneous Pneumothorax

Spontaneous pneumothorax (SP) is usually an acute and sometimes life-threatening event, occurring in otherwise healthy individuals. SPs occur more often in tall, thin men and may be seen in individuals with certain underlying connective tissue disorders. Familial SP may be inherited as an autosomal dominant condition associated with subpleural blebs and bullae or may be a sporadic (nongenetic) occurrence (**Table 15**). For any child, teen, or adult with an SP, a focused physical examination and targeted family history may help uncover a connective tissue disorder or a heritable trait.

Pulmonary Arterial Hypertension

Pulmonary arterial hypertension (PAH) is characterized by widespread obstruction and obliteration of the smallest pulmonary arteries. Although pulmonary hypertension frequently results from other systemic problems, heritable PAH may occur as a mendelian disorder (both autosomal dominant and autosomal recessive) as well as part of other well-described genetic syndromes.[30] A heritable PAH gene has been identified, which codes for the BMPR2 protein. **Table 16** summarizes genetic conditions associated with PAH.

Pulmonary Embolism

People with genetic disorders that increase their risk for thrombosis are considered to have thrombophilia. Deficiencies of protein S, protein C, or antithrombin are

Table 15
Genetic conditions associated with spontaneous pneumothorax

Syndrome	Clinical Features	Inheritance
Marfan syndrome	Spontaneous pneumothorax Pulmonary blebs Tall stature Severe myopia Aortic root dilatation Pectus deformity Kyphosis or scoliosis Joint hypermobility	AD ~1/4 due to new or de novo mutations
Primary spontaneous pneumothorax	Spontaneous pneumothorax Subpleural blebs and bullae More common in tall, thin men	AD
Birt-Hoge-Dube syndrome	Spontaneous pneumothorax Lung cysts	AD
Ehlers-Danlos syndrome, type IV (Vascular)	Spontaneous pneumothorax Pulmonary capillary hemangiomatosis Easy bruising, prominent veins Joint hypermobility	AD
Ehlers-Danlos syndrome, type VII (dermatosparaxis)	Spontaneous pneumothorax Micrognathia Joint and skin laxity and fragility	AR

Adapted from Pletcher, BA. Pulmonary Manifestations of Genetic Diseases in Turcios and Fink, editors. Pulmonary Manifestations of Pediatric Diseases. Philadelphia, PA Elsevier (2009). p 295-338; with permission.

Table 16
Genetic conditions associated with idiopathic pulmonary hypertension

Syndrome	Clinical Features	Inheritance
Primary pulmonary hypertension (PPH), types 1–4	PPH Arterial hypoxemia Right ventricular hypertrophy and failure Increase PA pressure and PVR Arterial fibrosis and medial hypertrophy	AD ~ 6% of PPH are genetic Females > Males
Primary pulmonary hypertension	Same as PPH	AR
Familial persistent pulmonary hypertension of the newborn	Neonatal pulmonary hypertension Abnormal pulmonary lobules Increased muscular wall in arterioles	AR
Lymphedema and cerebral arteriovenous anomaly	PPH AVM Cranial bruit Lymphedema	AD
Familial pulmonary capillary hemangiomatosis	PPH Pulmonary capillary hemangiomatosis	AR
Familial cirrhosis	PPH Congenital or childhood liver cirrhosis	AR
VATER-like defects, pulmonary hypertension, laryngeal webs, & growth deficiency	Pulmonary hypertension Laryngeal webs Pectus excavatum Rib and vertebral anomalies	AR
Severe congenital neutropenia	Pulmonary hypertension (some)	AR
Ischiocoxopodopatellar syndrome	Pulmonary hypertension Pelvic, patellar, and foot defects	AD

Abbreviations: PA, pulmonary artery; PVR is pulmonary vascular resistance; AVM is arteriovenous malformation.

Adapted from Pletcher, BA. Pulmonary Manifestations of Genetic Diseases in Turcios and Fink, editors. Pulmonary Manifestations of Pediatric Diseases. Philadelphia, PA Elsevier (2009). p 295-338; with permission.

thrombophilic. The *Arg*506 to *Gln*506 mutation in factor V (factor Leiden) poses a significant risk for thrombosis in individuals heterozygous for the disorder. This risk is much higher when factor Leiden is present in the homozygous state. Mutation in factor Leiden is present in about 5% of white people. Similarly, a relatively common mutation in the prothrombin gene is the factor II polymorphism, known as 20210G>A, present in about 2% of this population, causes a modest increased risk for deep venous thrombosis (DVT) and pulmonary embolism (PE). Individuals who carry 1 copy of the factor V Leiden mutation *and* 1 prothrombin mutation have a much more significant risk of developing a DVT and/or PE. Infants who are homozygous for protein C or antithrombin III mutations are at high risk for neonatal thrombosis and PE and may die in the newborn period, if untreated.

Surfactant Deficiency Syndromes and Miscellaneous Genetic Conditions

Surfactant protein (SP) deficiencies are now recognized to be a rare genetic cause of lung disease in infants and adults. Infants with SP-B deficiency and *NKX2-1/TTF1* may

Table 17
Genetic disorders causing surfactant dysfunction

	SFTPB	SFTPC	ABCA3	*NKX2-1/TTF1*
Mode of inheritance	Autosomal recessive	Autosomal dominant, de novo	Autosomal recessive	Autosomal dominant, de novo
Pulmonary presentations	Neonatal respiratory distress syndrome	Childhood interstitial lung disease Adult interstitial lung disease Neonatal respiratory distress syndrome	Neonatal respiratory distress syndrome Childhood interstitial lung disease	Neonatal respiratory distress syndrome Childhood interstitial lung disease Recurrent infection No pulmonary involvement
Course	Neonatal lethal	Highly variable Survival until sixth decade reported	Neonatal lethal Variable severity in childhood	Neonatal lethal Variable severity in childhood
Treatment options described in literature	Supportive lung transplant	Supportive corticosteroids hydroxychloroquine azithromycin Lung transplant	Supportive corticosteroids hydroxychloroquine lung transplant	Supportive

Reproduced with permission from: Nogee LM, Gower A. Genetic disorders of surfactant dysfunction. In: UpToDate, Post TW (Ed), UpToDate, Waltham, MA. (Accessed on [Date].) Copyright © 2020 UpToDate, Inc. For more information visit http://www.uptodate.com" www.uptodate.com.

Table 18
Genetic conditions associated with miscellaneous pulmonary findings

Syndrome	Clinical Features	Inheritance
Tuberous sclerosis complex	Pulmonary lymphangiomatosis Cardiac rhabdomyomas Facial angiofibromas Hypopigmented "ash-leaf" spots	AD de novo mutations in 80% of TSC1 & 60% TSC2
Diffuse panbronchiolitis	Micronodular pulmonary lesions Chronic sinobronchial infections	AD in affected East Asian patients
Familial Mediterranean fever	Pleuritis/pericarditis Episodic fevers Hepatosplenomegaly	AD or AR common among Sephardic Jews
Hereditary pancreatitis	Hemorrhagic pleural effusions Pancreatitis	AD
Alveolar capillary dysplasia with misalignment of the pulmonary veins	Neonatal pulmonary hypertension Abnormal lung lobulation Malposition of pulmonary arteries	AD (de novo)

present with severe respiratory failure at birth along with pulmonary hypertension. Respiratory disease is progressive, and death usually results from respiratory failure, Those infants with ABCA 3 deficiency may have a milder initial course within the first weeks after birth. The natural history of those with SP-C deficiency is variable (**Table 17**). In addition to the genetic conditions previously discussed, there are a few outliers that defy classification into specific categories of lung disease (**Table 18**).

Inborn Errors of Metabolism

Although one would not typically associate IEMs with pulmonary problems, many storage and biochemical disorders cause respiratory complications. Because most of these conditions are systemic, virtually all organs may be involved to a greater or lesser degree. Interstitial or restrictive lung disease may be seen in some of the lysosomal storage disorders. This topic is further discussed in Alexander Broomfield and colleagues' article, "Pulmonary Manifestations of Endocrine and Metabolic Diseases in Children," in this issue.

SUMMARY

Numerous pulmonary complications have been identified as associated with both cytogenetic and mendelian disorders. Lung development in early embryologic life is a complex process that is closely tied to the development of the GI tract. Intrinsic or extrinsic factors that impair lung expansion within the fetal thorax may lead to significant respiratory distress at birth. The degree of pulmonary compromise often predicts long-term survival despite aggressive intervention at birth. Most pulmonary defects are isolated occurrences, but children born with lung anomalies should be evaluated for additional malformations and syndromic features. Identification of additional anomalies or the diagnosis of a specific syndrome may provide guidance for medical management and important long-term prognostic information. Making a syndromic diagnosis may also provide essential information to the parents and extended family about recurrence risks and may guide family planning decisions.

With advances in molecular technologies, we are now able to provide better diagnostic information to patients with suspected genetic syndromes. Identification of specific gene mutations are likely to be more closely tied to therapeutic strategies over time. This approach to pulmonary disease will surely improve the quality of life for many children and adults, leading to risk reduction for pulmonary complications and enhanced pulmonary function.

WEB-BASED RESOURCES FOR TABLES

Gene Clinics and Gene Reviews: http://www.geneclinics.org.

Online Mendelian Inheritance in Man (OMIM): http://www.ncbi.nlm.nih.gov.

CLINICAL CARE POINTS

- Prenatal pulmonary malformations (both isolated and in concert with multiple defects) may have an underlying genetic etiology.
- Work-up for genetic causes of lung malformations might include cytogenetic testing incorporating microarray analysis, as well as testing for suspected single gene disorders utilizing next generation sequencing.
- Diagnostic testing for causative genetic disorders is best focused on optimizing medical management such as: avoiding unnecessary testing, selecting the best therapeutics, developing focus surveillance and interventional strategies, as well as informing family planning decisions.
- Genetic testing may also be indicated for a host of conditions that result in secondary pulmonary effects; cutting edge treatments may mitigate the deleterious effects of certain neuromuscular disorders, inborn errors of metabolism, storage disorders and other genetic conditions such as cystic fibrosis.

DISCLOSURE

The authors have nothing to disclose.

REFERENCES

1. Annunziata F, Bush A, Borgia F, et al. Congenital lung malformations: unresolved issues and unanswered questions. Front Pediatr 2019;7:239.
2. Mardini MK, Nyhan WL. Agenesis of the lung: report of four patients with unusual anomalies. Chest 1985;87:522–7.
3. Karolak JA, Vincent M, Deutsch G, et al. Complex compound inheritance of lethal lung developmental disorders due to disruption of the TBX-FGF pathway. Am J Hum Genet 2019;104:213–28.
4. Langer R, Kaufman HJ. Primary (isolated) bilateral pulmonary hypoplasia: a comparative study of radiologic findings and autopsy results. Pediatr Radiol 1986;16:175–9.
5. Sadler TW. Body cavities. In: Langman's medical embryology. 9th edition. Baltimore (MD): Lippincott, Williams & Wilkins; 2004. p. 211–21.
6. Slavotinek A, Lee SS, Davis R, et al. Fryns syndrome phenotype caused by chromosome microdeletions at 15q26.2 and 8p23.1. J Med Genet 2005;42:730–6.
7. Pober BR, Lin A, Russell M, et al. Infants with Bochdalek diaphragmatic hernia: sibling recurrence and monozygotic twin discordance in a hospital-based malformation surveillance program. Am J Med Genet 2005;138A:81–8.
8. Youssoufian H, Chance P, Tuck-Miller CM, et al. Association of a new chromosomal deletion [del (1)(q32q42)] with diaphragmatic hernia: assignment of a human ferritin gene. Hum Genet 1988;78:267–70.

9. Shapiro AJ, Davis SD, Ferkol TF, et al. Laterality defects other than situs inversus totalis in primary ciliary dyskinesia: insights into heterotaxy. Chest 2014;146: 1176–86.
10. Bush A, Abel RM, Chitty LS, et al. Congenital lung disease. In: Wilmott RW, Deterding RR, Li A, et al, editors. Kendig's disorders of the respiratory tract in children. 9th edition. Philadelphia: Elsevier; 2019. p. 289–337.
11. Durell J, Lakhoo K. Congenital cystic lesions of the lung. Early Hum Dev 2014;90: 935–9.
12. Casagrande A, Pederiva F. Association between congenital lung malformations and lung tumors in children and adults: a systematic review. J Thorac Oncol 2016;11:1837–45.
13. Sadler TW. The respiratory system. In: Langman's medical embryology. 9th edition. Baltimore (MD): Lippincott, Williams & Wilkins; 2004. p. 275–84.
14. Levy J, Levy-Carrick. Pulmonary complications of gastrointestinal disorder. Paediatr Respir Rev 2012;13:16–22.
15. Holland AJ, Fitzgerald DA. Oesophageal atresia and trachea-oesophageal fistula: current strategies and complications. Paediatr Respir Rev 2010;11(2):100–7.
16. Turcios, NL Recurrent pneumonia caused by diverticulum at the site of TEF repair. Consultant for pediatricians 2012;11(8):246
17. Reiterer F, Grossauer K, Morris N, et al. Congenital pulmonary lymphangiectasis. Paediatr Respir Rev 2014;15(3):275–80.
18. Connell FC, Gordon K, Brice G, et al. The classification and diagnostic algorithm for primary lymphatic dysplasia: an update to include molecular findings. Clin Genet 2013;84:303–14.
19. Schotland H, Denstaedt S. Hereditary hemorrhagic telangiectasia. N Engl J Med 2019;381:2552.
20. Stoltz DA, Meyerholz DK, Welsh MJ. Origins of cystic fibrosis lung disease. N Engl J Med 2015;372:351–62.
21. Rubin BK. Cystic fibrosis: myths, mistakes, and dogma. Paediatr Respir Rev 2014;15:113–6.
22. Garcia AM, Dorsey J. Nonpulmonary manifestations of cystic fibrosis. In: Wilmott RW, Deterding RR, Li A, et al, editors. Disorders of the respiratory tract in children. 9th edition. Philadelphia: Elsevier; 2019. p. 788–99.
23. Farrell PM, White TB, Ren CL, et al. Diagnosis of cystic fibrosis: consensus guidelines from the Cystic Fibrosis Foundation. J Pediatr 2017;181(Suppl 4):S4–15.
24. Afzelius BA. A human syndrome caused by immotile cilia. Science 1976;193: 317–9.
25. Leigh MW, Ferkol TW, Davis SD, et al. Clinical features and associated likelihood of primary ciliary dyskinesia in children and adolescents. Ann Am Thorac Soc 2016;13:1305–13.
26. Zariwala MA, Knowles, MR and Leigh MW. Primary ciliary dyskinesia GeneReviews (internet) Dec 5, 2019. Available at: https://www.ncbi.nih.gov/books/NBK1122/.
27. Boucher RC. Muco-obstructive lung diseases. N Engl J Med 2019;380:1941–53.
28. Li AM, Sonnappa S, Lex C, et al. Non-CF bronchiectasis: does knowing the aetiology lead to changes in management? Eur Respir J 2005;26(1):8–14.
29. Strnad P, McElvaney NG, Lomas DA. Alpha-1 antitrypsin deficiency. N Engl J Med 2020;382:1443–55.
30. Austin, ED, Loyd, JE, and Phillips, JA. Heritable pulmonary arterial hypertension. GeneReviews June 11, 2015. Available at: https://www.ncbi.nih.gov/books/NBK1485/.

Pulmonary Manifestations of Congenital Heart Disease in Children

Brandy N. Johnson, MD[a], Julie L. Fierro, MD[b], Howard B. Panitch, MD[c,*]

KEYWORDS

- Central airway obstruction • Aberrant (anomalous) vasculature
- Pulmonary mechanics • Abnormal pulmonary blood flow • Pulmonary edema
- Pulmonary hypertension • Exercise intolerance • Lymphatic system dysfunction

KEY POINTS

- Airways can be compressed by abnormally formed great vessels (rings and slings) or by normally formed but engorged, hypertensive ones.
- Cardiac lesions with decreased pulmonary blood flow are associated with pulmonary hypoplasia, which can improve with restoration of pulmonary blood flow.
- Cardiac lesions with increased pulmonary blood flow cause a decrease in lung compliance and an increase in resistance, both of which improve with corrective surgery.
- Congenital heart disease is the most common codiagnosis in pediatric pulmonary arterial hypertension.
- Cardiac lesions that impair normal lymphatic drainage can lead to plastic bronchitis, which may be corrected when normal lymphatic drainage is restored.

INTRODUCTION

Congenital heart disease (CHD) is one of most common major birth anomalies, with a mean estimated prevalence of 9.41 per thousand births.[1] In 2000, the number of pediatric and adult patients with severe CHD were nearly equal, with an increasing prevalence in the adult population.[2] Congenital and acquired cardiac lesions can affect airway and pulmonary parenchymal function, predispose toward the development of pulmonary hypertension, cause exercise limitation, and lead to abnormalities of

[a] Pediatric Pulmonology, Division of Pulmonary Medicine, Children's Hospital of Philadelphia, 3501 Civic Center Boulevard, Philadelphia, PA 19104, USA; [b] Division of Pulmonary Medicine, The Perelman School of Medicine at the University of Pennsylvania, Children's Hospital of Philadelphia, 3501 Civic Center Boulevard, Philadelphia, PA 19104, USA; [c] Technology Dependence Center, Division of Pulmonary Medicine, The Perelman School of Medicine at the University of Pennsylvania, Children's Hospital of Philadelphia, 3501 Civic Center Boulevard, Philadelphia, PA 19104, USA
* Corresponding author.
E-mail address: panitch@email.chop.edu

Pediatr Clin N Am 68 (2021) 25–40
https://doi.org/10.1016/j.pcl.2020.09.001 pediatric.theclinics.com

lymph flow. This review summarizes some of the more common pulmonary manifestations of congenital heart disease and abnormalities of the great vessels, and details clinical and physiologic findings that arise from pulmonary involvement in patients with CHD.

CENTRAL AIRWAYS

The close relationship of the heart and great vessels to the central airways accentuates the impact of anomalous cardiac structures on the architecture and function of the trachea and main bronchi. Cardiomegaly, chamber dilation, enlargement of normal vessels secondary to increased pulmonary blood flow (IPBF), and abnormally formed vessels all are recognized as causes of airway compromise.

Airway and Vessel Development

The trachea and main bronchi form approximately between 4 weeks and 6 weeks postconception.[3,4] The conducting airways all are formed by 16 weeks of gestation.[5] Development of the great vessels is completed by the seventh week of gestation (**Fig. 1**).[6–8] Throughout this timeframe, branchial arch pairs demonstrate patterns of persistence and regression and ultimately form the normal left aortic arch and pairs of major associated arteries.[9]

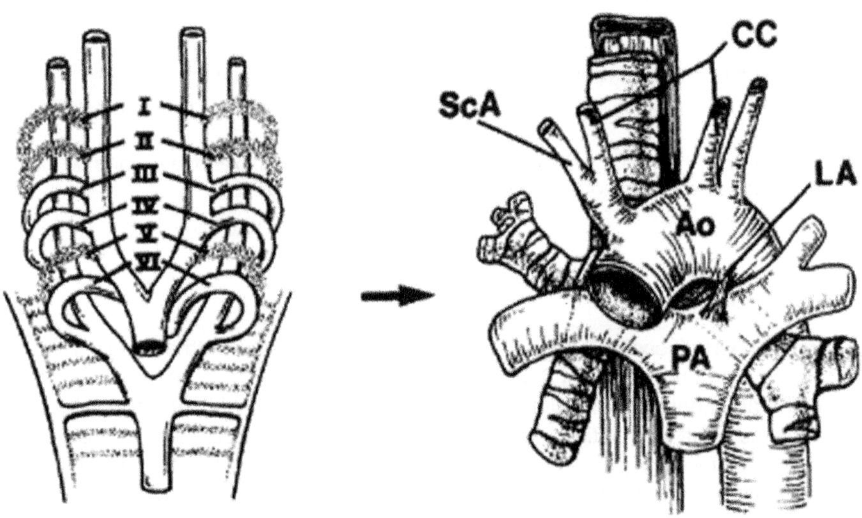

Fig. 1. Development of the great vessels. Branchial arches and paired ventral and dorsal aortae are shown on the left; their future structures are shown on the right. Under normal conditions, arches I, II, and V regress; arch III becomes the common carotid arteries (CC) (regression depicted as stippled structures). The aorta (Ao) is formed in 3 parts: the aortic root forms from fusion of the ventral aortae, the aortic arch from the left IV branchial arch, and the descending aorta from the left dorsal aorta whereas the right IV arch regresses. The subclavian artery (ScA) is formed from the right IV branchial arch and the seventh intersegmental artery. The proximal right and left VI arches give rise to the right and left central pulmonary arteries (PA), whereas the right distal VI arch regresses and the left distal VI arch becomes the ductus arteriosus and eventually the ligamentum arteriosum (LA). Anatomic abnormalities arise when vessels that normally are supposed to persist regress or those that should regress persist. (*From* McLaughlin RB, Jr., Wetmore RF, Tavill MA, Gaynor JW, Spray TL. Vascular anomalies causing symptomatic tracheobronchial compression. Laryngoscope. 1999;109(2 Pt 1):312-319; with permission.)

Abnormal Vasculature

Deviations at any point from this developmental pathway can distort normal anatomic relationships. For instance, failure of the right branchial fourth arch and right dorsal aorta to regress in combination with the normal persistence of a left arch results in one type of vascular ring, a double aortic arch (**Fig. 2**). Vascular rings are among the most frequently occurring great vessel malformations and the double aortic arch is the most common type of ring.[7] Some rings cause obstruction at the midtrachea and also impair swallowing by encircling both the trachea and esophagus. There also are cases in which rings are incomplete or involve only the trachea or esophagus.[10]

The pulmonary artery sling is the only lesion in which a great vessel travels between the trachea and esophagus (**Fig. 3**).[11] The anomalous left pulmonary artery compresses the right main bronchus and right distal trachea and forms an anterior indentation on the esophagus.[12] Approximately 50% of patients with pulmonary slings also have tracheal stenosis with complete cartilaginous rings.[7] Less frequently, the pulmonary artery sling is associated with a bridging bronchus, where the right middle and lower lobes and, in some instances, the entire right lung are supplied by a bronchus that originates from the left sided airways.[13]

One of the most common aberrant vessels to cause airway compression is the anomalous innominate (brachiocephalic) artery, where it crosses the trachea (**Fig. 4**). For unclear reasons, not all subjects with a leftward origin of the innominate artery develop symptoms.[14] Intraluminal compression of a pulsatile tracheal lesion with a rigid bronchoscope, which results in cessation of the right radial pulse (Waterston sign), confirms the presence of airway narrowing by an anomalous innominate artery.[15]

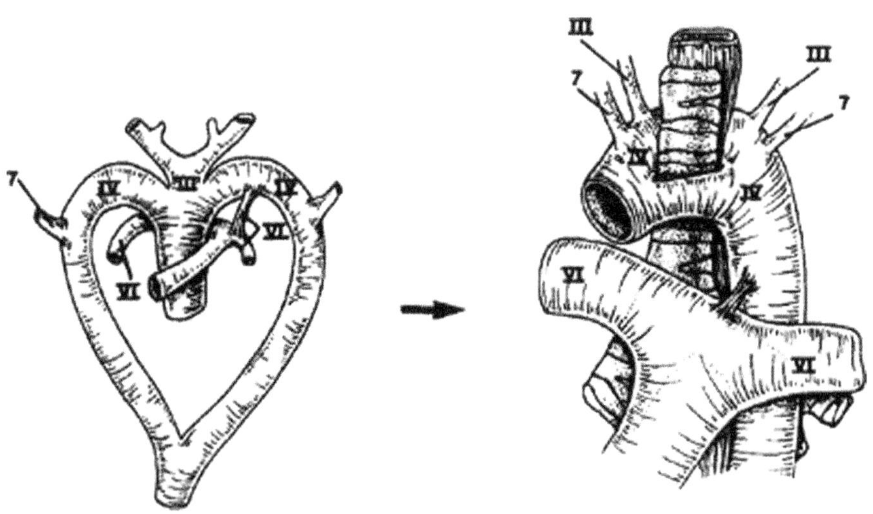

Fig. 2. A double aortic arch arises when both pairs of aortic roots and IV branchial arches persist, when the right IV branchial artery and right aortic root normally regress. The vascular ring encircles both the trachea and esophagus. (*From* McLaughlin RB, Jr., Wetmore RF, Tavill MA, Gaynor JW, Spray TL. Vascular anomalies causing symptomatic tracheobronchial compression. Laryngoscope. 1999;109(2 Pt 1):312-319; with permission.)

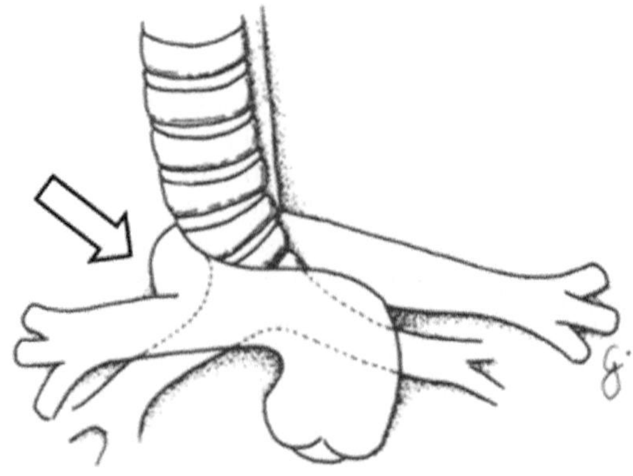

Fig. 3. A pulmonary artery sling occurs when the left pulmonary artery arises from the right pulmonary artery (*arrow*) rather than from the main pulmonary artery. It then traverses above the right main bronchus and between the trachea and esophagus toward the left lung. (*Adapted from* Marmon LM, Bye MR, Haas JM, Balsara RK, Dunn JM. Vascular rings and slings: long-term follow-up of pulmonary function. J Pediatr Surg. 1984;19(6):683-692; with permission.)

Enlarged Cardiac and Vascular Structures

Even when the great vessels form normally, airway compression still can arise from dilated pulmonary arteries. Normal mean pulmonary artery pressure (PAP) is insufficient to compress airways. At higher pressures, however, pulmonary vessels can

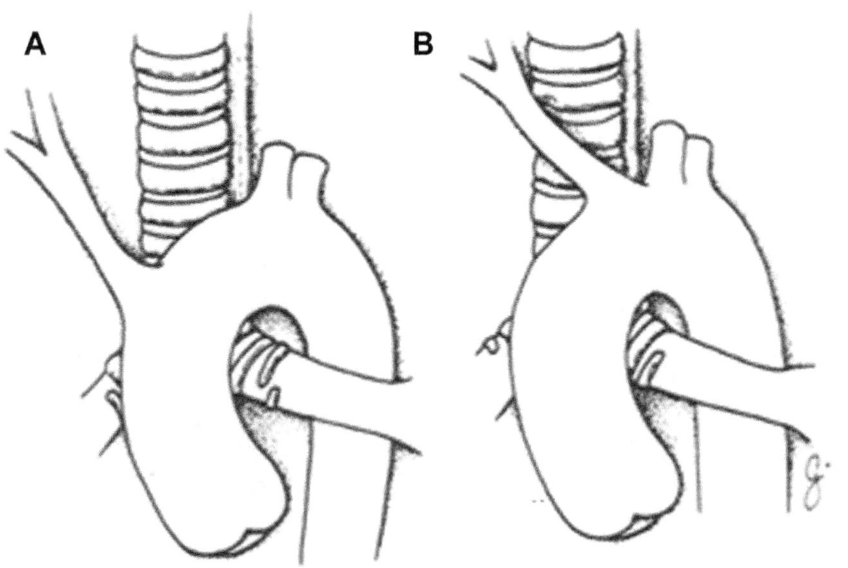

Fig. 4. (*A*) Normal takeoff of the innominate artery. (*B*) The anomalous innominate arises to the left of the trachea and crosses over to the right, causing a right anterolateral compression. (*From* Marmon LM, Bye MR, Haas JM, Balsara RK, Dunn JM. Vascular rings and slings: long-term follow-up of pulmonary function. J Pediatr Surg. 1984;19(6):683-692; with permission.)

become distended and stiff. Large left-to-right shunts that increase the ratio of pulmonary blood flow to systemic blood flow (Qp:Qs) cause pulmonary arterial hypertension (PAH). These shunts include atrioventricular canal defects, ventricular and atrial septal defects as well as patent ductus arteriosus. Hemodynamically significant defects occur when Qp:Qs is greater than 1.5.[16] Additionally, aneurysmal enlargement of the main and proximal branch pulmonary arteries can occur in patients with tetralogy of Fallot (TOF) with absent pulmonary valve, presumably resulting from excessive turbulence of blood flow just after the stenotic pulmonary valve ring.[17]

Enlarged pulmonary vessels cause compression where they juxtapose airways (**Fig. 5**).[18] The left main bronchus has the highest rate of compression in cases of CHD with pulmonary overflow.[19,20] Massive cardiomegaly or chamber enlargement can also cause airway compression. Other common patterns of compression by the pulmonary arteries are depicted in **Fig. 5**.

Complications of Unrepaired Anomalies

Localized vascular compression can be associated with fixed or dynamic (tracheomalacia or bronchomalacia) narrowing of the central airway.[21,22] Depending on the degree of obstruction, areas of either atelectasis or overinflation can result. Focal obstruction also impairs mucociliary clearance, creating trapped respiratory secretions and chronic inflammation. This can lead to recurrent infections and the development of bronchiectasis. Unfortunately, compromised airway structure and strength can persist past correction of the vascular lesion.[23]

When engorgement of the left pulmonary artery causes medial displacement of the aorta into the left lateral tracheal wall, the recurrent laryngeal nerve can become entrapped as it courses between the aorta and trachea (see **Fig. 5**A). This results in

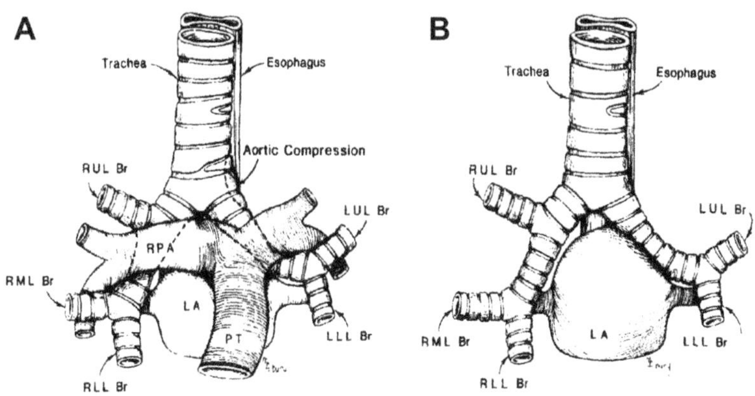

Fig. 5. (*A*) Enlargement of the left pulmonary artery (LPA) can compress the left main bronchus (LMB) anteriorly, whereas the left lower lobe artery courses behind the left upper lobe bronchus (LUL Br) and can compress the superior aspect of the LMB and LUL Br. The right pulmonary artery (RPA) crosses over the junction of the bronchus intermedius and right middle lobe bronchus (RML Br) and can compress those structures when it is dilated. The normal aortic compression on the left side of the trachea, which typically is minimal, can be exaggerated as a dilated LPA displaces the aorta medially. (*B*) The left atrium (LA) is positioned just below the tracheal bifurcation; when enlarged it elevates the LMB and compresses the LMB from below while an enlarged LPA can compress the airway from above and magnify the effect on the airway. PT, pulmonary trunk. (*From* Berlinger NT, Long C, Foker J, Lucas RV, Jr. Tracheobronchial compression in acyanotic congenital heart disease. Ann Otol Rhinol Laryngol. 1983;92(4 Pt 1):387-390; with permission.)

left vocal cord paralysis, or cardiovocal syndrome, which manifests as hoarseness that sometimes is difficult to discern during infancy.[24] There also is increased risk of aspiration associated with the paralyzed vocal cord, which can lead to subsequent parenchymal damage. Correcting the left-to-right shunt restores normal vocal cord function and re-establishes airway protection.[24]

Diagnosis and Management of Congenital Heart Disease–Related Central Airway Lesions

Symptoms of vascular airway compression can include an abnormal cry, stridor, homophonous or monophonic wheeze, chronic cough, cyanosis, apneic events, or recurrent lower respiratory tract infections.[25] Tighter rings present in early infancy with stridor and dysphagia secondary to concomitant esophageal entrapment. Feeding difficulty occasionally is the earliest presenting symptom.[7] In one review, diagnosis of vascular anomalies causing symptoms of tracheal compression occurred at a median age of 8 months.[9] Some children remain asymptomatic when vascular rings are less confining.

Several imaging techniques can be used to determine the cause and magnitude of central airway problems related to CHD (**Table 1**). Each technique has its own inherent risks and benefits, and the choice of modality for imaging often is determined by availability of equipment, cost, and local expertise. Computed tomography (CT) and magnetic resonance imaging (MRI) techniques are employed to achieve 3-dimensional definition of the vascular structure(s) when surgical planning dictates the need. Direct visualization of the airways via flexible or rigid bronchoscopy augments the clinical investigation initiated by these imaging techniques. Intraoperatively, bronchoscopy also allows for evaluation of airway complications or effects of procedures like aortopexy on luminal patency.

Occasionally, surgical correction of vascular anomalies causes acquired airway compression, especially in cases of arch reconstruction.[19,20] In one series, newly detected airway compression was noted in one-third of patients who underwent arch repair.[20]

Table 1
Evaluation of cardiovascular anomalies affecting the airway

Modality	Attributes	Detractions
Anterior-posterior and lateral plain films	Widely available Low radiation burden Gross structures visualized	Less sensitive for evaluation of the soft tissues and vasculature
Barium esophogram	Widely available	Increased radiation exposure
CT	Rapid acquisition time Improved visualization of the airway and soft tissue structures Dynamic evaluation possible	Increased ionizing radiation burden
MRI	No radiation exposure	Longer acquisition time Requires sedation in uncooperative patients
Rigid and flexible bronchoscopy	Structural and dynamic airway evaluation Allows for intraoperative/postoperative evaluation	Requires sedation and often mechanical ventilation

ALTERATIONS IN PULMONARY BLOOD FLOW

Several intracardiac shunts affect pulmonary blood flow (PBF) and ultimately have an impact on function of the respiratory system. Left-to-right shunts increase PBF whereas right-to-left shunts decrease PBF.

Reduced Pulmonary Blood Flow

The most common CHD associated with reduced PBF is TOF.[26] Other lesions include pulmonary valve stenosis and tricuspid valve abnormalities consisting of tricuspid atresia/stenosis and tricuspid valve displacement (Ebstein anomaly).[27] The reduction in PBF is accompanied by shunting through an atrial or ventricular septal defect, because blood is prevented from traveling through the pulmonary arteries because of obstruction or defect at the level of a right-sided valve, vessel, or chamber.

Parenchymal and pulmonary vasculature relationships

Postmortem examination of patients with CHD lesions associated with decreased PBF (CHD-DPBF) typically demonstrate lung volumes that are below normal for age or body surface area, reduced alveolar number, and a reduction in the size of intraacinar arteries.[28–30] Whether these findings represent primarily effects of reduced PBF on postnatal lung growth when rapid alveolarization occurs or are the result of alterations in prenatal lung development remains unclear.

Throughout gestation, the pulmonary circulation receives less than 25% of the combined ventricular output.[31] Lesions that cause additional reduction in flow are thought to disrupt normal pulmonary vascular development and alveolarization. Sonographically estimated lung volumes of fetuses with CHD-DPBF were smaller than those of controls.[32] Similarly, aborted fetuses who had CHD with right outflow tract obstruction had significantly lower lung weight, lung weight corrected for body weight, and evidence of pulmonary hypoplasia compared with fetuses having CHD with left outflow tract obstruction, transposition of the great vessels, or other types of CHD.[33] Lack of correlation of pulmonary hypoplasia with size of the pulmonary arteries, however, suggested that pulmonary hypoplasia occurred independent of perfusion mechanisms.[33] In contrast, postnatal surgical enhancement of perfusion can improve lung growth, resulting in children with normal or near-normal lung volumes.[30]

Pulmonary mechanics and reduced pulmonary blood flow

Infants and children with CHD-DPBF may appear cyanotic, but they typically do not have signs of altered lung or chest wall mechanics like retractions or accessory muscle use. That is because respiratory mechanics of CHD-DPBF patients are closer to normal compared with mechanics of patients with CHD-IPBF.[34,35] As a result, resting respiratory rate is lower in infants with CHD-DPBF than in those with CHD-IPBF.[34]

Children with TOF (CHD-DPBF) had normal airways resistance (R_{aw}) preoperatively and it did not change statistically following restoration of PBF.[35] Tissues of the respiratory system stiffened postoperatively, but the authors speculated this was more of an effect of cardiopulmonary bypass than of restoration of blood flow to the lungs. Other children with TOF demonstrated a slightly lower functional residual capacity (FRC) preoperatively compared with published normal values.[36] There was a gradual and statistically significant increase in R_{aw} and in tissue elastance between preoperative and postoperative conditions. Postoperatively, FRC decreased and the lung clearance index increased, reflecting greater ventilatory inhomogeneity. Perioperative changes in mechanics were minimized when values were corrected for the change in FRC, suggesting that the airway narrowing reflected in the increased R_{aw} was the result of a decrease in lung volume.

Acute cessation of PBF by balloon occlusion of the pulmonary artery during valvuloplasty in children with pulmonary valvular stenosis decreased tidal volume and dynamic respiratory system compliance (C_{RS}), and increased respiratory system resistance.[37] The investigators reasoned that the changes in mechanics reflected a loss of erectile function of small peribronchiolar vessels that help to maintain airway patency. They speculated that such changes contribute to the development of stiff and difficult-to-ventilate lungs that occur during acute pulmonary hypertensive crises.

In summary, subjects with CHD-DPBF demonstrate near-normal specific pulmonary mechanics at baseline, although lung volume is decreased slightly. PBF is important in maintaining the architecture of alveoli and bronchioles, and in providing a tethering effect of alveoli on the airways.

Chronic hypoxemia/polycythemia

Right-to-left shunts are characterized by chronic hypoxemia. Long-standing oxygen deprivation impairs mitochondrial respiration. Subsequent repair of cyanotic CHD then exposes affected tissue, notably the myocardium, to reperfusion injury from free radicals generated during acute reoxygenation. In an animal model of chronic hypoxia, acute exposure to normoxia during reperfusion resulted in decreased ventricular compliance and reduced contractilty.[38] One adaptive mechanism of chronic hypoxemia is polycythemia, which may increase oxygen-carrying capacity of the blood and oxygen delivery to tissues. The increase in hematocrit, however, can cause hyperviscosity, thrombosis, and an increase in pulmonary vascular resistance (PVR). Formation of major collateral vessels also may enhance perfusion to hypoxic pulmonary tissues. These abnormal vessels, however, can be a source of potentially life-threatening pulmonary hemorrhage.

Increased Pulmonary Blood Flow

Cardiac lesions that include left-to-right shunts increase PBF. The increase in PBF also can be accompanied by an increase in PAP, depending on PVR. The effects of coexisting increased PAP may influence pulmonary mechanics to a greater degree than those of IPBF alone.

Pulmonary mechanics and increased pulmonary blood flow

Infants with CHD-IPBF typically demonstrate tachypnea, intercostal retractions, and increased breathing effort.[34,39,40] These clinical manifestations reflect underlying alterations in lung mechanics. Infants and young children with CHD-IPBF studied preoperatively had normal FRC.[34,39,41] In contrast, pulmonary compliance or C_{RS} usually was below normal.[34,37,39–41] Whether reduced compliance was caused by IPBF or increased PAP was less clear. In 1 study, all subjects who had increases in both PBF and PAP demonstrated a reduction in specific lung compliance (sC_L) (lung compliance/FRC), whereas those who had either IPBF or increased PAP alone had sC_L that was not statistically decreased.[41] Another study showed that the reduction in sC_L did not correlate with the magnitude of the left to right shunt, but it did correlate with the mean PAP.[34] The investigators reasoned that the increase in PAP was primarily responsible for the alteration in elastic properties of the lung, and speculated that the higher pressure caused stiffening of the pulmonary vasculature. Other investigators showed that only those infants with CHD-IPBF and concurrent elevated PAP had low C_{RS}.[39] In addition, those infants with both IPBF and elevated PAP demonstrated a significant (50%) increase in C_{RS} within 10 days of cardiac repair; there was no postoperative change in C_{RS} among those infants with elevated PBF but normal PAP.[39] Echocardiographic estimates of shunt size and PAP confirm the observations that the combination of elevated PAP and IPBF or an increase in PAP alone, but not IPBF alone are responsible for the decrease in lung compliance in patients with CHD-IPBF.[40]

Some studies show that subjects with unrepaired CHD-IPBF also have elevated lung, airway or respiratory system resistance at baseline,[34,40,42] whereas others describe normal resistance values.[39,41] Regardless, correction of IPBF results in a reduction in resistance.[35,36,42] Unlike findings in children with CHD-DPBF, reduction in airways resistance persists even after normalization for lung volume, indicating improvement in airway function.[36] The postoperative change in resistance could result from reduction in size or pressure of vessels compressing airways. Alternately, IPBF causes engorgement of the outer airway wall, leading to uncoupling of the airway from surrounding alveolar tethering; this would lead not only to narrowing of the airway lumen at baseline but also to increased reactivity of airway smooth muscle.[43]

Pulmonary edema

Although alveoli are surrounded by blood within the pulmonary capillary network, the intersitium under normal circumstances is fairly dry.[44] Traditionally, the Starling equation has described the balance of forces that results in a small net flow of fluid from the pulmonary capillaries into the intersititum.[45] An increase in pulmonary hydrostatic pressure in children with CHD is the predominant perturbation that overcomes the lymphatic system's ability to remove fluid from the interstitium.[45] Fluid crosses the capillary endothelium and initially occupies the perivascular and peribronchial spaces.[46] An increase in lymphatic flow can compensate for this at first, but eventually the lymphatic reserves become overwhelmed and edema fluid moves from the perivascular and peribronchial interstitium to the periphery of the alveolar membrane, where it disrupts the alveolar wall and eventually causes alveolar flooding.[46]

Pulmonary edema occurs because of increased pulmonary vascular congestion resulting from IPBF, pulmonary venous obstruction or left ventricular failure.[45,47] Increases in right-sided cardiac pressures also impair effective drainage of interstitial fluid. Tachypnea and increased work of breathing are among the earliest signs of pulmonary edema, representing decreased lung compliance and can be present without other clinical findings.[48] Auscultatory findings can include wheezing (cardiac asthma) or crackles. Interstitial edema can contribute to compression of the airways and airway wall edema, producing an obstructive process on spirometry.[49] Progression of edema ultimately causes a loss of lung volume and restrictive pattern.[49] Diffusion capacity of carbon monoxide can become impaired, which worsens baseline hypoxemia.[49] Chest radiographs demonstrate accumulation of fluid in the perivascular spaces, lung fissures, or pleural space.

PULMONARY HYPERTENSION AND CONGENITAL HEART DISEASE

CHD is the most common codiagnosis in pediatric PAH, with natural history studies suggesting that approximately 10% of patients with CHD develop PAH.[50] PAH associated with CHD most commonly is a result of a significant left-to-right shunt. The associated increased blood flow leads to pulmonary vascular remodeling and elevated PVR. This sequence of events eventually results in a reversal of blood flow known as Eisenmenger syndrome, defined as "pulmonary hypertension due to a high PVR with reversed or bidirectional shunt at the aortopulmonary, ventricular, or atrial level."[51,52]

In the presence of a large communication between the right and left ventricles or aorta and pulmonary artery, changes in the pulmonary arteries occur because of an increase in blood flow and pressure. Increases in pressure and PVR trigger a cascade of endothelial cell dysfunction, abnormal shear stress, and circumferential wall stretch in the pulmonary arteries, causing vasoconstriction and remodeling of the pulmonary vessel wall.[53] Initial changes in pulmonary vasculature may be reversible if surgical correction is completed early.[54,55]

The risk of developing Eisenmenger syndrome varies and depends on the underlying heart defect, the size of the defect, and the degree of shunting. Patients with pre-tricuspid shunts tend to present with PAH later in life whereas those with post-tricuspid shunts can present as early as infancy.[56] Approximately 10% of patients with an unrepaired atrial septal defect (pretricuspid lesion) develop Eisenmenger syndrome, whereas 50% of patients with a large unrepaired ventricular septal defect (post-tricuspid lesion) develop Eisenmenger syndrome. Approximately 90% of patients with an unrepaired AV septal defect and nearly all of those with truncus arteriosus develop Eisenmenger syndrome.[54,57] The development of Eisenmenger syndrome in patients with complex CHD is associated with increased mortality compared with those with simple lesions.[58]

The World Health Organization (WHO) classification system for pulmonary hypertension classifies CHD as a group 1 disease.[59,60] Group 2 encompasses postcapillary pulmonary hypertension (PH) due to left heart disease. This includes congenital conditions such as coarctation of the aorta, pulmonary vein stenosis, or left-sided valvular disease. PAH, or precapillary pulmonary hypertension, is defined by the WHO as a mean pulmonary arterial pressure (PAP) greater than 20 mm Hg, a pulmonary capillary wedge pressure less than or equal to 15 mm Hg, and PVR greater than 3 index Wood units.[60] At the 5th World Symposium on Pulmonary Hypertension, a classification system for PAH associated CHD was put forth (**Box 1**).[61]

General symptoms of PAH include dyspnea, chest pain, syncope, and sudden death. Exercise intolerance is a common feature of patients with PAH associated with CHD. Patients who develop Eisenmenger syndrome develop cyanosis, which can lead to hematologic, renal, and hepatic dysfunction, resulting in significant morbidity.[54] Physical examination findings of PAH include an accentuated pulmonary component or single second heart sound and, in some cases, an early diastolic murmur consistent with pulmonary regurgitation. Palpation of the chest for a right ventricular heave is indicative of severe PAH. Severe disease also is associated with hepatic congestion, resulting in hepatomegaly. Long-standing cyanotic disease also leads to digital clubbing, or edema in the setting of heart failure.[62]

Diagnostic imaging includes chest radiograph, transthoracic echocardiography, and less commonly MRI and CT scans. Cardiac catheterization with vasodilator testing is the gold standard in diagnosing PAH. The 6-minute walk test can be used to determine exercise capacity and exercise-related desaturation. Treatment of

Box 1
World Health Organization Classification of pulmonary arterial hypertension–congenital heart disease

Group 1. Large systemic-to-pulmonary shunts that lead to elevated PVR and bidirectional/reversal of blood flow (Eisenmenger syndrome).

Group 2. Left-to-right shunts causing mild–moderate increases in PVR with preserved systemic-to-pulmonary shunting.

Group 3. PAH with coincidental CHD (the cardiac lesion is not felt to contribute to PAH development).

Group 4. PAH that recurs or persists after surgical correction of the cardiac lesion.

PAH-associated CHD consists of PAH-targeted drug treatment directed toward 3 pathways involved in the pulmonary vasoactive response: the endothelin pathway (endothelin receptor antagonists), NO-cGMP pathway (PDE5 inhibitors and soluble guanylate cyclase stimulators), and prostacyclin pathway (prostaglandins).[62]

EXERCISE INTOLERANCE

Limited exercise capacity is a hallmark of CHD patients with both types of altered PBF, however different explanations exist for each situation. Following repair of cyanotic heart lesions, patients with CHD-DPBF demonstrate lower systolic blood pressure and impaired chronotropy during exercise compared with healthy controls.[63] Postulated mechanisms include surgical damage to the cardiac autonomic nervous system, intraoperative ischemia, and chronic tissue hypoxia.[63] The reduction in heart rate variability correlates with an observed reduction in maximal oxygen consumption and functional capacity.[64] Fontan procedure patients cannot regulate PBF normally during exercise, so vascular resistance cannot be reduced.[65]

Conversely, patients with CHD-IPBF who have a large, unrepaired left-to-right shunt are limited primarily by reduced systemic perfusion.[66] Following repair, improvement in left ventricular stroke volume and cardiac output allow for improved peak oxygen consumption; however, values remain below that of healthy controls.[66,67] Again, impaired heart rate and inappropriate regulation of PBF likely explain the persistent deficit in exercise performance.[68]

The tendency to develop restrictive lung disease that further limits exercise is common to patients with both types of altered PBF. Impairment of lung function correlates with the complexity of cardiac disease, surgical history, and degree of scoliosis.[69] One study found a direct correlation between the number of thoracotomies required for correction of a cardiac defect and the degree of restrictive disease.[70] Although there was not a direct correlation between number of thoracotomies and exercise limitation, the investigators noted that for every percentage point increase in vital capacity the probability of impaired exercise capacity decreased.

LYMPHATIC DISORDERS

When cardiac failure or low flow states exist, the lymphatics serve to reduce cardiac pressures and avoid overload by acting as a highly efficient reservoir. Under normal conditions, the difference between the lower central venous and higher pulmonary arteriolar and wedge pressures maintains normal flow and fluid resorption. Processes that distort this differential make natural drainage impossible, because lymph would then be expected to drain toward a pressure that exceeds that at which it is produced.[71] Children with single-ventricle physiology are at risk for developing this abnormal lymphatic flow. The repair diverts the systemic blood flow to the pulmonary circulation, making pressure at the thoracic duct higher than or similar to the pressure at the capillary level where lymph is formed. Types of lymphatic dysfunction include a central lymphatic flow disorder with effusions in more than 1 compartment and dermal backflow through abdominal lymphatic channels, pulmonary lymphatic perfusion syndrome, and traumatic leak (**Box 2**).[71]

Impaired lymph drainage can lead to the formation of cohesive and branching casts within the airways, known as plastic bronchitis. Elevated venous pressures not only compromise the flow of lymph but also breach the integrity of airway mucosa. Proposed mechanisms for plastic bronchitis include hypersecretion of the mucous glands, leakage of proteinaceous fluid into the airway, and lymphobronchial fistula

Box 2
Complications of lymphatic dysfunction

Pulmonary edema

Pleural effusion

Spontaneous chylothorax

Atelectasis

Decreased pulmonary tissue compliance

Local tissue inflammation

Immunodeficiency

Plastic bronchitis

Lymphedema

Protein losing enteropathy

formation.[72,73] In cases of CHD, cast composition predominantly is mucin-containing debris.[74]

Increased lymphatic pressures also can lead to spontaneous chylothoraces. Chylothorax can occur in association with traumatic disruption of the thoracic duct during thoracic surgery as well. Leaking of lymphatic fluid into the pleural cavity leads to effusion, atelectasis, and impaired lung compliance unless evacuated.

There are a variety of specialized mapping techniques being used to evaluate the functional anatomy of the lymphatic system. These investigations can identify the specific etiology of dysfunction and guide approach to treatment.[75]

SUMMARY

Alterations in cardiovascular anatomy and function can impair airways, respiratory mechanics, the pulmonary vascular system, and the lymphatic system. A dynamic interplay between each altered aspect of the pulmonary system, as well as between the pulmonary and systemic circulations, dictates the clinical course of patients with CHD. A basic understanding of how various disorders of the cardiovascular system affect pulmonary physiology can help clinicians anticipate problems and address functional impairments.

CLINICS CARE POINTS

- It is important to assess the response to bronchodilator administration in wheezing infants and children with IPBF. If the cause is small airway wall edema, bronchodilators may improve the patient's status. If the cause is from large airway compression, wheezing and obstruction can worsen.
- The younger an infant with symptoms of a vascular ring presents, the more severe will be the degree of airway and/or esophageal narrowing.
- Surgical correction of lesions that cause hemodynamically significant IPBF and PAP will typically improve pulmonary mechanics; mechanics changes after correction of lesions causing DPBF reflect alterations in resting lung volume rather than primary airway or parenchymal characteristics.
- Increased PAP is likely the most important factor causing a reduction in lung compliance. IPBF alone probably does not reduce lung compliance.

- Symptoms of dyspnea, syncope, or chest pain, and findings of a single or accentuated second heart sound in a child with CHD-IPBF should raise a concern for PAH.

DISCLOSURE

The authors have nothing to disclose.

REFERENCES

1. Liu Y, Chen S, Zuhlke L, et al. Global birth prevalence of congenital heart defects 1970-2017: updated systematic review and meta-analysis of 260 studies. Int J Epidemiol 2019;48(2):455–63.
2. Marelli AJ, Mackie AS, Ionescu-Ittu R, et al. Congenital heart disease in the general population: changing prevalence and age distribution. Circulation 2007; 115(2):163–72.
3. Hislop AA. Airway and blood vessel interaction during lung development. J Anat 2002;201(4):325–34.
4. Jeffrey PK. The development of large and small airways. Am J Respir Crit Care Med 1998;157(5 Pt 2):S174–80.
5. Bucher U, Reid L. Development of the intrasegmental bronchial tree: the pattern of branching and development of cartilage at various stages of intra-uterine life. Thorax 1961;16:207–18.
6. Kau T, Sinzig M, Gasser J, et al. Aortic development and anomalies. Semin Intervent Radiol 2007;24(2):141–52.
7. Kussman BD, Geva T, McGowan FX. Cardiovascular causes of airway compression. Paediatr Anaesth 2004;14(1):60–74.
8. Stojanovska J, Cascade PN, Chong S, et al. Embryology and imaging review of aortic arch anomalies. J Thorac Imaging 2012;27(2):73–84.
9. McLaughlin RB Jr, Wetmore RF, Tavill MA, et al. Vascular anomalies causing symptomatic tracheobronchial compression. Laryngoscope 1999;109(2 Pt 1): 312–9.
10. Loomba RS. Natural History of Asymptomatic and Unrepaired Vascular Rings: Is Watchful Waiting a Viable Option? A New Case and Review of Previously Reported Cases. Children (Basel) 2016;3(4).
11. Berdon WE, Baker DH. Vascular anomalies and the infant lung: rings, slings, and other things. Semin Roentgenol 1972;7(1):39–64.
12. Rogers DJ, Cunnane MB, Hartnick CJ. Vascular compression of the airway: establishing a functional diagnostic algorithm. JAMA Otolaryngol Head Neck Surg 2013;139(6):586–91.
13. Wells TR, Gwinn JL, Landing BH, et al. Reconsideration of the anatomy of sling left pulmonary artery: the association of one form with bridging bronchus and imperforate anus. Anatomic and diagnostic aspects. J Pediatr Surg 1988; 23(10):892–8.
14. Benjamin B. Tracheomalacia in infants and children. Ann Otol Rhinol Laryngol 1984;93(5 Pt 1):438–42.
15. Ardito JM, Ossoff RH, Tucker GF Jr, et al. Innominate artery compression of the trachea in infants with reflex apnea. Ann Otol Rhinol Laryngol 1980;89(5 Pt 1): 401–5.
16. Marin Rodriguez C, Sanchez Alegre ML, Lancharro Zapata A, et al. What radiologists need to know about the pulmonary-systemic flow ratio (Qp/Qs): what it is, how to calculate it, and what it is for. Radiologia 2015;57(5):369–79.

17. Lakier JB, Stanger P, Heymann MA, et al. Tetralogy of Fallot with absent pulmonary valve. Natural history and hemodynamic considerations. Circulation 1974;50(1):167–75.
18. Berlinger NT, Long C, Foker J, et al. Tracheobronchial compression in acyanotic congenital heart disease. Ann Otol Rhinol Laryngol 1983;92(4 Pt 1):387–90.
19. An HS, Choi EY, Kwon BS, et al. Airway compression in children with congenital heart disease evaluated using computed tomography. Ann Thorac Surg 2013;96(6):2192–7.
20. Jhang WK, Park JJ, Seo DM, et al. Perioperative evaluation of airways in patients with arch obstruction and intracardiac defects. Ann Thorac Surg 2008;85(5):1753–8.
21. Gross RE. Surgical relief for tracheal obstruction from a vascular ring. N Engl J Med 1945;233:586–90.
22. Sprague HB, Ernlund CH, Albright F. Clinical Aspects of Persistent Right Aortic Root. Trans Am Clin Climatol Assoc 1933;49:83–94.
23. Hysinger EB, Panitch HB. Paediatric Tracheomalacia. Paediatr Respir Rev 2016;17:9–15.
24. Condon LM, Katkov H, Singh A, et al. Cardiovocal syndrome in infancy. Pediatrics 1985;76(1):22–5.
25. Marmon LM, Bye MR, Haas JM, et al. Vascular rings and slings: long-term follow-up of pulmonary function. J Pediatr Surg 1984;19(6):683–92.
26. Ossa Galvis MM, Bhakta RT, Tarmahomed A, et al. Cyanotic heart disease. In: StatPearls [Internet]. Treasure Island (FL): StatPearls Publishing; 2020.
27. Waldman JD, Wernly JA. Cyanotic congenital heart disease with decreased pulmonary blood flow in children. Pediatr Clin North Am 1999;46(2):385–404.
28. Haworth SG, Reid L. Quantitative structural study of pulmonary circulation in the newborn with pulmonary atresia. Thorax 1977;32(2):129–33.
29. Johnson RJ, Haworth SG. Pulmonary vascular and alveolar development in tetralogy of Fallot: a recommendation for early correction. Thorax 1982;37(12):893–901.
30. Rabinovitch M, Herrera-deLeon V, Castaneda AR, et al. Growth and development of the pulmonary vascular bed in patients with tetralogy of Fallot with or without pulmonary atresia. Circulation 1981;64(6):1234–49.
31. Gao Y, Raj JU. Regulation of the pulmonary circulation in the fetus and newborn. Physiol Rev 2010;90(4):1291–335.
32. Guo Y, Liu X, Gu X, et al. Fetal lung volume and pulmonary artery changes in congenital heart disease with decreased pulmonary blood flow: Quantitative ultrasound analysis. Echocardiography 2018;35(1):85–9.
33. Ruchonnet-Metrailler I, Bessieres B, Bonnet D, et al. Pulmonary hypoplasia associated with congenital heart diseases: a fetal study. PLoS One 2014;9(4):e93557.
34. Bancalari E, Jesse MJ, Gelband H, et al. Lung mechanics in congenital heart disease with increased and decreased pulmonary blood flow. J Pediatr 1977;90(2):192–5.
35. Habre W, Schutz N, Pellegrini M, et al. Preoperative pulmonary hemodynamics determines changes in airway and tissue mechanics following surgical repair of congenital heart diseases. Pediatr Pulmonol 2004;38(6):470–6.
36. von Ungern-Sternberg BS, Petak F, Hantos Z, et al. Changes in functional residual capacity and lung mechanics during surgical repair of congenital heart diseases: effects of preoperative pulmonary hemodynamics. Anesthesiology 2009;110(6):1348–55.

37. Schulze-Neick I, Penny DJ, Derrick GP, et al. Pulmonary vascular-bronchial interactions: acute reduction in pulmonary blood flow alters lung mechanics. Heart 2000;84(3):284–9.
38. Corno AF, Milano G, Samaja M, et al. Chronic hypoxia: a model for cyanotic congenital heart defects. J Thorac Cardiovasc Surg 2002;124(1):105–12.
39. Baraldi E, Filippone M, Milanesi O, et al. Respiratory mechanics in infants and young children before and after repair of left-to-right shunts. Pediatr Res 1993; 34(3):329–33.
40. Yau KI, Fang LJ, Wu MH. Lung mechanics in infants with left-to-right shunt congenital heart disease. Pediatr Pulmonol 1996;21(1):42–7.
41. Howlett G. Lung mechanics in normal infants and infants with congenital heart disease. Arch Dis Child 1972;47(255):707–15.
42. Stayer SA, Diaz LK, East DL, et al. Changes in respiratory mechanics among infants undergoing heart surgery. Anesth Analg 2004;98(1):49–55, table of contents.
43. Uhlig T, Wildhaber JH, Carroll N, et al. Pulmonary vascular congestion selectively potentiates airway responsiveness in piglets. Am J Respir Crit Care Med 2000; 161(4 Pt 1):1306–13.
44. Ingbar DH. Cardiogenic pulmonary edema: mechanisms and treatment - an intensivist's view. Curr Opin Crit Care 2019;25(4):371–8.
45. Uejima T. General pediatric emergencies. Acute pulmonary edema. Anesthesiol Clin North Am 2001;19(2):383–9, viii.
46. Assaad S, Kratzert WB, Shelley B, et al. Assessment of Pulmonary Edema: Principles and Practice. J Cardiothorac Vasc Anesth 2018;32(2):901–14.
47. Rudolph AM. Diagnosis and Treatment: Respiratory Distress and Cardiac Disease in Infancy. Pediatrics 1965;35:999–1002.
48. Lowe K, Alvarez DF, King JA, et al. Perivascular fluid cuffs decrease lung compliance by increasing tissue resistance. Crit Care Med 2010;38(6):1458–66.
49. Remetz MS, Cleman MW, Cabin HS. Pulmonary and pleural complications of cardiac disease. Clin Chest Med 1989;10(4):545–92.
50. Kidd L, Driscoll DJ, Gersony WM, et al. Second natural history study of congenital heart defects. Results of treatment of patients with ventricular septal defects. Circulation 1993;87(2 Suppl):I38–51.
51. Eisenmenger V. Die angeborenen Defecte der Kammerscheidewand des Herzens. Z Klin Med 1897;32:1–28.
52. Wood P. The Eisenmenger syndrome or pulmonary hypertension with reversed central shunt. Br Med J 1958;2(5099):755–62.
53. Adatia I, Kothari SS, Feinstein JA. Pulmonary hypertension associated with congenital heart disease: pulmonary vascular disease: the global perspective. Chest 2010;137(6 Suppl):52S–61S.
54. D'Alto M, Mahadevan VS. Pulmonary arterial hypertension associated with congenital heart disease. Eur Respir Rev 2012;21(126):328–37.
55. Humbert M, Sitbon O, Simonneau G. Treatment of pulmonary arterial hypertension. N Engl J Med 2004;351(14):1425–36.
56. Moceri P, Kempny A, Liodakis E, et al. Physiological differences between various types of Eisenmenger syndrome and relation to outcome. Int J Cardiol 2015;179: 455–60.
57. Beghetti M, Galie N. Eisenmenger syndrome a clinical perspective in a new therapeutic era of pulmonary arterial hypertension. J Am Coll Cardiol 2009;53(9): 733–40.

58. Diller GP, Dimopoulos K, Broberg CS, et al. Presentation, survival prospects, and predictors of death in Eisenmenger syndrome: a combined retrospective and case-control study. Eur Heart J 2006;27(14):1737–42.
59. Barst RJ, McGoon MD, Elliott CG, et al. Survival in childhood pulmonary arterial hypertension: insights from the registry to evaluate early and long-term pulmonary arterial hypertension disease management. Circulation 2012;125(1):113–22.
60. Simonneau G, Montani D, Celermajer DS, et al. Haemodynamic definitions and updated clinical classification of pulmonary hypertension. Eur Respir J 2019; 53(1):1801913.
61. Simonneau G, Gatzoulis MA, Adatia I, et al. Updated clinical classification of pulmonary hypertension. J Am Coll Cardiol 2013;62(25 Suppl):D34–41.
62. Frank DB, Hanna BD. Pulmonary arterial hypertension associated with congenital heart disease and Eisenmenger syndrome: current practice in pediatrics. Minerva Pediatr 2015;67(2):169–85.
63. Ohuchi H, Hasegawa S, Yasuda K, et al. Severely impaired cardiac autonomic nervous activity after the Fontan operation. Circulation 2001;104(13):1513–8.
64. Schaan CW, Macedo ACP, Sbruzzi G, et al. Functional Capacity in Congenital Heart Disease: A Systematic Review and Meta-Analysis. Arq Bras Cardiol 2017;109(4):357–67.
65. Shachar GB, Fuhrman BP, Wang Y, et al. Rest and exercise hemodynamics after the Fontan procedure. Circulation 1982;65(6):1043–8.
66. Cervi E, Giardini A. Exercise tolerance in children with a left to right shung. J Cardiol Ther 2015;2(1):244–9.
67. Reybrouck T, Rogers R, Weymans M, et al. Serial cardiorespiratory exercise testing in patients with congenital heart disease. Eur J Pediatr 1995;154(10): 801–6.
68. Reybrouck T, Vangesselen S, Gewillig M. Impaired chronotropic response to exercise in children with repaired cyanotic congenital heart disease. Acta Cardiol 2009;64(6):723–7.
69. Alonso-Gonzalez R, Borgia F, Diller GP, et al. Abnormal lung function in adults with congenital heart disease: prevalence, relation to cardiac anatomy, and association with survival. Circulation 2013;127(8):882–90.
70. Muller J, Ewert P, Hager A. Number of thoracotomies predicts impairment in lung function and exercise capacity in patients with congenital heart disease. J Cardiol 2018;71(1):88–92.
71. Kreutzer J, Kreutzer C. Lymphodynamics in Congenital Heart Disease: The Forgotten Circulation. J Am Coll Cardiol 2017;69(19):2423–7.
72. Madsen P, Shah SA, Rubin BK. Plastic bronchitis: new insights and a classification scheme. Paediatr Respir Rev 2005;6(4):292–300.
73. Hug MI, Ersch J, Moenkhoff M, et al. Chylous bronchial casts after fontan operation. Circulation 2001;103(7):1031–3.
74. Brogan TV, Finn LS, Pyskaty DJ Jr, et al. Plastic bronchitis in children: a case series and review of the medical literature. Pediatr Pulmonol 2002;34(6):482–7.
75. Dori Y, Keller MS, Rome JJ, et al. Percutaneous Lymphatic Embolization of Abnormal Pulmonary Lymphatic Flow as Treatment of Plastic Bronchitis in Patients With Congenital Heart Disease. Circulation 2016;133(12):1160–70.

Pulmonary Manifestations of Gastrointestinal, Pancreatic, and Liver Diseases in Children

Emily R. Le Fevre, MBBS[a],
Kathleen H. McGrath, MBBS, BSc(Med), FRACP[b],
Dominic A. Fitzgerald, MBBS, PhD, FRACP[a,c,*]

KEYWORDS

- Gastroesophageal reflux • Crohn disease • Ulcerative colitis • Pancreatitis
- Hepatopulmonary syndrome • Portopulmonary hypertension
- Alpha1-antitrypsin deficiency • Respiratory complications

KEY POINTS

- Gastroesophageal reflux is commonly seen in infants, including those who present with a brief resolved unexplained event, but may not be the cause of the event.
- Hepatopulmonary syndrome is associated with a poor prognosis and high mortality. Typical symptoms include platypnea and orthodeoxia. A bubble echocardiogram may be used to make the diagnosis.
- Obesity is an increasing problem worldwide. Weight management improves lung function (vital capacity and expiratory flows), improves exercise capacity, and reduces medication requirements in children with asthma.

SUMMARY

Pulmonary manifestations of gastrointestinal (GI) diseases are often subtle and underlying disease may precede overt symptoms. A high index of suspicion and a low threshold for consultation with a pediatric pulmonologist is warranted in common GI tract conditions. This article outlines the pulmonary manifestations of different GI, pancreatic, and liver diseases in children, including gastroesophageal reflux disease (GERD), inflammatory bowel disease (IBD), pancreatitis,

[a] Department of Respiratory Medicine, The Children's Hospital at Westmead, Locked Bag 4001, Westmead, New South Wales 2145, Australia; [b] Department of Gastroenterology and Clinical Nutrition, The Royal Children's Hospital, 50 Flemington Road, Parkville, Victoria 3052, Australia; [c] Faculty Health Sciences, University of Sydney, Sydney, New South Wales, Australia
* Corresponding author. Department of Respiratory Medicine, the Children's Hospital at Westmead, Locked Bag 4001, Westmead, New South Wales 2145, Australia.
E-mail address: Dominic.fitzgerald@health.nsw.gov.au

Pediatr Clin N Am 68 (2021) 41–60
https://doi.org/10.1016/j.pcl.2020.09.002 pediatric.theclinics.com

alpha1-antitrypsin deficiency, nonalcoholic fatty liver disease (NAFLD), and complications of chronic liver disease (hepatopulmonary syndrome [HPS] and portopulmonary hypertension).

GASTROESOPHAGEAL REFLUX DISEASE

Gastroesophageal reflux (GER) refers to the involuntary passage of gastric contents into the esophagus.[1,2] This process is a normal physiologic event commonly seen in childhood,[1] particularly during infancy because of the largely milk-based diet, recumbent positioning, and immaturity of the gastroesophageal junction.[2] Manifestations may include feeding difficulties, unsettled behaviors, back arching, and sleeping disturbance.[1,2] Infants may also present with respiratory symptoms, such as recurrent pneumonia, chronic cough, and wheezing.[2] Most patients resolve spontaneously by 1 year of age[1,3] and do not require any investigation or pharmacologic treatment.[1]

In contrast, GERD refers to reflux that results in symptoms severe enough to warrant medical treatment (eg, poor weight gain and dental erosions) and/or complications (esophageal or extraesophageal).[1,2] Conditions predisposing to GERD include cerebral palsy, CHARGE (coloboma, heart abnormalities, choanal atresia, retardation of growth, genital and ear anomalies) syndrome, global developmental delay, laryngeal cleft, and achalasia.[4–7] Children with esophageal atresia and tracheoesophageal fistula have a high rate of GERD as a result of esophageal dysmotility caused by deficient esophageal innervation or surgical nerve injury and anastomotic stricturing.[8,9] GERD is a common complication in infants who have had a repaired congenital diaphragmatic hernia, affecting up to 84% in the first year of life.[9–11] The current evidence base on the respiratory manifestations of gastroesophageal reflux in children is poor.[12]

Diagnosis

A thorough clinical history and physical examination may be sufficient to make the diagnosis of GERD. If the diagnosis is uncertain, a 24-hour impedance probe may be helpful. Barium swallow studies may be used to rule out structural abnormalities but are not useful in diagnosing GERD itself.[13] Nuclear medicine studies or pH probes may also be useful when attempting to distinguish incoordination of swallowing from GER, especially with pulmonary aspiration.[14] Pepsin has been identified as a potential biomarker in reflux-related lung disease. It is produced in the stomach and is used as a marker of gastric contents in the airways.[15] Studies in preterm infants with bronchopulmonary dysplasia (BPD) have found that pepsin in the airways may be associated with a more severe course of BPD.[15]

Management

Upright positioning after a feed may be used as initial management. Changes to feeding regimens may be beneficial, such as introducing small, frequent feeds, or thickened formula. Continuous (transpyloric) enteral tube feeding may be considered temporarily in refractory GERD not responding to positioning, simple measures, and medical management.

Proton pump inhibitors (PPIs), typically a course of 4 to 8 weeks, are used as the first-line treatment of reflux-related erosive esophagitis.[3,13] Histamine-2 receptor antagonists may be used when PPIs are not available or contraindicated; however, patients may develop tolerance.[13]

Laparoscopic fundoplication is widely used when medical treatment fails for GERD, and is a popular intervention thought to benefit patients with respiratory complications from GERD.[13,16] However, this assumption has not yet been extensively studied.

Children with neurocognitive impairment who may have difficulties with both managing oropharyngeal secretions and swallowing, in addition to GER, must be assessed carefully as to their suitability for a fundoplication and whether insertion of a gastrostomy tube should be an isolated procedure without concurrent fundoplication.[16,17]

Pulmonary manifestations

GERD has been linked to several pulmonary manifestations. Retrospective studies have revealed significantly higher rates of sinusitis, laryngitis, asthma, aspiration pneumonia, and bronchiectasis among neurologically normal children with GERD.[18]

Brief Resolved Unexplained Events

A brief resolved unexplained event (BRUE), previously known as apparent life-threatening episodes, may be defined as an episode that is frightening to the observer, with apnea, color change, altered muscle tone, choking, or gagging.[19] GERD is a common codiagnosis in infants presenting with BRUEs, with estimates ranging from 49% to 80%.[19,20] However, it may be unclear whether GER is a causative or an associated phenomenon. Performing an impedance pH probe study may be useful to assess for a correlation between episodes of reflux and apnea and assist in directing further management.[13]

Recurrent Aspiration Pneumonia

Recurrent pneumonia, as a result of aspirated gastric contents, is a well-reported complication of GERD.[13] Gastric contents are thought to induce lung injury because of their acidity.[21] One pediatric study found a 3 times higher rate of pneumonia in patients with GERD compared with controls.[18] However, other causes of recurrent bronchitis and pneumonia, including structural abnormalities or genetic abnormalities, such as cystic fibrosis and immunodeficiency, should be considered. Further, swallowing dysfunction should be considered as a possible differential cause of aspiration pneumonia, particularly in children with neurologic disability.

Cryptogenic Organizing Pneumonia

Cryptogenic organizing pneumonia (COP), also known as bronchiolitis obliterans organizing pneumonia, is a rare inflammatory lung disease affecting the bronchioles and surrounding alveoli.[22] Its characteristic feature is granulation tissue that extends into the alveolar ducts and alveoli.[22] GERD has been described as a possible cause of COP in pediatric patients. The mechanism behind this is thought to be gastric contents inducing hypoxemia through the destruction and dilution of surfactant, as well as causing pulmonary edema.[23] More commonly, there may be an underlying alternative diagnosis of postinfective bronchiolitis obliterans, which has been well described following adenoviral infections and mycoplasma.[24,25] Although there are no clear practice guidelines, patients are typically managed with a confirmatory lung biopsy before treatment is initiated with PPIs and anti-inflammatory agents, including low-dose azithromycin and corticosteroids.[23,25]

Chronic Cough

Chronic cough (>4 weeks duration) is a common complaint often linked to GERD. Studies are unable to describe a clear causal relationship between GERD and cough. However, both acidic and alkaline reflux may precede coughing episodes.[2,26] Factors contributing to reflux-triggered cough may include aspiration of gastric contents into the upper airways, gastric contents in the esophagus triggering a vagal-mediated cough, and the sensitization of the central cough reflex.[2,27] Recent guidelines recommend a 2 week course of appropriate antibiotics for chronic wet cough (eg, amoxicillin/clavulanic acid)[28] followed by further investigations such as flexible bronchoscopy and bronchoalveolar lavage looking for lipid-laden macrophages (and a sample for bacterial culture), chest computed tomography (CT) scans and immune function tests if the cough does not resolve.[28]

Asthma

Children who experience respiratory symptoms with their GERD are more likely to have asthma than those with GI symptoms alone.[2] It is been suggested that children with asthma with heartburn, nocturnal symptoms, or steroid-dependent asthma that is difficult to control should be considered for investigation of GERD because their asthma control may improve with the use of regular PPIs.[13] However, the evidence base for this is poor and response to therapy is variable.[12] Randomized controlled trials have found no significant difference in asthma control or improvement in forced expiratory volume in 1 second (FEV_1) in children treated with long-term PPIs.[29]

Cystic Fibrosis

Studies have identified a higher prevalence rate of GERD in children with cystic fibrosis (CF) compared with the general population.[30,31] One series suggested almost half of patients with CF have acid GER, and almost a quarter have delayed gastric emptying.[32] Possible explanations for this include medications that reduce the muscle tone of the lower esophageal sphincter making reflux more likely with frequent cough, forced expiration associated with chest physiotherapy maneuvers, and a high-fat diet resulting in delayed gastric emptying.[31] However, impedance monitoring in adults may show significant reflux in the absence of symptoms.[33] With advanced lung disease, and after lung transplant, there is a higher incidence of GERD, which in adults is estimated to be around 90%.[34] GERD has also been linked to earlier *Pseudomonas aeruginosa* and *Staphylococcus aureus* acquisition in young children, as well as poorer lung function.[30]

Gastroesophageal Reflux Disease Medication–Related Pulmonary Complications

Long-term use of PPIs is associated with more frequent lower respiratory tract infections[3,35,36] as well as a minimal increase in asthma exacerbations.[3] In particular, acid suppression therapy may place immune-deficient children at risk for the development of lower respiratory tract infections.[3,29] A literature review investigating the adverse effects of GERD treatment in the pediatric population found that patients prescribed lansoprazole experienced higher rates of asthma exacerbations and pneumonia.[3] Other studies have found that patients on ranitidine or omeprazole experienced significantly higher rates of pneumonia compared with controls up to 4 months after medication cessation.[37]

INFLAMMATORY BOWEL DISEASE

IBD is a chronic inflammatory condition resulting in damage to the intestinal wall.[38] IBD has a peak incidence in early adulthood,[39] with global incidence rates increasing.[40] The underlying cause of IBD is not understood; however, it is thought to result from an inappropriate immune response to gut flora in a genetically susceptible host.[41] Other environmental factors, including diet, may play a role in the pathogenesis.[41]

IBD is classified into Crohn disease (CD), ulcerative colitis (UC), and IBD unclassified.

CD is characterized by transmural inflammation and skip lesions that can occur anywhere along the GI tract, with the terminal ileum and colon most commonly affected.[38,42] Patients usually present with diarrhea, abdominal pain, or systemic features such as fever, fatigue, and weight loss.[39] In contrast, UC is characterized by mucosal inflammation, usually starting distally in the rectum,[43] and extending into the colon.[38] The presenting symptoms commonly include rectal bleeding, diarrhea, abdominal pain, and urgency associated with defecation.[39] IBD unclassified is diagnosed in approximately 10% of patients with IBD,[41] where there are no features to successfully differentiate between UC and CD.

Diagnosis

Any child with suspected IBD should have lower (plus or minus upper) GI endoscopy performed to assess for characteristic macroscopic and microscopic changes to confirm the diagnosis of IBD. In patients with CD, small bowel imaging using magnetic resonance enterography or small bowel ultrasonography may help identify small intestinal involvement and define its extent.[43]

Management

Exclusive parenteral nutrition is considered first-line therapy to induce remission in children with CD with active luminal inflammation.[44] In children with UC, options for induction therapy include 5-aminosalicylic acids (5-ASA) therapy and glucocorticoids, depending on the severity and extent of disease.[45] Immune modulators, such as azathioprine, mercaptopurine, and methotrexate, or biologic agents such as anti–tumor necrosis factor-alpha (TNF-α) may be used as maintenance agents to preserve remission in CD or more severe UC with selection dependent on disease severity, response to previous medications, and local prescribing guidelines. Surgical resection may be performed when disease is refractory to maximal medical management.[38]

Pulmonary Manifestations

It is estimated that nearly 30% of pediatric patients with IBD experience at least 1 extraintestinal manifestation.[46] Pulmonary manifestations are described in 10% of patients with UC or CD.[47] They may occur in active disease, independent of disease activity, as well as in postcolectomy patients.[47,48]

The pathogenesis of IBD leading to pulmonary abnormalities is not fully understood. It may be explained by the shared embryologic origin of the colonic and respiratory epithelia, as well as by them both playing a similar role in host mucosal defense, being subject to inflammation as a result of inhaled and ingested antigens.[41,48,49] Furthermore, it is thought that activated inflammatory cells in bowel tissue result in the production of circulating cytokines, such as interleukins and TNF-α, that may damage the lung parenchyma.[48] The sputum lymphocytosis that is seen in patients with IBD is thought to support this hypothesis.[49]

Interstitial lung disease

In adults, interstitial lung disease may precede bowel symptoms by several years, and occasionally is present in latent disease.[41] The most frequent type is COP.[46] Clinical features include cough, shortness of breath, and fever.[42,46] Imaging usually reveals either patchy or diffuse opacities on radiograph and unilateral or bilateral areas of consolidation on CT scan.[46] COP may be managed with inhaled or systemic corticosteroids.[42,46] There are few meaningful data in children.

Airway disease Abnormalities of the airways from the glottis to the small airways have been reported in IBD.[48,50] Large airways disease is the most common pulmonary manifestation, more typically associated with UC than CD.[42,48,50] Chronic bronchitis may also occur and is the second most common pulmonary manifestation.[42,46] Bronchiectasis occurs, presenting with chronic moist cough and copious secretions.[42] In contrast with regular so-called postinfective bronchiectasis, it is usually more steroid responsive.[42] Diagnosis is made with a high-resolution CT scan, which reveals dilated airways and bronchial wall thickening.[46] Smaller airway disease typically presents in younger patients earlier in the disease course.[51] Tracheitis and subglottic stenosis are the main upper airway complications.[46,48] Granulomatous inflammatory lesions, similar to those observed in CD in the GI tract, lead to airway narrowing that results in subglottic and tracheal strictures.[50] Symptoms may include shortness of breath, dysphonia, and cough.[42,48]

Fistulas

Enteric-pulmonary fistulas have occasionally been reported in patients with CD. These fistulas include colobronchial, ileobronchial, and esophageal-bronchial fistulas.[41,42,52]

Drug induced

Medications used in IBD may also lead to pulmonary complications (**Table 1**). The pattern of onset may vary, with reactions being dose related or idiosyncratic. Pulmonary manifestations may resolve on cessation of the drug (eg, sulfasalazine-based reactions).[52]

Asthma

Adult studies have revealed higher rates of asthma in patients with IBD, but pediatric studies have been inconsistent, perhaps owing to the small sample sizes.[54] More severe IBD has been linked with higher prevalence rates of asthma.[54] Furthermore, more severe asthma may be seen in UC, with a 20% lower FEV_1 compared with individuals with asthma alone.[51] Increased mast cell activity and levels of TNF-α have been suggested as a possible link.[51] Alternatively, given the high doses of systemic corticosteroids used in some patients, metabolic dysregulation, systemic inflammation, and obesity-related asthma may be other factors.[55]

Pulmonary function test abnormalities

Abnormal pulmonary function tests have been reported in up to 60% of asymptomatic patients with IBD.[41,42] Abnormalities are most often identified with active IBD disease, and may persist through remission.[49] Restrictive, obstructive, and mixed spirometry patterns may occur.[56] Reduced diffusion capacity in the lung for carbon monoxide (DLco) has also been reported, although the mechanism for this is unclear.[42,49,56]

Table 1
Respiratory complications of medications used to treat inflammatory bowel disease

Medication	Respiratory Complication
Sulfasalazine	Lower lobe opacities Interstitial pneumonitis COP
Azathioprine and 6-mercaptopurine	Infectious pneumonia Interstitial pneumonitis
Methotrexate	Hypersensitivity pneumonitis Pulmonary fibrosis
Biologics (eg, TNF-α inhibitors)	Infectious pneumonia Reactivation of latent tuberculosis Diffuse alveolar hemorrhage

Data from Refs.[41,50,52,53]

Fractional exhaled nitric oxide level is also frequently increased in asymptomatic individuals.[41]

Thromboembolic disease

IBD is an independent risk factor for venous and arterial thromboembolism, mainly when the disease is active.[42] Venous thromboembolism has also been known to occur up to 2 years after colectomy[51] and during remission.[48]

Diagnostic approach to pulmonary manifestations in inflammatory bowel disease

Pulmonary manifestations of IBD often go unnoticed by patients and clinicians. Plain chest radiographs may miss diagnoses and so high-resolution CT is often needed to diagnose important conditions such as fistulae, bronchiectasis, and drug-induced complications. Pulmonary function tests may also reveal abnormalities, even in the absence of reported symptoms. Spirometry should be considered in all school-aged children with IBD.[57]

PANCREATITIS

Although gallstones and alcohol consumption predominate in acute pancreatitis (AP) in adults,[58] causes in the pediatric population are numerous (**Table 2**). Infants and younger children may have an atypical presentation with nonspecific symptoms of nausea, vomiting, and irritability.[59]

Pathophysiology

Pancreatitis is thought to occur from autodigestion from pancreatic duct obstruction, resulting in acinar cell injury and local tissue damage.[59,62] As autodigestion occurs, chemokines and cytokines are released into the circulation, leading to multiorgan dysfunction.[51] Pulmonary manifestations are thought to occur as a result of these recruiting activated cellular mediators, leading to changes in the alveolar endothelium and pulmonary vasculature.[51]

Diagnosis

AP is defined by any 2 of acute upper abdominal pain, increased serum amylase and/or lipase levels greater than 3 times the upper limit of normal range, and abdominal imaging (ultrasonography, MRI, or CT scanning) consistent with the diagnosis.[58] Imaging of the abdomen can also be used to identify complications of AP, such as fluid collections, necrosis, and hemorrhage.[59]

AP usually resolves without complications; however, 15% to 35% of affected children go on to have recurrent pancreatitis,[59] characterized by persistent inflammation, chronic pain, loss of endocrine or exocrine function, and irreversible morphologic changes.[63] Children with recurrent or chronic pancreatitis are more likely to have underlying gene mutations (**Box 1**), with the most common being a mutation in the cystic fibrosis transmembrane conductance regulator (CFTR) gene.[59,64] Genetic testing is recommended.[65] If CFTR genetic abnormalities are detected, patients should have a sweat chloride test to further evaluate for CF as opposed to a CFTR metabolic syndrome.[59,66]

Management

Management involves supportive care with aggressive early fluid administration for resuscitation, careful monitoring, adequate analgesia, and provision of early oral or enteral nutrition when no contraindication exists.[65]

Table 2
Causes of pancreatitis in children

Idiopathic (20%–30%)	
Structural/ anatomic	Choledochal cysts Sphincter of Oddi dysfunction Annular pancreas
GI	Gallstones IBD
Infections	Viral: mumps, Coxsackie B, cytomegalovirus, varicella zoster, hepatitis A/B, human immunodeficiency virus Bacterial: *Salmonella typhi, Mycoplasma pneumoniae* Parasitic: ascaris species, cryptosporidium Sepsis
Medication	Azathioprine 6-Mercaptopurine Sulfasalazine Asparaginase Valproic acid Antiretrovirals Furosemide Thiazides
Metabolic	Hyperparathyroidism Hypercalcemia Hyperlipidemia
Hereditary conditions	Cystic fibrosis Hereditary pancreatitis Alpha1-antitrypsin deficiency

Data from Refs.[51,59–61]

Pulmonary Manifestations

Respiratory complications seen in AP range from mild abnormalities, such as pleural effusion and atelectasis, to severe respiratory failure.[67] Adult studies have estimated a respiratory complication in up to 29% of patients with AP.[67]

Pleural effusion

Small, left-sided pleural effusions occur in 4% to 17% of adult patients with AP and are thought to result from a chemically induced diaphragm-pleural inflammatory reaction.[68] Patients may present with epigastric pain and shortness of breath on exertion, with an effusion evident on chest radiograph. Most effusions resolve spontaneously as

Box 1
Genes associated with pancreatitis

CFTR (cystic fibrosis transmembrane regulator)

SPINK1 (serine protease inhibitor Kazal type 1)

PRSSI (cationic trypsinogen)

CPA1 (carboxypeptidase 1)

Data from Refs.[59,65]

the pancreatic inflammatory process resolves.[68] Decent prevalence data in children with AP and pleural effusions are lacking.

Acute lung injury/pneumonia

Acute lung injury (ALI) and acute respiratory distress syndrome are common complications of AP in adults. ALI occurs in 10% to 25% of acute pancreatitis in adults, and is reported to be the cause of up to 60% of all pancreatitis-associated deaths.[69] Pancreatitis may lead to mild lung injury that quickly resolves; however, with a secondary infection (ie, ventilator-associated or bacterial pneumonia), it may progress to severe respiratory dysfunction and death.[69] Appropriate prevalence data in children with AP and ALI are lacking.

Cystic fibrosis

The CFTR gene is associated with pancreatitis.[70,71] Rarely, pancreatitis may be the first manifestation of pancreatic-sufficient CF. CFTR modulators, such as ivacaftor and tezacaftor, are known to improve lung function and reduce pulmonary exacerbations of CF by improving the production, intracellular processing, and function of the defective CFTR protein.[72] Recent adult studies have found reduced rates of recurrent pancreatitis with CFTR modulators, even in the absence of respiratory symptoms.[72,73] Studies in the pediatric population are awaited.

COMPLICATIONS OF CHRONIC LIVER DISEASE

Hepatopulmonary Syndrome

HPS has been reported in up to 29% of children with liver cirrhosis or severe portal hypertension.[74,75] It is defined as the triad of chronic liver disease, arterial hypoxemia, and the formation of abnormal intrapulmonary vascular dilatations.[74,76] HPS has been hypothesized to be the result of progressive pulmonary vasodilation secondary to chronic liver failure.[77] The presence of HPS is synonymous with a poorer prognosis and quality of life compared with patients with the same degree of liver cirrhosis without HPS.[78] Mortalities worsen with more severe HPS.[78]

Pathophysiology

The exact pathophysiology is not fully understood. However, animal studies have suggested that abnormal liver function results in vasodilatory mediators (such as nitric oxide, TNF-α, and endothelin-1) entering the pulmonary circulation to cause vasodilatation. This process leads to hypoxemia as a result of ventilation-perfusion mismatch with right to left pulmonary arteriovenous shunting.[74,76,78,79]

Clinical manifestations

Patients with early-stage HPS may be asymptomatic.[79] As the condition progresses, the A-a gradient increases, leading to dyspnea, hypoxemia, and cyanosis. Approximately 25% of patients experience platypnea (dyspnea on standing) and orthodeoxia (hypoxemia on standing).[76,78,79] Digital clubbing and cyanosis are typically seen late in the disease process.[80] Most patients have normal chest radiographs. However, CT scans may reveal bibasilar nodules or reticulonodular opacities.[78] Pulmonary function tests often reveal decreased DLco.[81]

Diagnosis

The diagnosis of HPS is based on evidence of shunting in the lungs and impaired oxygenation in the presence of chronic liver disease.[74] Impaired oxygenation may be suggested by reduced SpO_2, confirmed by an increased A-a gradient of greater than or equal to 15 mm Hg, or PaO_2 less than 80 mm Hg in ambient air.[75,78,80] Severity is then graded by the degree of hypoxemia (**Table 3**).

The presence of shunting is confirmed on a bubble echocardiogram.[74,80] This test is performed using 10 mL of intravenous agitated saline, which produces sonographically visible microbubbles.[81] In a normal study, the microbubbles are visualized in the right ventricle within seconds, and then absorbed in the alveoli.[81] An abnormal test occurs when the microbubbles are not visualized in the left cardiac chambers until at least 3 cardiac cycles after they reach the right heart.[75,80] Although bubble echocardiograms are more sensitive in the detection of HPS,[75] lung perfusion scans with technetium-99 macroaggregated albumin may also be used to detect shunting.[74,80] This test is considered positive with more than 6% uptake in the brain.[74]

Management

Supplemental oxygen may be provided to improve hypoxemia. However, there is only a partial response because of the nature of the pathophysiology.[80] Liver transplant is currently the only effective treatment option.[74,78] Transplant results in complete resolution or significant improvement in gas exchange in up to 85% of patients.[81,82] Oxygenation typically normalizes within weeks to months,[76] reinforcing the notion that HPS is the result of functional changes of the pulmonary vasculature.[51]

PORTOPULMONARY HYPERTENSION

Portopulmonary hypertension (POPH) is a potentially fatal complication of chronic liver disease,[83] and is characterized by the presence of pulmonary artery hypertension in the setting of portal hypertension.[78] However, it may also occur in patients with portal hypertension without cirrhosis, such as with portosystemic shunts.[77,84] In a study examining pediatric autopsies, pulmonary hypertension was identified in 5.2% of patients with portal hypertension.[85] Another study of pediatric patients identified the prevalence as 0.9%.[86] Interestingly, there is no correlation between the severity of underlying liver disease and the development of POPH.[87]

Pathophysiology

The pathophysiology of POPH is likely multifactorial. It is proposed that the higher cardiac output seen in chronic liver disease[79] results in increased blood flow within the pulmonary vasculature.[77] This increased blood flow results in shear forces and damage in the pulmonary vascular walls.[79] In addition, endotoxins and cytokines (such as serotonin, prostacyclin, and endothelin-1) released as a result of splanchnic vasculature overload bypass the liver where they are usually metabolized.[83] These

Table 3
Grading severity of hepatopulmonary syndrome

Grade	PaO_2 (mm Hg)
Mild	≥80
Moderate	60–79
Severe	50–59
Very severe	<50

Data from Krowka M, Fallon M, Kawut S, et al. International liver transplant society practice guidelines: Diagnosis and management of hepatopulmonary syndrome and porto-pulmonary hypertension. Transplantation 2016;100(7):1440-1452.

inflammatory mediators enter the pulmonary circulation, resulting in further damage to the arterial walls.[79,88] Progressive remodeling and thickening of small pulmonary artery walls lead to vasoconstriction and/or vascular obstruction,[79] resulting in pulmonary arterial hypertension and right heart failure.[76] Findings on histopathology include vasoconstriction, endothelial and smooth muscle proliferation, and fibrosis, consistent with the findings in idiopathic pulmonary arterial hypertension.[78]

Clinical features

It is estimated that approximately 60% of patients with POPH are asymptomatic,[84] and POPH may be severe by the time diagnosis is made.[88] Presenting symptoms include dyspnea, chest pain, hemoptysis, fatigue, syncope, weakness, or light headedness, whereas others may present as an incidental finding on screening.[86,89] Clinical signs may include a systolic murmur, loud second heart sound, jugular venous distension, and edema.[80] An electrocardiogram may reveal signs of right ventricular hypertrophy, right axis deviation, and right atrial enlargement.[80]

Diagnosis

Pediatric studies have identified the utility of using brain natriuretic peptide (BNP) as a screening tool for POPH to promote early detection, and have found significantly higher levels in patients with POPH compared with chronic liver disease without POPH.[88] Serum BNP has been used in children more than 5 years of age as a noninvasive screening tool before echocardiogram and cardiac catheterization.[88]

Transthoracic echocardiography is a well-recognized screening tool, and may show increased right heart pressures, as well as pulmonary hypertension in the pulmonary artery.[84] However, the diagnosis of POPH can be missed in up to a third of patients.[80] Thus, right heart catheterization is required to confirm the diagnosis. Diagnostic criteria include the presence of increased mean pulmonary arterial pressure (>25 mm Hg) secondary to increased pulmonary vascular resistance (>3 Wood units), in the setting of a normal pulmonary arterial wedge pressure (<15 mm Hg).[78,86,87] Severity is then based on the grading of mean pulmonary arterial pressure (**Table 4**).

Management

Left untreated, POPH has a poor prognosis.[86] Up to 40% of patients with POPH die within 15 months of diagnosis.[88] Efficacy of treatment depends on the degree of increased pulmonary pressure, making early diagnosis of POPH essential.[86] Liver transplant remains the only treatment to definitively reduce pulmonary pressures and peripheral vascular resistance.[86] Studies have revealed an increased mortality following liver transplant in patients with higher pulmonary pressures,[86] caused by

Table 4
Grading severity of portopulmonary hypertension

Grade	mPAP (mm Hg)
Normal	<25
Mild	25–35
Moderate	35–45
Severe	≥45

Abbreviation: MPAP, mean pulmonary arterial pressure.

Data from Karrer F, Wallace B, Estrada A. Late complications of biliary atresia: hepatopulmonary syndrome and portopulmonary hypertension. Pediatr Surg Int 2017;33:1335-1340.

postoperative heart failure.[88] The current recommendations include liver transplant for patients with mild POPH,[86] but liver transplant is contraindicated in those with severe pulmonary hypertension.[90] Patients with moderate or severe POPH should be medically managed to reduce the pulmonary pressure and improve right ventricular function before transplant.[80,84,88] Pharmacologic management includes prostacyclins (eg, epoprostenol, treprostinil), phosphodiesterase-5 enzyme inhibitors (eg, sildenafil, tadalafil), and endothelin receptor antagonists (eg, bosentan, macitentan). These medications may be used alone or in combination and are usually continued for several months to years after liver transplant.[83]

ALPHA1-ANTITRYPSIN DEFICIENCY

Alpha1-antitrypsin (AAT) deficiency is a hereditary condition (autosomal recessive) that results in decreased circulating AAT protein (serine protease inhibitor), which is synthesized in the liver and secreted into serum.[91,92] It plays a role in protecting lung tissue, namely alveoli, from the neutrophil elastase that is secreted by leukocytes during times of inflammation.[93]

Gene mutations (SERPINA 1 gene) may either result in defective AAT that is unable to perform its role in protecting lung tissue, or may lead to retention of AAT in the endoplasmic reticulum of hepatocytes, preventing appropriate secretion of AAT into the bloodstream.[94] Accumulation of AAT in the liver may lead to chronic liver disease, including cirrhosis and liver failure.[91] The homozygous ZZ mutation is the most likely (10%) mutation to result in more severe liver and lung disease.[91,95]

Clinical features

Liver disease associated with AAT deficiency may present at any age, and signs and symptoms vary with age of presentation. The typical pediatric presentation is with prolonged neonatal cholestatic jaundice.[92] Older children may present with failure to thrive, abdominal distension, hepatosplenomegaly, ascites, or GI bleeding. However, some children are asymptomatic and identified by incidental finding of increased liver function tests.[96] Lung disease usually presents in adulthood but may rarely be seen in adolescence.

Diagnosis

Liver function tests reveal increased transaminase and bilirubin levels. Serum AAT level may also be used as initial screening; however, because AAT is an acute phase reactant, false-negative results may occur.[96] Polymerase chain reaction genotyping (PI typing) or gene sequencing should be obtained to confirm the diagnosis.[92,94] Liver biopsy is not required to make the diagnosis, but it can provide information regarding severity and progression of liver disease.[92,96]

Management

Management of AAT deficiency involves supportive care, monitoring for complications, and avoiding further injury to the liver and lungs (eg, hepatitis vaccination, avoiding alcohol/smoking, and maintaining a healthy weight).[96] AAT deficiency remains the second most common cause of liver transplant in children, after biliary atresia.[94] Five-year survival rates following liver transplant are excellent, being up to 92% in recent studies.[97]

Pulmonary manifestations

Chronic obstructive pulmonary disease

The classic clinical description of lung disease associated with AAT deficiency is of early-onset chronic obstructive lung disease (typically ages 40–50 years) and panacinar emphysema affecting mainly the lower lobes.[29,94,97] Although this lung damage is known to be linked to AAT's antiprotease activity, it is also suggested that it may be linked to an anti-inflammatory effect of AAT.[98] Cigarette smoking and environmental factors such as pollution accelerate the rate and severity of chronic obstructive pulmonary disease and should be avoided.[99]

Augmentation therapy with inhaled or intravenous AAT has been shown in various studies to reduce lung parenchymal loss, although it does not reverse the damage already done and may not reduce pulmonary exacerbation rates.[94,100–102]

Recurrent infections

AAT deficiency has been associated with recurrent pulmonary infections. However, it remains unclear whether infections are a direct result of AAT deficiency.[91] Infections may be an important exacerbating factor in progression of underlying lung disease and age-appropriate vaccinations, including annual influenza vaccine, should be administered.[94]

Asthma

Increased rates of asthma have been linked to some AAT deficiency genotypes, although the exact relationship remains unclear.[91,103,104]

OBESITY AND NONALCOHOLIC FATTY LIVER DISEASE

NAFLD is currently the most common cause of pediatric chronic liver disease.[105] It is defined as the histologic evidence of at least 5% hepatic steatosis, in the absence of other causes of liver fat accumulation.[105] Obesity has been closely linked to the development of NAFLD, with studies showing significantly higher rates of NAFLD in obese children (34.2%), compared with those of normal body habitus (7.6%).[105]

Diagnosis

NAFLD is diagnosed by the presence of hepatic steatosis with exclusion of alternative causes for hepatic steatosis or chronic liver disease. Liver biopsy should be considered in children at risk of nonalcoholic steatohepatitis or where the diagnosis is unclear or if multiple conditions coexist.[106] Alanine aminotransferase (ALT) may be used as a screening tool for NAFLD in children with risk factors.[106]

Management

Lifestyle modification to improve diet and increase physical activity is the first-line treatment of NAFLD in children. Further research is needed to delineate the role for pharmaceutical options.

Pulmonary manifestations of obesity

There are various mechanisms by which obesity affects the respiratory system, including decreased respiratory system compliance, increased airway resistance, reduced lung volumes, and altered ventilation and gas exchange.[107]

Pulmonary function test abnormalities

Obesity may result in various abnormalities in pulmonary function tests. Adults typically present with a restrictive spirometry pattern. However, children have been known to have restrictive or obstructive patterns on spirometry.[107] A large recent meta-analysis revealed a marked decline in FEV_1/forced vital capacity (FVC) ratio, and mid-expiratory flows (forced expiratory flow at 25%–75% [FEF_{25-75}]), consistent with an obstructive picture on spirometry.[107]

Asthma

Obesity has been linked to an increased risk of asthma. Studies have found a higher risk of developing asthma in infants of mothers who were obese during pregnancy.[108] Obese children with asthma tend to have a more severe course with poor control of symptoms and increased exacerbations. Spirometry shows a lower FEV_1 and FEV_1/FVC ratio compared with their normal-weight counterparts.[108] There is also a more marked decline in FEF_{25-75} in individuals with asthma compared with obesity alone.[107] Weight loss improves lung function, asthma symptoms, and medication requirements.[108,109]

Obstructive sleep apnea

Obstructive sleep apnea (OSA) is defined by prolonged partial upper airway obstruction and/or intermittent complete upper airway obstruction that disrupts ventilation during sleep.[110] The prevalence of OSA has increased over time because of increased rates of obesity, with current estimates that OSA affects up to 5.7% of children.[111] There are significant medical implications for children with OSA, including high post-operative respiratory complication risks, cardiovascular effects (including hypertension, pulmonary hypertension, and right heart failure), and neurocognitive effects (including reduced intelligence quotient, behavioral problems, and effects on concentration and memory).[111] Current management includes weight management, adenotonsillectomy where indicated, and the use of noninvasive ventilation.

CLINICS CARE POINTS

- GORD is commonly seen in infants, including those who present with a BRUE, but may not be the cause of the event.
- IBD is an increasingly common problem and may be associated with abnormalities on spirometry.
- Acute pancreatitis may result in a pleural effusion which is normally managed conservatively.
- HPS is associated with a poor prognosis and high mortality. Typical symptoms include platypnea and orthodeoxia. A bubble echocardiogram can be used to make the diagnosis.
- There is no correlation between the severity of liver disease and development of POPH. BNP can be used to screen in children over 5 years of age, with diagnosis made on echocardiogram and cardiac catheterizations.
- AAT deficiency typically presents as neonatal cholestatic jaundice. AAT is an acute phase reactant, thus serum measurement can give false-negative results. Definitive diagnosis is based on PCR.
- Obesity is a rising problem worldwide. Weight management improves lung function (vital capacity and expiratory flows), improves exercise capacity and reduces medication requirements in asthmatic children.

DISCLOSURE

The authors have nothing to disclose.

REFERENCES

1. Davies I, Burman-Roy S, Murphy M. Gastro-oesophageal reflux disease in children: NICE guidance. BMJ 2015;350:g7703.
2. Rybak A, Pesce M, Thapar N, et al. Gastro-esophageal reflux in children. Int J Mol 2017;18:1671.
3. Cohen S, Bueno de Mesquita M, Mimouni FB. Adverse effects reported in the use of gastroesophageal reflux disease treatments in children: A 10 years literature review. Br J Clin Pharmacol 2015;80(2):200–8.
4. Hudson A, Macdonald M, Friedman JN, et al. CHARGE syndrome gastrointestinal involvement: From mouth to anus. Clin Genet 2017;92(1):10–7.
5. Kim S, Koh H, Lee JS. Gastroesophageal reflux in neurologically impaired children: What are the risk factors? Gut Liver 2017;11(2):232–6.
6. Loh R, Phua M, Shaw CL. Diagnosis and management of type 1 laryngeal cleft: Systematic review. Aust J Otolaryngol 2019;2:5.
7. Yoshizaki K, Hachiya R, Tomobe Y, et al. MIRAGE syndrome with recurrent pneumonia probably associated with gastroesophageal reflux and achalasia: A case report. Clin Pediatr Endocrinol 2019;28(4):147–53.
8. Vergouwe F, van Wijk M, Spaander M, et al. Evaluation of gastroesophageal reflux in children born with esophageal atresia using pH and impedance monitoring. J Pediatr Gastroenterol Nutr 2019;69(5):515–22.
9. Marseglia L, Manti S, D'Angelo G, et al. Gastroesophageal reflux and congenital gastrointestinal malformations. World J Gastroenterol 2015;21(28):8508–15.
10. Leeuwen L, Walker K, Halliday R, et al. Growth in children with congenital diaphragmatic hernia during the first year of life. J Pediatr Surg 2014;49:1363–6.
11. Muratore CS, Utter S, Jaksic T, et al. Nutritional morbidity of survivors of congenital diaphragmatic hernia. J Pediatr Surg 2001;36:1171–6.
12. deBenedictus FM, Bush A. Respiratory manifestations of gastro-oesophageal reflux in children. Arch Dis Child 2018;103(3):292–6.
13. Rosen R, Vandenplas Y, Singendonk M, et al. Pediatric gastroesophageal reflux clinical practice guidelines: Joint recommendations of the North American society for pediatric gastroenterology, hepatology, and nutrition and the European society for pediatric gastroenterology, hepatology, and nutrition. J Pediatr Gastroenterol Nutr 2018;66(3):516–54.
14. Evbuomwan O, Momodu J, Purbhoo K, et al. Evaluation of technetium-99m metastable nanocolloid as an imaging agent for performing milk scans. Nucl Med Commun 2019;40(1):52–6.
15. Farhath S, He Z, Nakhla T, et al. Pepsin, a marker of gastric contents, is increased in tracheal aspirates from preterm infants who develop bronchopulmonary dysplasia. Pediatrics 2008;121(2):e253–9.
16. Wong K, Liu X. Perioperative and late outcomes of laparoscopic fundoplication for neurologically impaired children with gastro-esophageal reflux disease. Chin Med J 2012;125(21):3905–8.
17. Yap B, Nah S, Chen Y, et al. Fundoplication with gastrostomy vs gastrostomy alone: a systematic review and meta-analysis of outcomes and complications. Pediatr Surg Int 2017;33(2):217–28.
18. El-Serag H, Gilger M, Kuebeler M, et al. Extraesophageal associations of gastroesophageal reflux disease in children without neurologic defects. Gastroenterology 2001;121:1294–9.

19. Doshi A, Bernard-Stover L, Kuelbs C, et al. Apparent life-threatening event admissions and gastroesophageal reflux disease: The value of hospitalization. Pediatr Emerg Care 2012;28:17–21.
20. Macchini F, Morandi A, Cognizzoli P, et al. Acid gastroesophageal reflux disease and apparent life-threatening events: Simultaneous pH-metry and cardiorespiratory monitoring. Pediatr Neonatol 2017;58(1):43–7.
21. Laube B, Katz R, Loughlin G, et al. Quantification of the source, amount and duration of aspiration in the lungs of infants using gamma scintigraphy. Paediatr Respir Rev 2019;32:23–7.
22. Epler GR. BMJ best practice: Bronchiolitis obliterans organising pneumonia. 2018. Available at: https://bestpractice.bmj.com/topics/en-us/137. Accessed February 01 2020–.
23. Liu J, Xu X, Zhou C, et al. Bronchiolitis obliterans organizing pneumonia due to gastroesophageal reflux. Pediatrics 2015;136(6):e1510–3.
24. Kim J, Kim M, Sol I, et al. Quantitative CT and pulmonary function in children with post-infectious bronchiolitis obliterans. PLoS One 2019;14(4):e0214647.
25. Li Y, Liu L, Qiao H, et al. Post-infectious bronchiolitis obliterans in children: a review of 42 cases. BMC Pediatr 2014;14:238.
26. Blondeau K, Mertens V, Dupont L, et al. The relationship between gastroesophageal reflux and cough in children with chronic unexplained cough using combined impedance-pH-manometry recordings. Pediatr Pulmonol 2011;46(3): 286–94.
27. Borrelli O, Marabotto C, Mancini V, et al. Role of gastroesophageal reflux in children with unexplained chronic cough. J Pediatr Gastroenterol Nutr 2011;53(3): 287–92.
28. Chang A, Oppenheimer J, Weinberger M, et al. Management of children with chronic wet cough and protracted bacterial bronchitis CHEST guideline and expert panel report. Chest 2017;151(4):884–90.
29. Blake K, Teague WG. Gastroesophageal reflux disease and childhood asthma. Curr Opin Pulm Med 2013;19(1):24–9.
30. Duncan JA, Brown SM. The impact of co-morbidity in childhood cystic fibrosis. Paediatr Respir Rev 2018;26:13–5.
31. Brodzicki J, Trawińska M, Korzon M. Frequency, consequences and pharmacological treatment of gastroesophageal reflux in children with cystic fibrosis. Med Sci Monit 2002;8(7):CR529–37.
32. Hauser B, De Schepper J, Malfroot A, et al. Gastric emptying and gastro-oesophageal reflux in children with cystic fibrosis. J Cyst Fibros 2016;15(4): 540–7.
33. Blondeau KM, Dupont LJ, Mertens V, et al. Gastro-oesophageal reflux and aspiration of gastric contents in adult patients with cystic fibrosis. Gut 2008;57(8): 1049–55.
34. Mendez BM, Davis CS, Weber C, et al. Gastroesophageal reflux disease in lung transplant patients with cystic fibrosis. Am J Surg 2012;204(5):e21–6.
35. Orenstein S, Hassall E, Furmaga-Jablonska W, et al. Multicenter, double-blind, randomized, placebo-controlled trial assessing the efficacy and safety of proton pump inhibitor lansoprazole in infants with symptoms of gastroesophageal reflux disease. J Pediatr 2009;154(4):514–20.
36. De Bruyne P, Ito S. Toxicity of long-term use of proton pump inhibitors in children. Arch Dis Child 2018;103(1):78–82.

37. Canani R, Cirillo P, Roggero P, et al. Therapy with gastric acidity inhibitors increases the risk of acute gastroenteritis and community-acquired pneumonia in children. Pediatrics 2006;117(5):e817–20.
38. Casey G. Inflammatory bowel disease. Nurs New Zealand 2017;23(2):20–4.
39. Aziz D, Moin M, Majeed A, et al. Paediatric inflammatory bowel disease: Clinical presentation and disease location. Pak J Med Sci 2017;33(4):793–7.
40. Lopez R, Evans H, Appleton L, et al. Prospective incidence of paediatric inflammatory bowel disease in New Zealand in 2015: Results from the paediatric inflammatory bowel disease in New Zealand (PINZ) study. J Pediatr Gastroenterol Nutr 2018;66(5):e122–6.
41. Majewski S, Piotrowski W. Pulmonary manifestations of inflammatory bowel disease. Arch Med Sci 2015;11(6):1179–88.
42. Danve A. Thoracic manifestations of ankylosing spondylitis, inflammatory bowel disease, and relapsing polychondritis. Clin Chest Med 2019;40(3):599–608.
43. Lamb C, Kennedy N, Raine T, et al. British society of gastroenterology consensus guidelines on the management of inflammatory bowel disease in adults. Gut 2019;68:s1–106.
44. Lawley M, Wu JW, Navas-Lopez VM, et al. Global variation in use of enteral nutrition for pediatric crohn disease. J Pediatr Gastroenterol Nutr 2018;67(2):e22–9.
45. Turner D, Ruemmele FM, Orlanski-Meyer E, et al. Management of paediatric ulcerative colitis, part 1: Ambulatory care – an evidence-based guideline from European crohn's and colitis organization and European society of paediatric gastroenterology, hepatology and nutrition. J Pediatr Gastroenterol Nutr 2018;67(2):257–91.
46. Chams S, Badran R, Sayegh S, et al. Hajj Hussein I. Inflammatory bowel disease: Looking beyond the tract. Int J Immunopathol Pharmacol 2019;33:1–18.
47. Pillai S, Deshmukh F, Lentine J, et al. Pulmonary manifestations in children with inflammatory bowel disease. Am J Respir Crit Care Med 2018;197:A4943.
48. Ji X, Wang L, Lu D. Pulmonary manifestations of inflammatory bowel disease. World J Gastroenterol 2014;20(37):13501–11.
49. Ji X, Ji Y, Wang S, et al. Alterations of pulmonary function in patients with inflammatory bowel disease. Ann Thorac Med 2016;11(4):249–53.
50. Harbord M, Annese V, Vavricka S, et al. The first European evidence-based consensus on extra-intestinal manifestations in inflammatory bowel disease. J Crohns Colitis 2016;10(3):239–54.
51. Levy J, Levy-Carrick N. Pulmonary complications of gastrointestinal disorders. Paediatr Respir Rev 2012;13:16–22.
52. Casella G, Villanacci V, Di Bella C, et al. Pulmonary diseases associated with inflammatory bowel diseases. J Crohns Colitis 2010;4(4):384–9.
53. Mohamed-Hussein A, Mohamed N, Ibrahim M. Changes in pulmonary function in patients with ulcerative colitis. Respir Med 2007;101(5):977–82.
54. Wasielewska Z, Dolińska A, Wilczyńska D, et al. Prevalence of allergic diseases in children with inflammatory bowel disease. Postepy Dermatol Alergol 2019;36(3):282–90.
55. Rastogi D, Holguin F. Metabolic dysregulation, systemic inflammation, and pediatric obesity-related asthma. Ann Thorac Soc 2017;(Supplement_5):S363–7.
56. Songür N, Songür Y, Tüzün M, et al. Pulmonary function tests and high-resolution CT in the detection of pulmonary involvement in inflammatory bowel disease. J Clin Gastroenterol 2003;37(4):292–8.

57. El Amrousy DM, Hassan S, El-Ashry H, et al. Pulmonary function tests abnormalities in children with inflammatory bowel disease: Is it common? J Pediatr Gastroenterol Nutr 2018;67(3):346–50.
58. Nesvaderani M, Eslick G, Cox M. Acute pancreatitis: update on management. Med J Aust 2015;202(8):420–4.
59. Pohl J, Uc A. Paediatric pancreatitis. Curr Opin Gastroenterol 2015;31(5):380–6.
60. Shukla-Udawatta M, Madani S, Kamat D. An update on pediatric pancreatitis. Pediatr Ann 2017;46(5):e207–11.
61. Uretsky G, Goldschmiedt M, James K. Childhood pancreatitis. Am Fam Physician 1999;59(9):2507–12.
62. Lankisch P, Apte M, Banks P. Acute pancreatitis. Lancet 2015;386(9988):85–96.
63. Abu-El-Haija M, Lowe M. Pediatric pancreatitis - molecular mechanisms and management. Gastroenterol Clin North Am 2018;47(4):741–53.
64. Lucidi V, Alghisi F, Dall'Oglio L, et al. The etiology of acute recurrent pancreatitis in children: A challenge for pediatricians. Pancreas 2011;40(4):517–21.
65. Abu-El-Haija M, Kumar S, Quiros JA, et al. Management of acute pancreatitis in the pediatric population: A clinical report from the North American society for pediatric gastroenterology, hepatology and nutrition pancreas committee. J Pediatr Gastroenterol Nutr 2018;66:159–76.
66. Groves T, Robinson P, Wiley V, et al. Long term outcomes of children with intermediate sweat chlorides in infancy. J Pediatr 2015;166:1469–74.
67. Dombernowsky T, Kristensen M, Rysgaard S, et al. Risk factors for and impact of respiratory failure on mortality in the early phase of acute pancreatitis. Pancreatology 2016;16(5):756–60.
68. Ozbek S, Gumus M, Yuksekkaya H, et al. An unexpected cause of pleural effusion in paediatric emergency medicine. BMJ Case Rep 2013;2013. bcr2013009072.
69. Elder A, Saccone G, Dixon D. Lung injury in acute pancreatitis: Mechanisms underlying augmented secondary injury. Pancreatology 2012;12(1):49–56.
70. Iso M, Suzuki M, Yanagi K, et al. The CFTR gene variants in Japanese children with idiopathic pancreatitis. Hum Genome Var 2019;6:17.
71. Frossard J, Dumonceau J, Pastor C, et al. Concomitant autoimmune and genetic pancreatitis leads to severe inflammatory conditions. World J Gastroenterol 2008;14(16):2596–8.
72. Akshintala V, Kamal A, Faghih M, et al. Cystic fibrosis transmembrane conductance regulator modulators reduce the risk of recurrent acute pancreatitis among adult patients with pancreas sufficient cystic fibrosis. Pancreatology 2019;19(8):1023–6.
73. Johns J, Rowe S. The effect of CFTR modulators on a cystic fibrosis patient presenting with recurrent pancreatitis in the absence of respiratory symptoms: a case report. BMC Gastroenterol 2019;19:123.
74. De Jesus-Rojas W, McBeth K, Yadav A, et al. Severe hepatopulmonary syndrome in a child with caroli syndrome. Case Rep Pediatr 2017;2017:2171974.
75. Borkar V, Poddar U, Kapoor A, et al. Hepatopulmonary syndrome in children: A comparative study of non-cirrhotic vs. cirrhotic portal hypertension. Liver Int 2015;35:1665–72.
76. Gupta S, Krowka M. Hepatopulmonary syndrome. CMAJ 2018;190:E223.
77. Tingo J, Rosenzweig E, Lobritto S, et al. Portopulmonary hypertension in children: a rare but potentially lethal and under-recognized disease. Pulm Circ 2017;7(3):712–8.

78. Krowka M, Fallon M, Kawut S, et al. International liver transplant society practice guidelines: Diagnosis and management of hepatopulmonary syndrome and portopulmonary hypertension. Transplantation 2016;100(7):1440–52.
79. Lee WS, Wong SY, Ivy DD, et al. Hepatopulmonary syndrome and portopulmonary hypertension in children: Recent advances in diagnosis and management. J Pediatr 2018;196:14–21.
80. Karrer F, Wallace B, Estrada A. Late complications of biliary atresia: hepatopulmonary syndrome and portopulmonary hypertension. Pediatr Surg Int 2017;33: 1335–40.
81. Machicao V, Balakrishnan M, Fallon M. Pulmonary complications in chronic liver Disease. Hepatology 2014;59:1627–37.
82. Shah T, Isaac J, Adams D, et al. Development of hepatopulmonary syndrome and portopulmonary hypertension in a paediatric liver transplant patient. Pediatr Transplant 2005;9:127–31.
83. Serrano R, Subbarao G, Mangus R, et al. Combination therapy for severe portopulmonary hypertension in a child allows for liver transplantation. Pediatr Transplant 2019;5:e13461.
84. Savale L, Manes A. Pulmonary arterial hypertension populations of special interest: portopulmonary hypertension and pulmonary arterial hypertension associated with congenital heart disease. Eur Heart J Suppl 2019;21:K37–45.
85. Ridaura-Sanz C, Mejía-Hernández C, López-Corella E. Portopulmonary hypertension in children: A study in pediatric autopsies. Arch Med Res 2009;40(7): 635–9.
86. Ecochard-Dugelay E, Lambert V, Schleich J, et al. Portopulmonary hypertension in liver disease presenting in childhood. J Pediatr Gastroenterol Nutr 2015;61(3): 346–54.
87. Chen X, Zhu Z, Sun L, et al. Liver transplantation for severe portopulmonary hypertension: A case report and literature review. World J Clin Cases 2019;7(21): 3569–74.
88. Yoshimaru K, Matsuura T, Takahashi Y, et al. The efficacy of serum brain natriuretic peptide for the early detection of portopulmonary hypertension in biliary atresia patients before liver transplantation. Pediatr Transplant 2018;5:e13203.
89. Chen H, Xing S, Xu W, et al. Portopulmonary hypertension in cirrhotic patients: Prevalence, clinical features and risk factors. Exp Ther Med 2013;5(3):819–24.
90. Hollatz T, Musat A, Westphal S, et al. Treatment with sildenafil and treprostinil allows successful liver transplantation of patients with moderate to severe portopulmonary hypertension. Liver Transpl 2012;18:686–95.
91. Teckman JH, Rosenthal P, Abel R, et al. Baseline analysis of a young a-1-antitrypsin deficiency liver disease cohort reveals frequent portal hypertension. J Pediatr Gastroenterol Nutr 2015;61(1):94–101.
92. Comba A, Demirbaş F, Çaltepe G, et al. Retrospective analysis of children with α -1 antitrypsin deficiency. Eur J Gastroenterol Hepatol 2018;30:774–8.
93. Ruiz M, Lacaille F, Berthiller J, et al. Liver disease related to alpha1-antitrypsin deficiency in French children: The DEFI-ALPHA cohort. Liver Int 2019;39: 1136–46.
94. Torres-Durán MA, Lopez-Campos JL, Barrecheguren M, et al. Alpha-1 antitrypsin deficiency: Outstanding questions and future directions. Orphanet J Rare Dis 2018;13:114.
95. Lee WS, Yap SF, Looi LM. Alpha1-antitrypsin deficiency is not an important cause of childhood liver diseases in a multi-ethnic Southeast Asian population. J Paediatr Child Health 2007;43:636–9.

96. Feldman A, Sokol RJ. Alpha-1-antitrypsin deficiency: An important cause of pediatric liver disease. Lung Health Prof Mag 2013;4(2):8–11.
97. Townsend S, Edgar R, Ellis P, et al. Systematic review: the natural history of alpha-1 antitrypsin deficiency, and associated liver disease. Aliment Pharmacol Ther 2018;47:877–85.
98. Cosio MG, Bazzan E, Rigobello C, et al. Alpha-1 antitrypsin deficiency: Beyond the protease/antiprotease paradigm. Ann Am Thorac Soc 2016;13:S305–10.
99. Silverman GA, Pak SC, Perlmutter DH. Disorders of protein misfolding: Alpha-1 antitrypsin deficiency of prototype. J Pediatr 2013;163(2):320–6.
100. Gøtzsche P, Johansen H. Intravenous alpha-1 antitrypsin augmentation therapy for treating patients with alpha-1 antitrypsin deficiency and lung disease (Review). Cochrane Database Syst Rev CD007851, 2016;(9).
101. Sandhaus RA. Randomized, placebo-controlled trials in alpha-1 antitrypsin deficiency. Ann Am Thorac Soc 2016;13:S370–3.
102. Stolk J, Tov N, Chapman KR, et al. Efficacy and safety of inhaled α1-antitrypsin in patients with severe α1-antitrypsin deficiency and frequent exacerbations of COPD. Eur Respir J 2019;54(5):1900673.
103. Eden E, Strange C, Holladay B, et al. Asthma and allergy in alpha-1 antitrypsin deficiency. Respir Med 2006;100:1384–91.
104. McGee D, Schwarz L, McClure R, et al. Is PiSS alpha-1 antitrypsin deficiency associated with disease? Pulm Med 2010;2010:570679.
105. Di Sessa A, Cirillo G, Guarino S, et al. Pediatric non-alcoholic fatty liver disease: Current perspectives on diagnosis and management. Pediatric Health Med Ther 2019;10:89–97.
106. Shah J, Okubote T, Alkhouri N. Overview of updated practice guidelines for pediatric nonalcoholic fatty liver disease. Gastroenterol Hepatol 2018;14(7): 407–14.
107. Forno E, Han YY, Mullen J, et al. Overweight, obesity, and lung function in children and adults - a meta-analysis. J Allergy Clin Immunol 2017;6(2):570–81.
108. Peters U, Dixon AE, Forno E. Obesity and asthma. J Allergy Clin Immunol 2018; 141:1169–79.
109. da Silva PL, de Mello MT, Cheik NC, et al. Interdisciplinary therapy improves biomarkers profile and lung function in asthmatic obese adolescents. Pediatr Pulmonol 2012;47(1):8–17.
110. Ngiam J, Cistulli PA. Dental treatment for paediatric obstructive sleep apnea. Paediatr Respir Rev 2015;16(3):174–81.
111. Waters KA, Suresh S, Nixon GM. Sleep disorders in children. Med J Aust 2013; 199(8):S31–5.

Pulmonary Manifestations of Hematologic and Oncologic Diseases in Children

Lama Elbahlawan, MD[a,*], Antonio Moreno Galdo, MD[b], Raul C. Ribeiro, MD[c]

KEYWORDS

• Pulmonary complications • Hematopoietic stem cell transplant (HSCT) • Oncology • Pediatrics • Sickle cell disease • Immune compromised

KEY POINTS

- Pulmonary complications are common after hematopoietic stem cell transplant (HSCT); some occur early (eg, idiopathic pneumonia syndrome and diffuse alveolar hemorrhage), and others occur later (eg, cryptogenic organizing pneumonia and bronchiolitis obliterans syndrome).
- Children with malignancies or those receiving HSCT are susceptible to pneumonia. Prophylactic antibiotics may reduce the incidence of some infections.
- Children with sickle cell disease are frequently hospitalized because of acute chest syndrome or wheezing. Pulmonary hypertension may occur later and may require further cardiology evaluation.
- Chemotherapy and radiation, which are used to treat many of these malignancies or as preparative regimen for HSCT, may also induce lung injury.

INTRODUCTION

Pulmonary involvement is common at diagnosis, relapse, and during or after treatment of malignant neoplasms in pediatric patients. In many patients, pulmonary compromise may progress to rapid respiratory deterioration and death. Anatomic regions likely involved are mediastinal structures, airways (trachea and bronchus), alveolar-capillary units, lung parenchyma, pleura, diaphragm, and chest wall.[1] Recognizing the clinical manifestations and understanding the various consequences of neoplastic involvement in the respiratory system may facilitate the appropriate treatment based

[a] Division of Critical Care, Department of Pediatrics, St. Jude Children's Research Hospital, MS 620, 262 Danny Thomas Place, Memphis, TN 38105-3678, USA; [b] Pediatric Pulmonology Section, Hospital Vall d'Hebron, Universitat Autònoma de Barcelona, Barcelona, Spain; [c] Leukemia/Lymphoma Division, International Outreach Program, Department of Oncology, St. Jude Children's Research Hospital, Memphis, TN, USA
* Corresponding author.
E-mail address: lama.elbahlawan@stjude.org

Pediatr Clin N Am 68 (2021) 61–80
https://doi.org/10.1016/j.pcl.2020.09.003

on the physiopathology of underlying processes.[2] Given the complexity of presenting manifestations, heterogeneity of the diseases, and potentially life-threatening complications, an evidence-based, multidisciplinary team integrating expertise from intensive care, pulmonology, cardiology, oncology, surgery, and anesthesiology is an essential approach.[3]

PULMONARY COMPLICATIONS OF HEMATOLOGIC NEOPLASMS

Leukemias and lymphomas account for approximately 40% of all pediatric neoplasms. Pulmonary complications in children with leukemia include pulmonary leukostasis, leukemic infiltration, and leukemic cell lysis pneumopathy. Lymphoma may cause airway compression or lead to the superior vena cava (SVC) syndrome.

Hyperleukocytosis/Leukostasis

Hyperleukocytosis in leukemia is defined as a white blood cell (WBC) count greater than 100×10^9/L for acute lymphoblastic leukemia (ALL) and chronic myeloid leukemia in the chronic phase; greater than 50×10^9/L for acute myeloid leukemia (AML), and greater than 10×10^9/L for acute promyelocytic leukemia (APL). Lymphoid blasts tend to be more pliable and smaller and have less metabolic activity and tissue-invasive properties than do myeloid blasts.[4,5] Patients with APL presenting with WBC count greater than or equal to 10×10^9/L or a rapidly increasing count after treatment with all-*trans* retinoic acid (ATRA) or arsenic trioxide (ATO) are at risk of developing pulmonary infiltrates, pleural effusion, and respiratory distress (differentiation syndrome).[6]

Manifestations of hyperleukocytosis/leukostasis syndrome have been observed in patients with AML with relatively low counts, and rarely in patients with ALL with counts less than 300×10^9/L.[7] The mechanism of leukostasis is poorly understood and is likely related to the WBC count and also to leukemia cell contents, deformability, and interactivity with the vascular endothelium during blood flow.[8] Hyperleukocytosis increases blood viscosity and occludes the pulmonary microvasculature, resulting in tissue hypoperfusion and tissue damage. Inflammatory mediators produced in response to proliferating blasts and tissue damage contribute to this process, including pulmonary hemorrhage.

In addition to pulmonary complications, hyperleukocytosis is commonly associated with disseminated intravascular coagulopathy (DIC), systemic inflammatory response syndrome (SIRS), and tumor lysis syndrome (TLS). Intensive AML therapy or deep sedation for procedures may precipitate acute respiratory distress syndrome (ARDS), particularly in patients with monoblastic or myelomonocytic leukemia. This syndrome, termed leukemic cell lysis pneumopathy, occurs within 24 to 48 hours of the start of chemotherapy.[9] Leukemia cell lysis with the release enzymes (elastase, lysozyme) and subsequent SIRS may cause sudden deterioration of respiratory function, leading to diffuse alveolar damage and ARDS.

Hyperleukocytosis in patients with leukemia is a medical emergency. Because the initial management of hyperleukocytosis differs by leukemia subtype, the first step is to determine the leukemia subtype. In patients suspected to have APL and WBC counts greater than or equal to 10×10^9/L, ATRA should be initiated immediately, even before confirming the diagnosis. To prevent the differentiation syndrome associated with ATRA or ATO, corticosteroids should also be initiated.[6] Management of myeloid leukemia with monocytic differentiation complicated by hyperleukocytosis is challenging because of associated DIC and multiorgan involvement (pulmonary, central nervous system, heart, and kidneys).[10–12] The unique combination of hypophosphatemia, hypokalemia, hypoalbuminemia, hyperuricemia, and acute renal failure is thought to be caused by the renal tubular filtration of leukemia cell–released lysozyme.[13–15]

Standard-dose induction chemotherapy is not recommended for patients with leukemia complicated with hyperleukocytosis, because high levels of lysozyme and other inflammatory mediators released during cell lysis may cause further multiorgan damage.[16] Hydroxyurea or low-dose cytarabine is used to slowly reduce the tumor burden. Dexamethasone has been reported to improve pulmonary function.[17,18] If the WBC count continues to increase despite the use of hydroxyurea or low-dose cytarabine, leukapheresis or exchange transfusion should be considered before administering more intensive chemotherapy.[19,20]

Mediastinal Compartment Syndromes

Benign or malignant mediastinal cystic and solid tumors are common in pediatrics (**Table 1**).

Depending on the tumor location and growth, patients may develop life-threatening complications. The least invasive technique is used to obtain tissue for diagnosis. In many patients, a peripheral blood or bone marrow aspirate obtained under topical anesthesia may be used to establish the diagnosis. If a pleural effusion is present, thoracentesis may be performed for diagnostic and therapeutic purposes.

Central Airway Compression Syndrome

Compression of the trachea or main bronchus frequently occurs in children with a mediastinal mass. Signs and symptoms of airway compression include dyspnea on exertion, orthopnea, stridor, chest pain, fatigue, nonproductive cough, cyanosis, decreased breath sounds, and persistent wheezing. Chest radiograph findings may

Table 1
Mediastinal tumors in children

Mediastinum	Structures	Conditions
Superior/anterior	Thymus, lymph nodes, trachea, esophagus, aortic arch, brachiocephalic trunk, left common carotid artery, superior vena cava, brachiocephalic veins, arch of the azygous, thoracic duct, left and right vagus, recurrent laryngeal nerves, cardiac nerve, left and right phrenic nerves	Non-Hodgkin lymphomas, Hodgkin disease, cystic hygroma, germ cell tumors, hemangioma, lymphangioma, teratoma, lipoma, thymoma, thymic cyst, retrosternal thyroid, parathyroid tumors, and metastatic tumors
Middle	Heart and its great vessel roots, SVC, pulmonary veins, pericardiophrenic veins, and phrenic, vagus, and sympathetic nerves	Bronchogenic cyst, lymphoma, pericardial cyst, mesothelial cyst, thoracic duct cyst, granuloma, and hamartoma
Posterior	Esophagus, thoracic aorta, azygos and hemiazygos veins, thoracic duct, and vagus nerve	Neuroblastoma, ganglioneuroma, primitive neuroectodermal tumor, neurofibroma, and other neurogenic tumors, chloroma, and non-Hodgkin lymphoma

include the anterior mediastinal mass, prominent hilar lymph nodes, a posteriorly deviated trachea, atelectasis, and pleural effusion. Patients unable to lie supine and/or showing compression of greater than or equal to 50% in the tracheal cross-sectional area on a computed tomography (CT) scan are considered at high risk of complete tracheal obstruction.[21–23] Total airway obstruction may occur during the induction of general anesthesia, tracheal intubation, and when positioning a patient in a supine or flexed position (for lumbar puncture). Echocardiography is used to evaluate myocardial function and tumor extension in the heart and great vessels. Chemotherapy should be started as soon as the oncologic diagnosis is established.

Superior Vena Cava Syndrome

Because the vena cava, a vessel of fragile wall and low intraluminal pressure, is in direct contact with relatively rigid anatomic structures, it may be easily compressed by mediastinal tumors. In children, T-cell ALL and lymphomas are the most common causes of mediastinal involvement. The intensity of symptoms depends on the flow of the venous return from the head, neck, and upper extremities, reflecting the severity of the SVC compression. In tumors with slow growth, partial compression of the vena cava promotes neovascularization. If the obstruction is superiorly located, collateral veins drain into the inferior vena cava via the azygous veins. If the blockage is below the azygous confluence, these collaterals drain via the hemizygous or chest wall veins and are rare.[24] Patients with SVC with near-complete compression may experience dizziness, headaches, facial hyperemia, and facial swelling. Physical findings include facial and periorbital edema, cyanosis, plethora, neck and chest vein distention, papilledema, edema of the upper extremities, and increased pulsus paradoxus. Diagnostic vascular imaging requires Doppler ultrasonography and echocardiography to evaluate flow through the great vessels and magnetic resonance venography to assess the venous obstruction.[25]

Management of children with SVC syndrome caused by a mediastinal mass is similar to that for central airway compression described earlier. Although hyperhydration has frequently been advocated for patients at high risk of TLS, it should be avoided in patients with SVC syndrome because of the risk of respiratory failure and the worsening of existent pleural effusion. In patients with SVC syndrome, venous access should be through the lower extremities. Infusion through veins of the upper extremities should be avoided.

Although the mediastinal mass does not per se increase the risk of thrombosis,[26] induction chemotherapy regimens for ALL and lymphoma regularly include corticosteroid and L-asparaginase, a thrombogenic drug combination, and the prophylactic use of low-molecular-weight heparin should be considered, particularly in patients showing signs of collateral circulation and having femoral inserted central lines. However, most importantly, prompt specific chemotherapy for the primary malignancy should be implemented as soon as the diagnosis is confirmed.

PULMONARY COMPLICATIONS OF HEMATOPOIETIC STEM CELL TRANSPLANT

Pulmonary complications are common and occur in 25% to 50% of children after hematopoietic stem cell transplant (HSCT).[27–31] Several pretransplant factors may adversely affect post-HSCT pulmonary status, including conditioning regimens, irradiation targeting the lung, pulmonary toxic chemotherapy (bleomycin, busulfan, or cyclophosphamide), immunologic status, lung infections (viral, fungal), thoracic surgical procedures, and graft-versus-host disease (GvHD), among a variety of other pre-HSCT factors.

It is essential that patients previously exposed to treatments that are potentially pneumotoxic have pre-HSCT pulmonary screening, including complete pulmonary function tests (volumes, flows, and diffusing capacity of the lung for carbon monoxide [DLco]). Monitoring of pulmonary function tests (PFTs) remains useful during the posttransplant period and may serve as an adjunct to radiographic evaluation of intercurrent illness affecting the lung. Recent reports suggest that pre-HSCT pulmonary function may predict post-HSCT pulmonary complications as well as survival.

Pulmonary complications may have infectious or noninfectious causes. Infections causing pneumonia or ARDS may occur at any stage during the HSCT course. However, noninfectious lung injury, depending on the cause, follows a more predictable timeline (**Table 2**). It is essential to recognize and treat these complications as soon as they are identified, because the mortality in children who develop acute respiratory failure (ARF) post-HSCT is as high as 60%.[35]

Idiopathic Pneumonia Syndrome

Idiopathic pneumonia syndrome (IPS), also known as idiopathic interstitial pneumonitis, is a constellation of pulmonary diseases characterized by alveolar injury with diffuse infiltrates on chest radiograph, and negative bronchoalveolar lavage (BAL) cultures for infectious pathogens. Lung injury may affect the pulmonary parenchyma, vascular endothelium, or airway epithelium. It may occur within weeks to months post-HSCT. Children may present with nonproductive cough, dyspnea, and hypoxemia. Incidence of IPS is nearly 10% with a high mortality (50%–75%).[36,37] Treatment usually includes corticosteroids with tumor necrosis factor (TNF) inhibitors such as etanercept. A multicenter clinical trial included 28 children with IPS who were given systemic corticosteroids plus etanercept. Seventy-one percent of patients experienced a complete response at a median of 10 days. Overall survival was 89% at day 28.[38]

SUBSETS OF IDIOPATHIC PNEUMONIA SYNDROME

Periengraftment Respiratory Distress Syndrome

Engraftment syndrome represents an inflammatory status after HSCT. It is mainly manifested by fever, rash, and noncardiogenic pulmonary edema occurring at the time of neutrophil recovery after HSCT.[39,40] Hepatic and renal failure are comorbidities, occurring in up to 25% of patients with this syndrome. A small number of patients experience transient encephalopathy. Children with periengraftment respiratory distress syndrome may present with progressive hypoxemia and respiratory distress that requires supplemental oxygen and noninvasive positive pressure ventilation or, less often, invasive conventional ventilation (mechanical ventilation).

Capillary leak leads to the development of pulmonary edema usually within 2 to 3 weeks posttransplant. Treatment usually involves aggressive diuresis to prevent fluid overload. In addition, a short course of systemic corticosteroids may help ameliorate the inflammatory response and reduce the increased pulmonary capillary leak.[41]

Diffuse Alveolar Hemorrhage

Diffuse alveolar hemorrhage (DAH) is an uncommon pulmonary complication with a mortality of up to 80% when associated with multiorgan dysfunction.[42] It usually presents early within 1 to 2 months post-HSCT. Children usually present with rapidly progressive dyspnea and hypoxemia. Chest radiographs reveal diffuse perihilar or

Table 2
Characteristics of pulmonary complications after hematopoietic stem cell transplant

Pulmonary Complication	Onset Post-HSCT	Symptoms	Characteristic Findings	Chest Radiograph	CT	Treatment
IPS	Within 120 d	Cough, hypoxia, dyspnea	Widespread alveolar injury	Bilateral infiltrates	—	Corticosteroids TNF inhibitors
PERDS	Within 5–7 d of neutrophil engraftment	Fever, rash, hypoxia	Noncardiogenic pulmonary edema	Bilateral infiltrates	—	Fluid overload prevention, diuretics, corticosteroids
DAH	Within 100 d	Cough, progressive hypoxia	Progressive bloody BAL	Diffuse, bilateral infiltrates	Bilateral ground-glass infiltrates	Platelet count >50,000, correct coagulopathy, corticosteroids, inhaled TXA/inhaled rFVII
BOS	3–24 m	Cough, dyspnea, wheezing	Obstructive lung disease: reduced FEV_1	Normal or hyperinflation	Mosaic lung attenuation, air trapping, centrilobular nodules, bronchiectasis	Corticosteroids, inhaled corticosteroids, azithromycin and montelukast
COP	2–12 m	Cough, dyspnea, fever, crackles	Restrictive lung disease: reduced TLC and DL_{CO}	Patchy infiltrates	Patchy air space consolidation, ground-glass attenuation, nodular opacities	Corticosteroids, macrolides

Abbreviations: BAL, bronchoalveolar lavage; BOS, bronchiolitis obliterans syndrome; COP, cryptogenic organizing pneumonia; DAH, diffuse alveolar hemorrhage; FEV_1, forced expiratory volume in 1 second; IPS, idiopathic pneumonia syndrome; PERDS, periengraftment respiratory distress syndrome; rFVIIa, recombinant factor VIIa; TLC, total lung capacity; TNF, tumor necrosis factor; TXA, tranexamic acid.

Data from Refs.[32–34]

bibasilar interstitial and/or alveolar infiltrates, which may precede the worsening of clinical condition by several days. Chest CT typically shows dense bilateral and diffuse ground-glass infiltrates (**Fig. 1**).

Pathogenesis of DAH involves injury of the endothelium of small blood vessels and thrombotic microangiopathy. Alveolitis and cytokine release (eg, TNF and/or interleukin-12) resulting from either acute GvHD or pulmonary inflammation associated with bone marrow recovery are confounding factors, and may explain the frequently observed timing of DAH early in the post-transplant period.[43] Ultimately, distal alveolar airspace is obliterated by blood, fibrin, and inflammatory cells, leading to severely impaired gas exchange and refractory hypoxemia. Diagnosis is usually confirmed by bronchoscopy with progressively bloody BAL.

Treatment includes maintaining platelet count greater than 50,000/μL and correcting coagulopathy. Corticosteroids are often empirically used, although studies have not confirmed their benefit. Hypoxemia and dyspnea may worsen rapidly, and many patients require mechanical ventilation. Recent studies have reported success with inhaled recombinant factor VIIa (rFVIIa) as well as tranexamic acid (TXA).[44,45] In a small cohort of 18 children with DAH, Bafahiq and colleagues[45] used a 2-step therapy protocol that included inhaled TXA every 6 hours followed by the addition of inhaled rFVIIa every 4 hours if the bleeding did not stop. Bleeding ceased in 10 children with inhaled TXA alone, and in 6 more children with the combined therapy (TXA plus rFVIIa).

Bronchiolitis Obliterans Syndrome

Bronchiolitis obliterans syndrome (BOS) also known as obliterative bronchiolitis a chronic lower airways obstruction, is a common late-onset pulmonary complication that may present 3 to 24 months post-HSCT.[46] It occurs almost exclusively in patients receiving allogeneic HSCT.[47] It is thought that donor T-helper cell alloreactivity causes distal airways epithelial cell injury leading to subepithelial fibrotic changes in the small airways. Presentation is usually insidious with dry cough and dyspnea, and occasional wheezing, but fever is usually absent.

PFTs are the diagnostic mainstay. PFTs reveal an obstructive pattern (decrease in both forced expiratory volume in 1 second [FEV_1] and in FEV_1/forced vital capacity [FVC] ratio) without reversibility. Decline in lung function is associated with poor survival: only 45% of patients with BOS survive for 2 years.[47] Disease severity usually

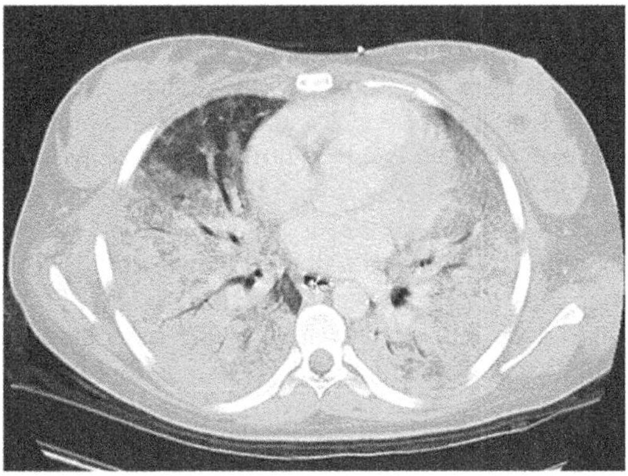

Fig. 1. CT of the chest in a patient with DAH after allogeneic HSCT. Findings include extensive and diffuse bilateral ground-glass pulmonary infiltrates.

correlates with the percentage reduction of FEV_1 from baseline before transplant.[48] Chest radiograph may be normal or show hyperinflation. Chest CT usually shows areas of patchy hyperaeration, bronchial dilatation, and other areas of increased density or hypoattenuation. These findings are often referred to as mosaic attenuation.[49] Lung biopsy may help confirm the diagnosis and to exclude other causes and usually shows small airway involvement with fibrinous obliteration of the lumen.[50]

Treatment of BOS remains challenging and aims at delaying further pulmonary function decline. Corticosteroids are usually used, although their prolonged use is associated with increased risk of infection and other side effects.[51,52] Other systemic steroid-sparing drugs have been introduced, such as inhaled fluticasone, azithromycin, and montelukast (FAM). The use of FAM and steroid pulse in 36 patients with BOS prevented further pulmonary decline in new-onset BOS in most patients and allowed reductions in corticosteroids.[53] Use of extracorporeal photopheresis may improve survival in patients receiving HSCT and reduce the rate of decline of FEV_1.[54] Novel antiinflammatory therapies such as ruxolitinib, a JAK1/2 inhibitor, are also emerging.

Cryptogenic Organizing Pneumonia

Cryptogenic organizing pneumonia (COP) is another uncommon chronic pulmonary complication post-HSCT. COP is a T-helper 1 inflammatory disease[29] and occurs almost exclusively after allogeneic HSCT. Children usually present 2 to 12 months post-HSCT with cough, dyspnea, fever, and inspiratory crackles on lung auscultation. PFTs are consistent with restrictive lung disease with normal FEV_1/FVC and reduced total lung capacity and DL_{CO}. Chest CT usually shows patchy air space consolidation, ground-glass attenuation, and nodular opacities, usually with a peripheral distribution pattern.[55–57] Lung biopsy is recommended to confirm the diagnosis. Histologic findings usually include patchy intraluminal fibrosis with granulation tissue consisting of fibroblast and collagen obliterating the distal airways, alveolar ducts, and peribronchial alveolar space.[58,59] The primary adverse consequence is effective loss of distal airspace and progressive impairment in gas exchange. COP often resolves after 1 to 3 months of steroid initiation; however, relapse may occur after discontinuing.

PULMONARY COMPLICATIONS OF SOLID NEOPLASMS

Primary lung tumors are rare in childhood, the most common being pleuropulmonary blastoma (chest masses) and carcinoid tumors (endobronchial obstruction).[60] However, pulmonary involvement is common in children with solid tumors. Malignant pleural effusion, mediastinal mass, interstitial lung disease, radiation-induced or chemotherapy-induced lung injury, or pulmonary hypertension may occur at presentation or during treatment. In addition, lungs are the most common site of metastasis. Osteosarcoma presents with metastasis (mostly pulmonary) at diagnosis in 20% of patients and similar percentage eventually develop metastasis. Other solid tumors associated with pulmonary metastasis include Wilms tumor (13%), hepatoblastoma (17%), rhabdomyosarcoma (16%), and Ewing sarcoma (10%). Pulmonary metastasis surgical resection increases survival in patients with osteosarcoma or hepatoblastoma, but not in patients with the other tumors mentioned earlier.[61]

INFECTIOUS PULMONARY COMPLICATIONS

Infections are so common in immune-compromised children that many patients are initiated on prophylactic antibiotics, antifungals, and antivirals. It is critical to know the immune dysfunction because it predicts the potential infectious pathogens. In children post-HSCT, the preengraftment period is dominated by neutropenia, compromised mucosal immunity as a result of preparative chemotherapy, and damaged skin barrier as a result of vascular access. Subsequently, in the early postengraftment period, cell-mediated immunity is impaired because of immunosuppression and acute GvHD and its treatments. Infections during the late postengraftment period usually are the result of impaired cell-mediated and humoral-mediated immunity,[62] with the exception that cluster of differentiation (CD) 4^+ T cells, lymphocyte subsets, and total lymphocyte counts recover within the first 2 to 3 months after transplant. However, despite numerical T-lymphocyte recovery, T-cell responses remain defective for a long time after transplant. In general, B-cell numbers normalize 6 months after autologous HSCT and 9 months after allogeneic HSCT.[63,64] However, antibody responses remain defective because of lack of T-cell interaction and GvHD and its treatments.[64,65] Neutropenia recovery may be associated with worsening hypoxemia in children with ARF, but survival improves.[66,67]

Bacterial Pneumonia

Children with hematologic malignancies as well as with some solid neoplasms receive chemotherapy that is associated with profound neutropenia and increased risk of bacterial pneumonia. In addition, bacterial pneumonia is common in the preengraftment phase (<30 days) post-HSCT. The most common gram-positive bacterial organisms are *Staphylococcus epidermidis* and *Streptococcus* spp, and the most common gram-negative organisms are *Pseudomonas aeruginosa* and *Klebsiella* spp.[68]

Stenotrophomonas maltophilia, a nonfermenting gram-negative bacillus, may cause pneumonia in children with hematologic malignancies or post-HSCT.[69,70] *S maltophilia* may cause a mostly fatal hemorrhagic pneumonia that usually leads to ARF. Patients suspected of having *S maltophilia* pneumonia should be started on trimethoprim-sulfamethoxazole (TMP-SMX). The prognosis is very poor in cases of hemorrhagic pneuomia..[69]

Pneumonias that occur later than 100 days post-HSCT are generally caused by encapsulated bacteria (eg, *S pneumoniae* and *H influenzae*), largely because of defects in cellular and humoral immunity. Other bacteria occurring during that phase include the genera *Legionella*, *Nocardia*, and *Actinomyces*.

Viral Pneumonia

Common viral pathogens, such as influenza A and B, parainfluenza viruses, respiratory syncytial virus (RSV), and human metapneumovirus, may cause lower respiratory tract infection and increased mortality in immune-compromised children. Lymphopenia is a risk factor for respiratory virus infection. Nasopharyngeal swabs or washings with cultures or enzyme immunoassays are the most commonly used diagnostic tools for most viral pathogens, including RSV.

Untreated RSV infection may be associated with mortalities as high as 80%. Aerosolized ribavirin and intravenous immunoglobulin may decrease mortality if treatment is initiated at the earliest stages of upper respiratory symptoms.[71] Palivizumab, a monoclonal antibody that targets the fusion protein of RSV, is used for prophylaxis in patients at risk of RSV infection.

Cytomegalovirus (CMV) pneumonia may occur secondary to reactivation of latent CMV, or may be acquired as a new infection or by blood transfusion (via infected WBCs), although the use of blood products from CMV-seronegative donors and leukocyte-depleted filtered blood have decreased that risk.[72,73] Preemptive and prophylactic antiviral therapy has markedly reduced the incidence and severity of CMV disease in children post-HSCT. The diagnosis of CMV pneumonia is usually made by demonstration of typical inclusions in lung tissue as well as a clinical picture consistent with CMV pneumonia. Treatment of CMV infection or reactivation includes ganciclovir, foscarnet, or cidofovir/brincidofovir.

Fungal Pneumonia

Profound neutropenia (absolute neutrophil count <500) and/or prolonged duration of neutropenia (>10 days) increase the risk of fungal infection.[74] The most clinically significant fungal pathogenic organisms include yeast (mainly *Candida*), molds (*Aspergillus*, zygomycetes, and other rare molds), endemic fungi, *Cryptococcus*, and *Pneumocystis*.

Fungal pneumonia may occur by direct lung invasion via inhalation of spores (eg, *Aspergillus*, *Cryptococcus*), or organisms that reach the lung from another site (*Aspergillus*, *Candida* spp), or systemic mycoses that lie dormant and reactivate in immunocompromised patients (*Coccidioides*, *Mucor*, and *Histoplasma* spp).[75] Because the outcomes of invasive fungal infection in immunocompromised patients are poor, prophylaxis with antifungal agents in high-risk patients and preemptive screening with galactomannan are essential.

Pneumocystis jiroveci is a fungal pathogen that does not respond to antifungal treatment. TMP-SMX prophylaxis is part of standard care for children with leukemia receiving chemotherapy. At present, *P jiroveci* pneumonia (PJP) may still occur as a result of noncompliance with TMP-SMX or a breakthrough event. The organism seems to attach to type I alveolar cells. This interaction leads to cell injury and altered permeability contributing to the development of pulmonary edema and altered gas exchange. Children with PJP present with cough, dyspnea, hypoxemia, and fever. Chest radiograph shows diffuse interstitial alveolar infiltrates, and chest CT shows a characteristic ground-glass pattern. BAL with immunofluorescent staining for PJP is the diagnostic gold standard. However, identifying *P jiroveci* DNA by polymerase chain reaction (PCR) assays in BAL fluid is more sensitive. These children may develop profound hypoxemia and require mechanical ventilation. Treatment includes administration of TMP-SMX as well as systemic corticosteroids.[76]

DIAGNOSTIC ROLE OF BRONCHOALVEOLAR LAVAGE

BAL is a valuable diagnostic tool to determine the cause and appropriate treatment of children with malignancy or post-HSCT presenting with pulmonary infiltrates on chest radiographs. Studies report a BAL diagnostic yield in 30% to 60% of immune-compromised children.[77–79] BAL yield is higher if bronchoscopy is done earlier in the course of illness. In a retrospective review of 501 nonintubated allogeneic HSCT recipients with new pulmonary infiltrates during the first 100 days after HSCT, the diagnostic yield of bronchoscopy more than doubled during the first 4 days after symptom onset.[80] Several adjuvants have recently been developed to improve the BAL diagnostic yield, such as multiplex PCR and metagenomic next-generation sequencing assays.

PULMONARY COMPLICATIONS OF SICKLE CELL DISEASE

Sickle cell disease (SCD) is the most common inherited disease affecting African and Caribbean populations. Pulmonary complications are common and may develop early in life, such as acute chest syndrome (ACS) or recurrent wheezing. Recurrent ACS is the most important risk factor for the development of sickle cell chronic lung disease (SCLD) and increased morbidity. Other complications, such as pulmonary hypertension, may have a more indolent course and present later in childhood to early adulthood.

ACUTE PULMONARY COMPLICATIONS

Acute Chest Syndrome

ACS is common in children with SCD. More than half of all children with homozygous SCD (HbSS) experience at least 1 episode of ACS in the first decade of life and recurrence is common.[81] The cause of ACS is often multifactorial. Proposed mechanisms include increased adhesion of sickle red cells to the pulmonary microvasculature in the presence of hypoxia. Risk factors for ACS include younger age, low fetal hemoglobin (HbF) and increased WBC count.[82] Clinical features include chest pain, productive cough, dyspnea, fever (>38.5°C), hypoxemia, and tachypnea. The spectrum of clinical manifestations ranges from mild respiratory illness to ARDS requiring mechanical ventilation. Chest radiograph usually shows new pulmonary infiltrates most commonly affecting the lower and middle lobes.

Infection is a common trigger for ACS. *Mycoplasma pneumoniae*, *Chlamydia pneumoniae*, RSV, *Staphylococcus aureus*, and pneumococci are the most common responsible pathogens. Infections caused by *S pneumoniae* have significantly decreased with the appropriate vaccination. Other proposed precipitating causes include pulmonary fat embolism. Infarction of the bony thorax or pain following abdominal surgery may cause splinting, hypoventilation, and atelectasis leading to hypoxia and intrapulmonary sickling. In addition, opioids prescribed for the pain may suppress respiratory drive, aggravating the hypoventilation.

Initial management of ACS starts with hydration, pain control, and broad-spectrum antibiotics that include macrolide and third-generation cephalosporin. Vancomycin is added in severely ill patients. Measures to prevent atelectasis include incentive spirometry or positive expiratory pressure devices, as well as supplemental oxygen to maintain Spo_2 greater than 95% (there may be poor correlation of Spo_2 with arterial blood gases). Simple transfusion is used to achieve a hemoglobin concentration of 9 to 11 g/dL or HbS levels of less than 30%.[83] If the patient has a high hematocrit, then exchange transfusion should be undertaken to avoid increasing blood viscosity. Exchange transfusion is also indicated in patients with rapidly worsening course of ACS. Indications for increasing respiratory support include worsening hypoxemia and dyspnea. Noninvasive ventilation may be initiated; if there is no improvement or rapid progression to ARF, conventional ventilation should be implemented. Bronchodilator therapy is recommended for patients with airway hyperreactivity or asthma.

Hydroxyurea is a key preventive intervention and patients must be carefully monitored. Hydroxyurea increases HbF level and reduces neutrophil and platelet counts, thereby ameliorating the abnormal cell adhesion inflammation pathways as well as correcting the nitric oxide (NO) deficiency state caused by SCD-associated hemolysis.[84] The use of antiinflammatory, antipolymerization, and antiadhesive medications offers potential beneficial approaches to treat ACS.

Asthma

Asthma is seen in 15% to 28% of patients with SCD and is associated with increased morbidity and mortality.[85] In a cohort of 521 children with SCD, those having asthma had higher incidence rates of ACS episodes (19 vs12 episodes per 100 patient years; $P = .02$) as well as more vasoocclusive pain episodes than those without asthma.[85] Bronchodilator inhalers are used in acute episodes. Oral corticosteroids are often used in the treatment of acute asthma; however, they are associated with an increased risk of rebound acute vasoocclusive pain and hospital readmission.[86,87] Up to 70% of children with SCD have airway hyperresponsiveness, even in those not having a clinical diagnosis of asthma.[88]

CHRONIC PULMONARY COMPLICATIONS

Sickle Chronic Lung Disease

SCLD is a progressive disease with hypoxemia, restrictive lung disease, cor pulmonale, and evidence of diffuse interstitial fibrosis on chest radiograph. Recurrent ACS episodes damage the lung parenchyma, resulting in restrictive lung disease.

Pulmonary Hypertension

Pulmonary arterial hypertension (PAH) is a common complication in children with SCD, with a steady increase in incidence with age. The prevalence of PAH in children with SCD is 10% to 35%.[89] Endogenous NO produced in the endothelium from arginine maintains patent vessel lumens. In patients with SCD, NO is consumed by plasma-free hemoglobin and degraded by arginase, which is released from hemolyzed sickle erythrocytes.[90] The resultant vascular dysfunction plays a prime role in the manifestations of stroke, pulmonary hypertension, leg ulceration, sickle nephropathy, and priapism. Evaluation by cardiology should be requested if diagnosis of PAH is suspected. The treatment of PAH in SCD is complex. Conventional therapies, such as sildenafil, may increase the risk of hospitalization for patients with vasoocclusive crisis. Other targeted therapies include prostacyclin agonists and endothelin receptor antagonists.[91] Prevention with early initiation of hydroxyurea is essential to reduce this complication.

CHEMOTHERAPY-INDUCED LUNG TOXICITY

Pulmonary tissue is particularly sensitive to chemotherapeutic agents.[92] Some adverse drugs reactions are cumulative, many are idiosyncratic, and others are triggered by concomitant treatments (eg, radiation therapy or oxygen).[93] Treatment includes discontinuation of the drug, glucocorticoid therapy in patients with severe pneumonitis or a histologic pattern suggesting good steroid response, and supportive care. In patients who have received bleomycin, high inspired oxygen should be avoided (**Table 3**).

RADIATION THERAPY

Lungs are very sensitive to the deleterious effects of ionizing radiation. However, modern treatment planning has significantly mitigated the risk of radiation pneumonitis.[101] Pulmonary complications include pneumonitis, fibrosis, and chest wall deformity. Treatment of radiation pneumonitis is supportive. In patients with moderate to severe symptoms, oral steroids are recommended.

LONG-TERM PULMONARY OUTCOME

Childhood cancer survivors experience long-term treatment-related pulmonary deficits. A cohort of 606 adult survivors of childhood cancer with a median elapsed time from diagnosis of 21.9 years was evaluated by PFT and a 6-minute walk. Restrictive lung disease was found in 31.2%, whereas obstructive lung disease was found in 0.8% of survivors. Abnormal PFTs were associated with decreased 6-minute walk distance.[102] The odds of restrictive lung defects may be 6.5 times higher in cancer survivors than in healthy controls.[103] Risk factors associated with restrictive lung disease include age younger than 16 years at diagnosis and exposure to more than 20 Gy of

Table 3
Clinical lung syndromes caused by antineoplastic agents

	Agents
Acute bronchoconstriction	Carboplatin, cyclophosphamide, etoposide, paclitaxel, rituximab, vinorelbine, vinblastine
Infusion reaction	Platinum drugs, paclitaxel, rituximab, L-asparaginase, carfilzomib, cytarabine, doxorubicin, etoposide
Alveolar hemorrhage	ATRA, bevacizumab, busulfan, crizotininb, docetaxel, erlotinib, etoposide, fludarabine, gefitinib, gemcitabine, irinotecan, lenalidomide, sorafenib, sunitinib
Noncardiogenic pulmonary edema	Cytarabine, bleomycin, doxorubicin, gemcitabine, interleukin-2, methotrexate, mitomycin, teniposide
Capillary leak syndrome	Docetaxel, interleukin-2
Acute lung injury, ARDS	Bleomycin, busulfan, cytarabine, dactinomycin, erlotinib, gemcitabine, mitomycin
Interstitial pneumonitis	Bleomycin, busulfan, carmustine, checkpoint immunotherapy, cyclophosphamide, gemcitabine, irinotecan, methotrexate, mitomycin, mitoxantrone, taxanes, procarbazine, rituximab, tyrosine kinase inhibitors (dasatinib, imatinib), everolimus, temsirolimus
Eosinophilic pneumonia	Bleomycin, lenalidomide, fludarabine, gemcitabine
Hypersensitivity pneumonitis	Bleomycin, methotrexate, cytarabine, dactinomycin
Pulmonary veno-occlusive disease	Bleomycin, carmustine, cisplatin, cyclophosphamide, gemcitabine, mitomycin
Pulmonary embolism	Asparaginase, bevacizumab, cisplatin, thalidomide
Radiation recall	Actinomycin-D, carmustine, doxorubicin, etoposide, gefitinib, gemcitabine, paclitaxel, trastuzumab
Bronchiolitis obliterans organizing pneumonia	Bleomycin, checkpoint immunotherapy, doxorubicin
Differentiation syndrome	ATRA
Long-term lung fibrosis	Asparaginase, bleomycin, busulfan, carmustine, cyclophosphamide, mitomycin-C, platinum agents

Data from Refs.[92–100]

chest radiation, pulmonary surgery, and bleomycin.[103,104] Therefore, preventing pulmonary complications while treating the underlying hematologic/oncologic disease is critical. This approach may be achieved by early detection and treatment of pulmonary complications as well as careful choice of cancer treatments with the best efficacy and the least toxicity.

CLINICS CARE POINTS

- Prophylactic antimicrobial therapy for CMV and fungal infection has reduced the infectious complications.
- BOS and COP, although sometimes confused together, are two different pathologic pulmonary complications post-HSCT. COP has a better survival rate than BOS.

- Childhood Caner survivors need close followup and monitoring for long term pulmonary complications.

ACKNOWLEDGEMENT

The authors thank Vani Shanker, PhD, ELS, for editing the manuscript.

DISCLOSURE

This research was funded by the American Lebanese Syrian Associated Charities (ALSAC).

REFERENCES

1. Lee EY. Pediatric thoracic oncology disorders. In: Cleveland R, Lee E, editors. Imaging in pediatric pulmonology. Cham (Switzerland): Springer; 2020. p. 293–323.
2. Schmidt JE, Tamburro RF, Sillos EM, Hill DA, Ribeiro RC, Razzouk BI. Pathophysiology-directed therapy for acute hypoxemic respiratory failure in acute myeloid leukemia with hyperleukocytosis. J Pediatr Hematol Oncol 2003;25(7): 569–71.
3. Kim MM, Barnato AE, Angus DC, Fleisher LA, Kahn JM. The effect of multidisciplinary care teams on intensive care unit mortality. Arch Intern Med 2010; 170(4):369–76.
4. Porcu P, Cripe LD, Ng EW, Bhatia S, Danielson CM, Orazi A, et al. Hyperleukocytic leukemias and leukostasis: a review of pathophysiology, clinical presentation and management. Leuk Lymphoma 2000;39(1-2):1–18.
5. Lowe EJ, Pui CH, Hancock ML, Geiger TL, Khan RB, Sandlund JT. Early complications in children with acute lymphoblastic leukemia presenting with hyperleukocytosis. Pediatr Blood Cancer 2005;45(1):10–5.
6. Sanz MA, Fenaux P, Tallman MS, Estey EH, LÃ¶wenberg B, Naoe T, et al. Management of acute promyelocytic leukemia: updated recommendations from an expert panel of the European LeukemiaNet. Blood 2019;133(15):1630–43.
7. Bunin NJ, Pui CH. Differing complications of hyperleukocytosis in children with acute lymphoblastic or acute nonlymphoblastic leukemia. J Clin Oncol 1985; 3(12):1590–5.
8. Stucki A, Rivier AS, Gikic M, Monai N, Schapira M, Spertini O. Endothelial cell activation by myeloblasts: molecular mechanisms of leukostasis and leukemic cell dissemination. Blood 2001;97(7):2121–9.
9. Tryka AF, Godleski JJ, Fanta CH. Leukemic cell lysis pneumonopathy. A complication of treated myeloblastic leukemia. Cancer 1982;50(12):2763–70.
10. Haferlach T, Schoch C, Schnittger S, Kern W, LÃ¶ffler H, Hiddemann W. Distinct genetic patterns can be identified in acute monoblastic and acute monocytic leukaemia (FAB AML M5a and M5b): a study of 124 patients. Br J Haematol 2002;118(2):426–31.
11. Liu LP, Zhang AL, Ruan M, Chang LX, Liu F, Chen X, et al. Prognostic stratification of molecularly and clinically distinct subgroup in children with acute monocytic leukemia. Cancer Med 2020;9(11):3647–55.
12. Azoulay E, Fieux F, Moreau D, Thiery G, Rousselot P, Parrot A, et al. Acute monocytic leukemia presenting as acute respiratory failure. Am J Respir Crit Care Med 2003;167(10):1329–33.

13. Osserman EF, Lawlor DP. Serum and urinary lysozyme (muramidase) in monocytic and monomyelocytic leukemia. J Exp Med 1966;124(5):921–52.
14. Perazella MA, Eisen RN, Frederick WG, Brown E. Renal failure and severe hypokalemia associated with acute myelomonocytic leukemia. Am J Kidney Dis 1993;22(3):462–7.
15. Aström M, Bodin L, Hörnsten P, Wahlin A, Tidefelt U. Evidence for a bimodal relation between serum lysozyme and prognosis in 232 patients with acute myeloid leukaemia. Eur J Haematol 2003;70(1):26–33.
16. Hijiya N, Metzger ML, Pounds S, Schmidt JE, Razzouk BI, Rubnitz JE, et al. Severe cardiopulmonary complications consistent with systemic inflammatory response syndrome caused by leukemia cell lysis in childhood acute myelomonocytic or monocytic leukemia. Pediatr Blood Cancer 2005;44(1):63–9.
17. Azoulay É, Canet E, Raffoux E, et al. Dexamethasone in patients with acute lung injury from acute monocytic leukaemia. Eur Respir J 2012;39(3):648–53.
18. Bertoli S, Picard M, Bérard E, Griessinger E, Larrue C, Mouchel PL, et al. Dexamethasone in hyperleukocytic acute myeloid leukemia. Haematologica 2018; 103(6):988–98.
19. Nguyen R, Jeha S, Zhou Y, Cao X, Cheng C, Bhojwani D, et al. The role of leukapheresis in the current management of hyperleukocytosis in newly diagnosed childhood acute lymphoblastic leukemia. Pediatr Blood Cancer 2016;63(9): 1546–51.
20. Stahl M, Shallis RM, Wei W, Montesinos P, Lengline E, Neukirchen J, et al. Management of hyperleukocytosis and impact of leukapheresis among patients with acute myeloid leukemia (AML) on short- and long-term clinical outcomes: a large, retrospective, multicenter, international study. Leukemia 2020.
21. Ernst A, Feller-Kopman D, Becker HD, Mehta AC. Central airway obstruction. Am J Respir Crit Care Med 2004;169(12):1278–97.
22. Anghelescu DL, Burgoyne LL, Liu T, Li CS, Pui CH, Hudson MM, et al. Clinical and diagnostic imaging findings predict anesthetic complications in children presenting with malignant mediastinal masses. Paediatr Anaesth 2007;17(11): 1090–8.
23. Ng A, Bennett J, Bromley P, Davies P, Morland B. Anaesthetic outcome and predictive risk factors in children with mediastinal tumours. Pediatr Blood Cancer 2007;48(2):160–4.
24. Mathew PM, Prangnell DR, Cole AJ, Hill FG, Shah KJ, Jones PH, et al. Clinical, haematological, and radiological features of children presenting with lymphoblastic mediastinal masses. Med Pediatr Oncol 1980;8(2):193–204.
25. Sonavane SK, Milner DM, Singh SP, Abdel Aal AK, Shahir KS, Chaturvedi A. Comprehensive imaging review of the superior vena cava. Radiographics 2015;35(7):1873–92.
26. Gartrell J, Kaste SC, Sandlund JT, Flerlage J, Zhou Y, Cheng C, et al. The association of mediastinal mass in the formation of thrombi in pediatric patients with non-lymphoblastic lymphomas. Pediatr Blood Cancer 2020;67(2):e28057.
27. Eikenberry M, Bartakova H, Defor T, Haddad IY, Ramsay NK, Blazar BR, et al. Natural history of pulmonary complications in children after bone marrow transplantation. Biol Blood Marrow Transplant 2005;11(1):56–64.
28. Park M, Koh KN, Kim BE, Im HJ, Seo JJ. Clinical features of late onset non-infectious pulmonary complications following pediatric allogeneic hematopoietic stem cell transplantation. Clin Transplant 2011;25(2):E168–76.

29. Lucena CM, Torres A, Rovira M, Marcos MA, de la Bellacasa JP, SÃ¡nchez M, et al. Pulmonary complications in hematopoietic SCT: a prospective study. Bone Marrow Transplant 2014;49(10):1293–9.
30. Elbahlawan L, Rains KJ, Stokes DC. Respiratory care considerations in the childhood cancer patient. Respir Care 2017;62(6):765–75.
31. Elbahlawan L, Srinivasan A, Morrison RR. A critical care and transplantation-based approach to acute respiratory failure after hematopoietic stem cell transplantation in children. Biol Blood Marrow Transplant 2016;22(4):617–26.
32. Rowan CM, McArthur J, Hsing DD, Gertz SJ, Smith LS, Loomis A, et al. Acute respiratory failure in pediatric hematopoietic cell transplantation: a multicenter study. Crit Care Med 2018;46(10):e967–74.
33. Sakaguchi H, Takahashi Y, Watanabe N, Doisaki S, Muramatsu H, Hama A, et al. Incidence, clinical features, and risk factors of idiopathic pneumonia syndrome following hematopoietic stem cell transplantation in children. Pediatr Blood Cancer 2012;58(5):780–4.
34. Sano H, Kobayashi R, Iguchi A, Suzuki D, Kishimoto K, Yasuda K, et al. Risk factor analysis of idiopathic pneumonia syndrome after allogeneic hematopoietic SCT in children. Bone Marrow Transplant 2014;49(1):38–41.
35. Yanik GA, Grupp SA, Pulsipher MA, Levine JE, Schultz KR, Wall DA, et al. TNF-receptor inhibitor therapy for the treatment of children with idiopathic pneumonia syndrome. A joint Pediatric Blood and Marrow Transplant Consortium and Children's Oncology Group Study (ASCT0521). Biol Blood Marrow Transplant 2015; 21(1):67–73.
36. Nishio N, Yagasaki H, Takahashi Y, Hama A, Muramatsu H, Tanaka M, et al. Engraftment syndrome following allogeneic hematopoietic stem cell transplantation in children. Pediatr Transplant 2009;13(7):831–7.
37. Schmid I, Stachel D, Pagel P, Albert MH. Incidence, predisposing factors, and outcome of engraftment syndrome in pediatric allogeneic stem cell transplant recipients. Biol Blood Marrow Transplant 2008;14(4):438–44.
38. Abongwa C, Abu-Arja R, Rumelhart S, Lazarus HM, Abusin G. Favorable outcome to glucocorticoid therapy for engraftment syndrome in pediatric autologous hematopoietic cell transplant. Pediatr Transplant 2016;20(2):297–302.
39. Ben-Abraham R, Paret G, Cohen R, Szold O, Cividalli G, Toren A, et al. Diffuse alveolar hemorrhage following allogeneic bone marrow transplantation in children. Chest 2003;124(2):660–4.
40. Soubani AO. Critical care considerations of hematopoietic stem cell transplantation. Crit Care Med 2006;34(9 Suppl):S251–67.
41. Park JA, Kim BJ. Intrapulmonary recombinant factor VIIa for diffuse alveolar hemorrhage in children. Pediatrics 2015;135(1):e216–20.
42. Bafaqih H, Chehab M, Almohaimeed S, Thabet F, Alhejaily A, AlShahrani M, et al. Pilot trial of a novel two-step therapy protocol using nebulized tranexamic acid and recombinant factor VIIa in children with intractable diffuse alveolar hemorrhage. Ann Saudi Med 2015;35(3):231–9.
43. Au BK, Au MA, Chien JW. Bronchiolitis obliterans syndrome epidemiology after allogeneic hematopoietic cell transplantation. Biol Blood Marrow Transplant 2011;17(7):1072–8.
44. Dudek AZ, Mahaseth H, DeFor TE, Weisdorf DJ. Bronchiolitis obliterans in chronic graft-versus-host disease: analysis of risk factors and treatment outcomes. Biol Blood Marrow Transplant 2003;9(10):657–66.

45. Estenne M, Maurer JR, Boehler A, Egan JJ, Frost A, Hertz M, et al. Bronchiolitis obliterans syndrome 2001: an update of the diagnostic criteria. J Heart Lung Transplant 2002;21(3):297–310.
46. Jung JI, Jung WS, Hahn ST, Min CK, Kim CC, Park SH. Bronchiolitis obliterans after allogenic bone marrow transplantation: HRCT findings. Korean J Radiol 2004;5(2):107–13.
47. Williams KM, Chien JW, Gladwin MT, Pavletic SZ. Bronchiolitis obliterans after allogeneic hematopoietic stem cell transplantation. JAMA 2009;302(3):306–14.
48. Even-Or E, Ghandourah H, Ali M, Krueger J, Sweezey NB, Schechter T. Efficacy of high-dose steroids for bronchiolitis obliterans syndrome post pediatric hematopoietic stem cell transplantation. Pediatr Transplant 2018;22(2).
49. Uhlving HH, Buchvald F, Heilmann CJ, Nielsen KG, Gormsen M. Bronchiolitis obliterans after allo-SCT: clinical criteria and treatment options. Bone Marrow Transplant 2012;47(8):1020–9.
50. Williams KM, Cheng GS, Pusic I, Jagasia M, Burns L, Ho VT, et al. Fluticasone, Azithromycin, and Montelukast Treatment for New-Onset Bronchiolitis Obliterans Syndrome after Hematopoietic Cell Transplantation. Biol Blood Marrow Transplant 2016;22(4):710–6.
51. Hefazi M, Langer KJ, Khera N, Adamski J, Roy V, Winters JL, et al. Extracorporeal photopheresis improves survival in hematopoietic cell transplant patients with bronchiolitis obliterans syndrome without significantly impacting measured pulmonary functions. Biol Blood Marrow Transplant 2018;24(9):1906–13.
52. Graham NJ, Müller NL, Miller RR, Shepherd JD. Intrathoracic complications following allogeneic bone marrow transplantation: CT findings. Radiology 1991;181(1):153–6.
53. Worthy SA, Flint JD, Müller NL. Pulmonary complications after bone marrow transplantation: high-resolution CT and pathologic findings. Radiographics 1997;17(6):1359–71.
54. Long NM, Plodkowski AJ, Schor-Bardach R, Geyer AI, Zheng J, Moskowitz CS, et al. Computed tomographic appearance of organizing pneumonia in an oncologic patient population. J Comput Assist Tomogr 2017;41(3):437–41.
55. Myers JL, Colby TV. Pathologic manifestations of bronchiolitis, constrictive bronchiolitis, cryptogenic organizing pneumonia, and diffuse panbronchiolitis. Clin Chest Med 1993;14(4):611–22.
56. Yoshihara S, Yanik G, Cooke KR, Mineishi S. Bronchiolitis obliterans syndrome (BOS), bronchiolitis obliterans organizing pneumonia (BOOP), and other late-onset noninfectious pulmonary complications following allogeneic hematopoietic stem cell transplantation. Biol Blood Marrow Transplant 2007;13(7):749–59.
57. Wells AU. Cryptogenic organizing pneumonia. Semin Respir Crit Care Med 2001;22(4):449–60.
58. Radzikowska E, Roży A, Jagus P, Polubiec-Kownacka M, Wiatr E, Chorostowska-Wynimko J, et al. Clarithromycin decreases IL-6 concentration in serum and BAL fluid in patients with cryptogenic organizing pneumonia. Adv Clin Exp Med 2016;25(5):871–8.
59. Patriarca F, Skert C, Sperotto A, Damiani D, Cerno M, Geromin A, et al. Incidence, outcome, and risk factors of late-onset noninfectious pulmonary complications after unrelated donor stem cell transplantation. Bone Marrow Transplant 2004;33(7):751–8.
60. Dishop MK, Kuruvilla S. Primary and metastatic lung tumors in the pediatric population: a review and 25-year experience at a large children's hospital. Arch Pathol Lab Med 2008;132(7):1079–103.

61. Heaton TE, Davidoff AM. Surgical treatment of pulmonary metastases in pediatric solid tumors. Semin Pediatr Surg 2016;25(5):311–7.
62. Wingard JR, Hsu J, Hiemenz JW. Hematopoietic stem cell transplantation: an overview of infection risks and epidemiology. Infect Dis Clin North Am 2010; 24(2):257–72.
63. Storek J. B-cell immunity after allogeneic hematopoietic cell transplantation. Cytotherapy 2002;4(5):423–4.
64. Small TN, Keever CA, Weiner-Fedus S, Heller G, O'Reilly RJ, Flomenberg N. B-cell differentiation following autologous, conventional, or T-cell depleted bone marrow transplantation: a recapitulation of normal B-cell ontogeny. Blood 1990;76(8):1647–56.
65. Storek J, Wells D, Dawson MA, Storer B, Maloney DG. Factors influencing B lymphopoiesis after allogeneic hematopoietic cell transplantation. Blood 2001; 98(2):489–91.
66. Elbahlawan LM, Morrison RR, Jeha S, Cheng C, Liu W, Fiser RT. Impact of neutrophil recovery on oxygenation in pediatric oncology patients with acute hypoxemic respiratory failure. J Pediatr Hematol Oncol 2011;33(7):e296–9.
67. Moffet JR, Mahadeo KM, McArthur J, Hsing DD, Gertz SJ, Smith LS, et al. Acute respiratory failure and the kinetics of neutrophil recovery in pediatric hematopoietic cell transplantation: a multicenter study. Bone Marrow Transplant 2020; 55(2):341–8.
68. Aguilar-Guisado M, Jiménez-Jambrina M, Espigado I, Rovira M, Martino R, Oriol A, et al. Pneumonia in allogeneic stem cell transplantation recipients: a multicenter prospective study. Clin Transplant 2011;25(6):E629–38.
69. Tada K, Kurosawa S, Hiramoto N, Okinaka K, Ueno N, Asakura Y, et al. Stenotrophomonas maltophilia infection in hematopoietic SCT recipients: high mortality due to pulmonary hemorrhage. Bone Marrow Transplant 2013;48(1):74–9.
70. Mori M, Tsunemine H, Imada K, Ito K, Kodaka T, Takahashi T. Life-threatening hemorrhagic pneumonia caused by Stenotrophomonas maltophilia in the treatment of hematologic diseases. Ann Hematol 2014;93(6):901–11.
71. Hynicka LM, Ensor CR. Prophylaxis and treatment of respiratory syncytial virus in adult immunocompromised patients. Ann Pharmacother 2012;46(4):558–66.
72. Ljungman P, Hakki M, Boeckh M. Cytomegalovirus in hematopoietic stem cell transplant recipients. Hematol Oncol Clin North Am 2011;25(1):151–69.
73. Ljungman P, Hakki M, Boeckh M. Cytomegalovirus in hematopoietic stem cell transplant recipients. Infect Dis Clin North Am 2010;24(2):319–37.
74. Young AY, Leiva Juarez MM, Evans SE. Fungal pneumonia in patients with hematologic malignancy and hematopoietic stem cell transplantation. Clin Chest Med 2017;38(3):479–91.
75. Shi JM, Pei XY, Luo Y, Tan YM, Tie RX, He JS, et al. Invasive fungal infection in allogeneic hematopoietic stem cell transplant recipients: single center experiences of 12 years. J Zhejiang Univ Sci B 2015;16(9):796–804.
76. Shankar SM, Nania JJ. Management of pneumocystis jiroveci pneumonia in children receiving chemotherapy. Paediatr Drugs 2007;9(5):301–9.
77. Nadimpalli S, Foca M, Satwani P, Sulis ML, Constantinescu A, Saiman L. Diagnostic yield of bronchoalveolar lavage in immunocompromised children with malignant and non-malignant disorders. Pediatr Pulmonol 2017;52(6):820–6.
78. Elbahlawan LM, Avent Y, Montoya L, Wilder K, Pei D, Cheng C, et al. Safety and benefits of bronchoalveolar lavage and lung biopsy in the management of pulmonary infiltrates in children with leukemia. J Pediatr Hematol Oncol 2016;38(8): 597–601.

79. Efrati O, Gonik U, Bielorai B, Modan-Moses D, Neumann Y, Szeinberg A, et al. Fiberoptic bronchoscopy and bronchoalveolar lavage for the evaluation of pulmonary disease in children with primary immunodeficiency and cancer. Pediatr Blood Cancer 2007;48(3):324–9.
80. Shannon VR, Andersson BS, Lei X, Champlin RE, Kontoyiannis DP. Utility of early versus late fiberoptic bronchoscopy in the evaluation of new pulmonary infiltrates following hematopoietic stem cell transplantation. Bone Marrow Transplant 2010;45(4):647–55.
81. Gill FM, Sleeper LA, Weiner SJ, Brown AK, Bellevue R, Grover R, et al. Clinical events in the first decade in a cohort of infants with sickle cell disease. Cooperative Study of Sickle Cell Disease. Blood 1995;86(2):776–83.
82. Castro O, Brambilla DJ, Thorington B, Reindorf CA, Scott RB, Gillette P, et al. The acute chest syndrome in sickle cell disease: incidence and risk factors. The Cooperative Study of Sickle Cell Disease. Blood 1994;84(2):643–9.
83. Yawn BP, Buchanan GR, Afenyi-Annan AN, Ballas SK, Hassell KL, James AH, et al. Management of sickle cell disease: summary of the 2014 evidence-based report by expert panel members. JAMA 2014;312(10):1033–48.
84. Thornburg CD, Files BA, Luo Z, Miller ST, Kalpatthi R, Iyer R, et al. Impact of hydroxyurea on clinical events in the BABY HUG trial. Blood 2012;120(22): 4304–10 [quiz: 448].
85. An P, Barron-Casella EA, Strunk RC, Hamilton RG, Casella JF, DeBaun MR. Elevation of IgE in children with sickle cell disease is associated with doctor diagnosis of asthma and increased morbidity. J Allergy Clin Immunol 2011; 127(6):1440–6.
86. Strouse JJ, Takemoto CM, Keefer JR, Kato GJ, Casella JF. Corticosteroids and increased risk of readmission after acute chest syndrome in children with sickle cell disease. Pediatr Blood Cancer 2008;50(5):1006–12.
87. Darbari DS, Fasano RS, Minniti CP, Castro OO, Gordeuk VR, Taylor JGt, et al. Severe vaso-occlusive episodes associated with use of systemic corticosteroids in patients with sickle cell disease. J Natl Med Assoc 2008;100(8):948–51.
88. Leong MA, Dampier C, Varlotta L, Allen JL. Airway hyperreactivity in children with sickle cell disease. J Pediatr 1997;131(2):278–83.
89. Lamina MO, Animasahun BA, Akinwumi IN, Njokanma OF. Doppler echocardiographic assessment of pulmonary artery pressure in children with sickle cell anaemia. Cardiovasc Diagn Ther 2019;9(3):204–13.
90. Bakshi N, Morris CR. The role of the arginine metabolome in pain: implications for sickle cell disease. J Pain Res 2016;9:167–75.
91. Klings ES, Machado RF, Barst RJ, Morris CR, Mubarak KK, Gordeuk VR, et al. An official American Thoracic Society clinical practice guideline: diagnosis, risk stratification, and management of pulmonary hypertension of sickle cell disease. Am J Respir Crit Care Med 2014;189(6):727–40.
92. Dietz AC, Chen Y, Yasui Y, Ness KK, Hagood JS, Chow EJ, et al. Risk and impact of pulmonary complications in survivors of childhood cancer: a report from the Childhood Cancer Survivor Study. Cancer 2016;122(23):3687–96.
93. Leger P, Limper AH, Maldonado F. Pulmonary toxicities from conventional chemotherapy. Clin Chest Med 2017;38(2):209–22.
94. Vahid B, Marik PE. Pulmonary complications of novel antineoplastic agents for solid tumors. Chest 2008;133(2):528–38.
95. Huang TT, Hudson MM, Stokes DC, Krasin MJ, Spunt SL, Ness KK. Pulmonary outcomes in survivors of childhood cancer: a systematic review. Chest 2011; 140(4):881–901.

96. Grace RF, Dahlberg SE, Neuberg D, Sallan SE, Connors JM, Neufeld EJ, et al. The frequency and management of asparaginase-related thrombosis in paediatric and adult patients with acute lymphoblastic leukaemia treated on Dana-Farber Cancer Institute consortium protocols. Br J Haematol 2011;152(4):452–9.
97. Josephson MB, Goldfarb SB. Pulmonary complications of childhood cancers. Expert Rev Respir Med 2014;8(5):561–71.
98. Possick JD. Pulmonary toxicities from checkpoint immunotherapy for malignancy. Clin Chest Med 2017;38(2):223–32.
99. Mahadeo KM, Khazal SJ, Abdel-Azim H, Fitzgerald JC, Taraseviciute A, Bollard CM, et al. Management guidelines for paediatric patients receiving chimeric antigen receptor T cell therapy. Nat Rev Clin Oncol 2019;16(1):45–63.
100. Maldonado FL, Limper AH, Cass AS, et al. Pulmonary toxicity associated with antineoplastic therapy: citotoxic agents. In: Flaherty KR, Savarese DMF, Hollingsworth H, editors. UpToDate [Internet]. Waltham (MA): UpToDate Inc; 2020.
101. Bledsoe TJ, Nath SK, Decker RH. Radiation pneumonitis. Clin Chest Med 2017; 38(2):201–8.
102. Green DM, Zhu L, Wang M, Ness KK, Krasin MJ, Bhakta NH, et al. Pulmonary function after treatment for childhood cancer. A Report from the St. Jude Lifetime Cohort Study (SJLIFE). Ann Am Thorac Soc 2016;13(9):1575–85.
103. Armenian SH, Landier W, Francisco L, Herrera C, Mills G, Siyahian A, et al. Long-term pulmonary function in survivors of childhood cancer. J Clin Oncol 2015;33(14):1592–600.
104. Mulder RL, Thönissen NM, van der Pal HJ, Bresser P, Hanselaar W, Koning CC, et al. Pulmonary function impairment measured by pulmonary function tests in long-term survivors of childhood cancer. Thorax 2011;66(12):1065–71.

Pulmonary Manifestations of Endocrine and Metabolic Diseases in Children

Alexander A. Broomfield, MBBS[a,*], Raja Padidela, MD[b,c], Stuart Wilkinson, MBChB[d]

KEYWORDS

- Restrictive lung disease • Obstructive lung disease • Inborn errors of metabolism
- Endocrinological disorders

KEY POINTS

- The improved phenotyping of inborn errors of metabolism and endocrinopathies is increasingly revealing the extent of the pulmonary involvement in these systemic disorders.
- Early recognition can enable potential disease modifying therapy to be initiated and prevent needless investigation.
- Although particular diseases may predominately manifest as restrictive or obstructive lung disease, often a combination of both exist.

INTRODUCTION

Advances in technology, methodology, and deep phenotyping are increasingly driving the understanding of the pathologic basis of disease. The resultant improvements in patient identification and treatment are in turn impacting survival and unmasking new aspects of disease. This is especially true in endocrinology and inborn errors of metabolism, where disease-modifying therapies continue to be developed. Inherent to this evolving picture is the increasing awareness of the respiratory manifestations of these rare diseases. This review updates clinicians on these manifestations, stratifying diseases principally spirometerically; short sections on pulmonary hypertension and diseases with a predisposition to recurrent pulmonary infection are also included.

[a] Willink Biochemical Genetics Unit, Manchester Centre for Genomic Medicine, St Mary's Hospital, Manchester University NHS Foundation Trust, Manchester, UK; [b] Department of Paediatric Endocrinology, Royal Manchester Children's Hospital, Manchester, UK; [c] Faculty of Biology, Medicine and Health, University of Manchester, Manchester, UK; [d] Respiratory Department Royal Manchester Children's Hospital, Manchester University, NHS Foundation Trust, Manchester Academic Health Science Centre, Manchester, UK
* Corresponding author.
E-mail address: Alexander.Broomfield@mft.nhs.uk

Pediatr Clin N Am 68 (2021) 81–102
https://doi.org/10.1016/j.pcl.2020.09.011 pediatric.theclinics.com

This division is, however, artificial with many diseases having multiple pathologic effects on respiration. Owing to considerations of space, this review does not cover the impact of obesity.

OBSTRUCTIVE DISEASE

The endocrine and metabolic causes of obstructive airway disease are principally owing to alterations of the upper airways, typically presenting as either stridor or snoring with or without obstructive sleep apnea (OSA). The clinical hallmarks of these diseases and the approach to their diagnosis is detailed in **Table 1**. Acute stridor is a feature of some B vitamin deficiencies. In biotinidase deficiency, a recycling defect of biotin (vitamin B_7), a laryngeal spasm unresponsive to steroids but responsive within hours to oral biotin supplementation, can occur.[1–3] Stridor is also a feature of Brown–Vialetto–Van Leadre (BVVL), a disorder of gastrointestinal riboflavin (vitamin B_2) uptake, owing to defects in the luminal B_2 transporters RFTVT2 or RFTVT3. Although the classical clinical triad suggestive of BVVL is sensorineural deafness, bulbar palsy and respiratory compromise caused by muscular weakness,[4,5] it is now recognized that up to 50% of patients with BVVL presenting before the age of 3 years do so with stridor. Stridor has also been seen in a closely linked disorder, multiple acyl-coenzyme A dehydrogenase deficiency. Here the proteins, electron transfer flavoprotein, and electron transfer flavoprotein ubiquinone oxidoreducatase for which riboflavin is a precursor, accept the electrons generated by the flavin adenine dinucleotide–linked dehydrogenases. Abnormalities in either protein will ultimately also cause inhibition of the same fatty acid dehydrogenases as affected by BVVL. Unlike in BVVL, only severe multiple acyl-coenzyme A dehydrogenase deficiency has been linked with recurrent stridor,[6] with it not seeming to occur in milder multiple acyl-coenzyme A dehydrogenase deficiency variants.[7] Acute laryngospasm is also a symptom of hypocalcemia, whose main cause is hypoparathyroidism,[8] which in just under 10% of cases has a genetic basis.[9] Although this condition can be isolated or part of as syndrome, most typically the 22q11 microdeletion responsible for DiGeorge syndrome, it has also be seen to be secondary to defects in mitochondrial energetics such as Kearns–Sayre, MELAS [Mitochondrial encephalomyopathy, lactic acidosis, and stroke-like episodes], and mitochondrial trifunctional protein deficiency.[10–12]

However, the majority of endocrine and metabolic upper airway problems result from progressive anatomic changes. The archetypical examples are the lysosomal storage disorders, where inherited deficiencies in the activity of the inherent catabolic enzymes result in excessive substrate accumulation, which in turn trigger localized and systemic inflammatory responses. This response is most prominently seen in the mucopolysaccharidoses, a group of inherited conditions of glycosaminoglycan (GAG) degradation.[13] However, given their multilevel airway disease, they are considered in their own section in this article. Other lysosomal disorders resulting in upper airway distortion include the non/minimally neurologically affected patients with Faber disease. They generally suffer from progressive joint deformation and contractures, subcutaneous nodules, and inflammatory granuloma formation,[14] the latter occurring anywhere in the respiratory tract[15] and potentially causing extensive upper airway obstruction.[16] The respiratory hallmarks are a hoarse voice and respiratory insufficiency secondary to obstruction or interstitial pneumonitis. The pneumonitis of itself leads to death in the third or fourth decade of life. The upper airway lesions have been successfully surgically resected, but these lesions can reoccur.[16]

Soft tissue changes, especially tongue enlargement, is a feature of hypothyroidism, although alteration in central respiratory drive, suppression of the hypercapnic

Table 1
Causes of obstructive lung disease

Disease	Main Presenting Features	Investigation
Biotindase	Insidious onset of lethargy hypotonia, seizures after 7 wk. Hearing loss, marked dermatitis, optic atrophy, developmental delay	Urine organic acids Acylcarnitines Biotindase red cell assay
Brown–Vialetto–Van– Leare	Progressive pontocerebellar palsy and deafness. RFTV2 often also have sensory ataxia followed by distal weakness with or without nystagmus RFVT3—normally PC in infancy with hypotonia Both types→ rapidly progressive bulbar palsy and respiratory failure	Urine organic acids Acylcarnitines genetics
Hypocalcemia syndromic: 1. DeGeorge type 1 + 2 2. CHARGE 3. Autoimmune polyendocrine syndrome type 1 4. Hypoparathyroidism, sensorineural deafness and renal disease (hdr) 5) Kenney–Caffey syndrome type 1 + 2 6. Snajad–Sakati syndrome 7. Gracile bone dysplasia Mitochondrial: 1. MELAS 2. Kearns–Sayre 3. Mitochondrial trifunctional protein Autosomal dominant hypocalcemia: Autosomal dominant hypocalcemia type 1 Autosomal dominant hypocalcemia type 2 Isolated hypoparathyroidism	Congenital heart defects, thymic hypoplasia, cleft palate, parathyroid hypoplasia, developmental delay, renal, laryngotracheoesophageal and skeletal abnormalities Coloboma, heart anomaly, choanal atresia, retardation, genital and ear anomalies Addison disease, hypoparathyroidism, and chronic mucocutaneous candidiasis Hypoparathyroidism, sensorineural deafness, renal dysplasia and occasional female genitourinary dysplasia Dwarfism, developmental delay (NB normal type 2) cortical thickening and medullary stenosis of long bones Intrauterine growth restriction at birth, microcephaly, congenital hypoparathyroidism, facial dysmorphism, mild intellectual delay Perinatally lethal condition, gracile bones with thin diaphyses, premature closure of basal cranial sutures, and microphthalmia Mitochondrial myopathy, encephalopathy, lactic acidosis, and stroke-like episodes, but multisystem disease	Genetic analysis of following genes, except where stated: DNA methylation MPLA CHD7 variants AIRE HDR TBCE/FAM111A TBCE FAM111A Mitochondrial DNA analysis: Most commonly mt point mutations 3243A-G, 8993T-G Mitochondrial DNA analysis: Acylcarntitines, HADHA HADHB gene analysis CASR/GNA11 GCM2/PTH/SOX3

(*continued on next page*)

Table 1
(continued)

Disease	Main Presenting Features	Investigation
	Progressive external ophthalmoplegia, pigmentary retinopathy, and onset before 20 y of age, plus at least one of the followings: heart block, cerebellar symptoms, or cerebral spinal fluid protein levels of >100 mg/dL. Neonatal/early onset hypotonia, cardiomyopathy, liver dysfunction, hypoketotic hypoglycemia. 50% of patients have mild or asymptomatic hypocalcemia; about 50% have paresthesias, carpopedal spasm, and seizures; about 10% have hypercalciuria with nephrocalcinosis or kidney stones; >35% have ectopic and basal ganglia calcifications	
Farber disease	Triad of subcutaneous nodules, arthritis, and laryngeal involvement Hepatosplenomegaly	Acid ceramidase levels ASAH1
Prader–Willi syndrome	Neonatal hypotonia, facial dysmorphism with bifrontal narrowing then philtrum and almond shaped palpebral fissures, poor suck leading to failure to thrive, decreased responsiveness, small gentiles → subsequent hyperphagia developmental delay and short stature.	Genetic first line DNA methylation-specific MLPA

response,[17] and diaphragmatic weakness[18] also contribute to the multiple causes of respiratory dysfunction. A meta-analysis suggested that up to 30% of patients with overt clinical hypothyroidism have OSA,[19] but the historical link with pleural effusions is debated.[19] It is to be noted that obstruction has also been noted to occur in neonatal autoimmune hyperthyroidism owing to thyromegaly.[20]

Although the association of acromegaly and OSA is well established in adults,[21] there is little evidence that it causes problems in childhood. However the relationship of growth hormone supplementation in Prader–Willi syndrome (PWS) (see **Table 1**) and sudden death has been questioned.[20] Classically, the respiratory problems in PWS include OSA, central sleep apnea, and hypoventilation. Sudden death in patients with PWS has been long recognized and largely attributed to acute respiratory illness in combination with these preexisting respiratory problems. Although the body mass index standard deviation score has been found to correlate with OSA in children with PWS, the PWS-related obesity alone does not explain the association with OSA. Comparison studies of polysomnography (PSG) with non-PWS obesity-matched controls showed that the PWS group had a significantly longer time with suboptimal oxyhemoglobin concentrations.[22] Poor upper airway tone, pharyngeal narrowing, micrognathia, adenoid hyperplasia, and decreased respiratory muscle strength all contribute, alongside an abnormal response to hypoxia and hypercapnia thought to be a result of hypothalamic dysfunction. Growth hormone deficiency is common in PWS, with an incidence of 40% to 100% reported. It is likely to contribute to the lower muscle mass, increased adipose tissue, and short stature found in PWS. In November 2000, growth hormone therapy was licensed in the UK for the indication "improvement of body composition and growth."[23] Growth hormone therapy is proposed to lead to adenotonsillar hyperplasia, which may lead to worsening OSA. Metabolic demand increases while on growth hormone therapy,[23] causing increased oxygen demand and leading to a relative state of hypoventilation. A preexisting decrease in hydration can be reversed while on GHT; this state may lead to a temporary increase in volume load and could also cause airway edema. All of these factors could contribute toward sudden death, especially in the context of an acute respiratory illness.

RESTRICTIVE DISEASE

The metabolic and endocrine causes of restrictive lung disease are principally caused by interstitial lung disease and musculoskeletal disease (**Table 2**).

Interstitial Disease

Many metabolic disorders can also manifest as interstitial lung disease. Indeed the European Childhood interstitial lung disease[24] and American[24] classifications have long recognized the potential for lysosomal storage disorders especially the sphingolipidoses to cause disease. However, it is becoming increasingly evident that, in addition to the lysosomal diseases identified, defects in other cellular biochemical pathways, such as amino acid transport and aminoacylation, can also result in diffuse chronic interstitial involvement.

The major pathologic mechanism underlying most metabolic causes of interstitial lung disease seems to be abnormal alveolar macrophage function. The presence of high concentrations lipid laden macrophages,[25] in the bronchoalveolar lavages of sphingolipid metabolic disorders such as Gaucher,[26,27] Niemann–Pick A, B, and C,[28] and animal models of lysosomal acid lipase[29] is extensively documented. In these disorders, it is the glycolipid accumulation within the macrophages and resultant interruption of normal intracellular vesicular cycling that result in the damaging proinflammatory cascades.[30–32] A number of disorders—that is Niemann–Pick A, B, and C, lysinuric protein intolerance, and methionyl tRNA synthetase, may also give rise to pulmonary alveolar proteinosis. In lysinuric protein intolerance, the alteration in intracellular arginine concentration is thought to impair macrophage Toll-like receptor function with resultant imbalance of proinflammatory and anti-inflammatory cytokines.[33] The mechanisms in methionyl tRNA synthetase are less well-defined, but global translational repression is thought to lead to the macrophage inflammatory response.[34]

Studies in lysinuric protein intolerance have shown infiltrative lung disease in approximately 2/two-thirds of patients when examined with high-resolution computed tomography (CT) scans.[35,36] However, a great degree of variability in respiratory presentation exists, even within families carrying the same mutation.[35] Thus, although patients can present with acute respiratory failure (16[37] to 60%[35]), some can be apparently clinically asymptomatic despite chronic radiologic changes.[36] There is extremely limited data on the efficacy of treatment, although the use of intravenous

Table 2
Causes of restrictive lung disease

Disease	Is Primary Presentation Pulmonary?	Main Presenting Features	Pulmonary Alveolar Proteinosis Seen	Investigation
NPA/B	Rarely	Common features: hepatosplenomegaly, growth restriction. and delayed bone age Raised triglycerides, low cholesterol Type A will typically have hypotonia and neurologic regression from 6 mo	Yes	Urine—oligosaccharides Blood—oxysterols white cell enzymology
Infantile-onset lysosomal acid lipase	No	Worsening gastrointestinal function then liver impairment <3 mo → death 6–12 mo Increasing hemophagocytic lymphohistiocytosis phenotype on investigation with worsening disease	Yes	Blood—oxysterols White cell enzymology
Niemann–Pick C	No	1. Neonatal liver disease 2. Incidental splenomegaly 3. Progressive neurologic ataxia/vertical gaze palsy/ seizures and eventual neuroregression	Yes	Blood—oxysterols + chitotriosidase = suggestive Fibroblast—Phillipin staining Genetics
Lysinuric protein intolerance	No	Acute hyperammonemia Chronic—failure to thrive, protein intolerance, renal insufficiency, developmental delay, occasional hepatosplenomegaly and pancytopenia	Yes	Urine/plasma amino acid ratio Blood—ammonia (can be normal)
Methionyl tRNA synthetase	Yes	Multiorgan involvement with liver dysfunction prominent, occasional lactic acidosis and hyperammonemia	Yes	Genetics
MPS 1	Yes, but mainly obstructive	Coarse facies, otitis media, hepatosplenomegaly, umbilical/inguinal hernias, dysostosis multiplex, cervical spine instability potential neurologic decline (Hurler), corneal clouding, joint stiffness, valvular heart disease. Recurrent upper airway symptoms- infections, rhinorrhea, snoring	No	Urine—MPS screen Blood—white cell enzymology

MPS 2	Yes, but mainly obstructive	As in MPS1, but no corneal clouding	No	Urine—MPS screen Blood—white cell enzymology
Gaucher	No	Common features hepatosplenomegaly, anemia, thrombocytopenia, acute painful crisis, failure to thrive, horizontal saccade initiation failure with progression to more severe oculomotor apraxia	No	White cell enzymology
HPP	No	Perinatal from foreshortened/limb deformation, caput memebanecum, osteogenic spurs in midshaft, period apnea ulnas, fibula skeletal hyopmineralization on radiographs Infantile—Pc before 6 mo, poor feeding, failure to thrive, hypotonia, rickets, with or without increased intracranial pressure, blue sclera, vitamin B_6-dependant epilepsy, hypercalcemia and hypercalciuria Childhood PC >6 mo premature deciduous tooth loss, rachiatic deformities of wrists, costocondrial junction and genu varus/valgum, skeletal pain and delayed walking. Marrow edema mimicking osteomyelitis, craniosynostosis, characteristic radiology	No	Liver function –alkaline phosphatase Genetics ALPL
OI		Type 1—non deforming autosomal dominant, blue sclera Type 2- severe perinatal lethal autosomal recessive Type 3- severe progressive deformity autosomal recessive Type 4-moderate severity autosomal dominant normal sclera Type 5-calcification of interosseous membranes ± hypertrophic callus NB hearing loss, dental involvement/joint hypermobility, increased cardiac valvular disease variable dependent on severity	No	80%–85% COL1A1 or COL1A2

(*continued on next page*)

Table 2
(continued)

Disease	Is Primary Presentation Pulmonary?	Main Presenting Features	Pulmonary Alveolar Proteinosis Seen	Investigation
Infantile-onset Pompe disease	Possible respiratory distress	Typically Pc <6 mo with respiratory distress, cardiomegaly, developmental delay, hypotonia, poor feeding and weight gain	No	White cell enzymology, urinary Glc4,
Phosphomannomutase-2 deficiency—CDG	No	Neonatal hypotonia, inverted nipples and unusual subcutaneous fat pads, ataxia, mental retardation apparent from later childhood while muscular atrophy and hypogonadism is seen in later life	No	Transferrin isoelctrofocusing

corticosteroids and whole lung lavages in established respiratory failure, was thought to be ineffective in the French cohort.[35] There is a single recorded heart–lung transplant[38] in a 3-year-old child with acute respiratory failure unresponsive to intravenous corticosteroids and lavage.

In methionyl tRNA synthetase, a number of case series have emphasized its impact on the lungs.[39,40] The largest of these was a retrospective cohort of 29 patients the median age of onset of respiratory symptoms was 2.5 months (range, 0.5–72.0 months), with 26 patients presenting before 1 year of age. Fibrosis was present in 19 of 28 patients (69%) who underwent lung biopsy.[41] An initial CT scan was available for 17 patients (median age, 10 months) and showed intralobular septal thickening (100%), ground glass opacities (94%), and consolidation (76%). In the 13 patients who had a repeat CT scan (median age, 10 years), the consolidation had resolved although in 12 signs of fibrosis were present. The restrictive pattern on pulmonary function testing mirrored this, whereas 15 of the 18 had a diffusing capacity of the lung for carbon monoxide of less than 80% of the predicted value.[41] Twenty-six patients were treated with lavages, 14 with steroids, and 1 underwent transplantation, with the latter showing no recurrence of pulmonary alveolar proteinosis 1 year after the transplant. There was no overall correlation between outcome and any of the treatment modalities. Twelve of the 29 patients died, the majority before 3 years of age; survivors were aged between 1.1 and 24.9 years.

The sphingolipid disorders have varying degrees of lung involvement being near universal in Niemann–Pick B, where the leading causes of death are respiratory and liver failure.[42] Ninety percent of a prospective series of 54 pediatric and adult patients had parenchymal changes on radiographs, which increased to 98% on CT scan.[43] The CT scans showed ground-glass opacities, interlobular septal thickening, and intralobular lines, mainly in the lower zones.[43] These changes, although not pathognomonic,[44] are, in the context of Niemann–Pick B, highly suggestive of pulmonary alveolar proteinosis. Cysts, thought to be secondary to air trapping[45] and even emphysematous changes,[46] have been described, but are rare.

Niemann–Pick C, a defect in lysosomal egress of unesterified cholesterol lipids,[47] tends to have a milder respiratory phenotype. Although overall 95% of cases are caused by defects in the NPC1 gene, those documented with severe lung manifestations have typically had defects in the NPC2 gene.[48–50] These cases typically develop respiratory failure within the first year of life,[49] with ground glass changes on chest radiographs and pulmonary alveolar proteinosis on autopsy.[50]

In the third of the sphingolipidoses, Gaucher's disease, pulmonary and overall severity have been correlated.[51] Patients have traditionally been divided into 3 major subgroups depending on the absence (type I) or presence (type II and III) of neurologic symptoms.[52] Although generally having milder visceral disease, the majority of enzyme replacement therapy (ERT)-naive type I patients still had abnormalities in pulmonary function, particularly a decrease in functional residual capacity and diffusing capacity of the lung for carbon monoxide, which preceded radiologic changes.[53] In the pre-ERT era, even patients with type I Gaucher could develop respiratory failure secondary to alveolar occlusion by Gaucher cells, most typically in splenectomized patients.[27,54] Autopsy findings also demonstrated Gaucher's cell invasion of the septal capillaries, fitting with reports of pulmonary hypertension.[55] Although ERT has decreased the degree of lung involvement even in those type 1 patients with severe initial disease,[56,57] in older patients, respiratory response may be minimal.[51] Respiratory complications, although similar in the chronic neuropathic form (type III) tend to be more prevalent[58] and also include pulmonary haemorrhage.[59] Although lavage[60] and even intrabronchial ERT have been tried, the combination of ERT and substrate reduction may be the best therapy for improving pulmonary function.[61] Lung transplantation has been successfully undertaken both in the pediatric and adult populations.[25,62]

Although pulmonary involvement has been seen in Wolmans disease, historically these patients presented with growth failure and liver dysfunction within the 1st months of life and typically died of ensuing liver failure by 4 months.[63] With the advent of ERT the respiratory complications have become more overt. These patients suffer from an interstitial lung disease,[64] which may not be surprising given the disruption in surfactant production seen in animal models.[65]

Within mucopolysaccharidosis (MPS), interstitial disease is predominately seen in neonates, before commencement of ERT, with both MPS1 (Hurler syndrome)[66] and MPS II (Hunter syndrome).[67] These patients all showed glycogen deposition on lung biopsy, leading to an initial misdiagnosis of pulmonary interstitial glycogenosis. However, interstitial lung disease has also been seen in patients who should, theoretically, have been provided with adequate replacement enzyme.[68,69] Although in both the lung disease was postulated to be multifactorial, the former responded to increased enzyme provision, whereas the latter responded to steroids after spinal surgery.

Although type 2 diabetes has been seen of itself, even when weight gain has been accounted for, to be a risk factor for restrictive lung disease in adults,[70] comparable studies in pediatrics have not yet been performed.

Musculoskeletal Causes

Although potentially all causes of impaired respiratory muscle function can cause a degree of restrictive lung disease, it is beyond the capacities of this review to expand on the multiple genetic defects that decrease the mitochondrial energy production interfering with either respiratory drive or muscle function. We concentrate on 3 disorders that typify this form of restriction.

Infantile-onset Pompe disease is an autosomal recessive lysosomal storage disorder is caused by a deficiency of the enzyme acid α-glucosidase.[71] The resulting accumulation of glycogen in lysosomes triggers inflammatory pathologic cascades[72] that principally affect skeletal and cardiac muscles. Patients typically present within the first few months of life, with a combination of cardiorespiratory insufficiency, hypotonia, and failure to thrive.[73,74] Untreated patients follow a rapid, progressive, and ultimately fatal course, dying typically between 7 and 9 months of age from cardiorespiratory failure.[73] The advent of ERT has markedly changed the overall survival; however, data from the UK and Germany suggest that ventilator-free survival was at best 40% in those treated on standard doses, because respiratory muscle failure still results in insufficiency in the majority of patients.[75,76]

Hypophosphatasia (HPP) is a rare disorder of bone mineralization caused by mutation in the *ALPL* gene, which codes for tissue-nonspecific alkaline phosphatase. Mineralization of the tissues is controlled by inhibitor of mineralization, inorganic pyrophosphate, which is deactivated by alkaline phosphatase dephosphorylation. In HPP, a low alkaline phosphatase concentration causes undermineralization of the skeleton and severe rickets. HPP is a heterogenous disorder with the most severe form, perinatal HPP, presenting with severe hypomineralization of the fetal skeleton; the moderately severe form, infantile HPP, presents within 6 months of age. Infants with perinatal and infantile HPP manifest with varying degree of respiratory failure secondary to undermineralized thoracic cage, hypoplastic lungs and hypotonia requiring respiratory support. Until recently, perinatal HPP was fatal with 100% mortality.[77] ERT with asfotase alfa significantly improves survival compared with historic controls and this result is secondary to improved mineralization of the thoracic skeleton, allowing these infants to survive with respiratory support.[78] Requirements for respiratory support are variable, with some children requiring it until 4 years of age.[79] A multidisciplinary team consisting of an intensivist, pulmonologist, physical rehabilitation therapist, and metabolic bone disease specialist is required for the management of neonates and infants with HPP manifesting with respiratory complications.[80] If prolonged respiratory support is predicted, a tracheostomy should be considered, and long-term home ventilation should be planned. Tracheobronchomalacia can complicate ventilatory requirements and duration and, therefore, if clinically indicated, tracheobronchoscopy should be performed.

Osteogenesis imperfecta (OI) refers to a group of disorders where abnormalities in collagen formation and/or deposition result in defective bone matrix formation. Most common forms of OI, types I to IV, are caused by autosomal dominant mutations in the *COL1A1* and *COL1A2* genes coding for type 1 collagen. The nosology of OI has, however, expanded, with multiple genes now identified which can cause autosomal dominant and autosomal recessive OIs.[81] OI clinically manifests with frequent nontraumatic fractures; whereas moderate to severe OI presents with limb deformities, thoracic deformities from rib and vertebral fractures, and hypoplastic lungs. Indeed, the most common cause of death is secondary to pulmonary diseases,[82] which may in part reflect the abundance of type 1 collagen in the connective tissues surrounding the alveoli structures. The risk of pulmonary disease is directly related to the severity of OI; neonates with severe OI (type III and autosomal recessive) may develop respiratory failure requiring ventilatory support from chest wall deformities and pulmonary hypoplasia.[83] In addition, kyphoscoliosis from vertebral collapses and rib deformities, pectus carinatum, decreased diaphragmatic movement (abdominal contents pressing on diaphragm), airway distortions, and restrictive pulmonary abnormalities can in combination significantly decrease alveolar ventilation.[84] Furthermore, ineffective clearance of secretion and infections can lead to bronchiectasis. Finally, soft skull and platybasia can cause basilar invagination that, in severe cases, may disturb respiratory function secondary to brain stem compression and hydrocephalus. There are reports of ventilatory requirements for this complication.[85] Although there is no specific disease-modifying therapy for OI type IV, bisphosphonates have been shown to prevent vertebral fractures, decrease the frequency of rib fractures, and prevent worsening of chest deformities, therefore contributing to improving respiratory function. Physical rehabilitation assists in positioning and effective clearance of secretions. Some children may require spinal surgeries for the correction of kyphoscoliosis, which also contributes to improving respiratory function. Yearly monitoring with lung function testing, imaging, and pulse oximetry can help in screening for respiratory complications.[84] In those infants with severe OI requiring ventilatory support, a global view must be taken because they normally also have developmental delay, neurologic complications, and multiple fractures, and are completely dependent on care givers. Therefore, the ethics of treatment, especially long-term ventilation, should be considered carefully, and palliative care should be offered after a discussion with the family.

It is to be noted that dysostosis multiplex like skeletal changes have been seen in the congenital disorders of glycosylation (CDGs).[86] These are a rapidly evolving field of disorders where defects in the normal post-translational glycosylation processes occurring in the endoplasmic reticulum and Golgi complex result in aberrant tertiary protein structure. By far the best described is phosphomannomutase-2 deficiency, which has been seen to have very similar thoracic changes to those described in the MPSs. This multisystem disease presents normally in infancy with hypotonia, inverted nipples, and unusual subcutaneous fat pads. However, patients often develop ataxia–mental retardation in childhood and muscular atrophy and hypogonadism in later life.[87] Diagnosis of the CDGs has been based on the glycosylation pattern of transferrin with differing glycosylation patterns occurring in differing groups of CDGs with these patterns being recognized using electrophoretic analysis. It is to be noted that this transferrin isoelectofocusing can give false-negative results in the first 3 months of life.[87]

Other causes of restrictive lung disease include disorders of thyroid transcription factor TITF1/NKX2.1, which is required for pulmonary development, with affected infants suffering from pulmonary hypoplasia.[88]

MIXED AIRWAY DISEASE

Mucopolysaccharidosis

Inherited defects in the catabolic pathways of the GAGs heparan, dermatan, and keratan sulfate have all been associated with obstructive symptoms.[13,89] At a cellular level, substrate accumulation results in a localized proinflammatory response.[90,91] Although the major impact of heparan sulfate is seen on neurologic tissue,[92] it is the accumulation of dermatan[93,94] and keratan moieties[95] that have the greatest effect on extracellular matrix structure and airway growth and caliber.

The impact of MPS on airway function can be seen from the fact that, despite the advances in diagnostics and therapeutics, respiratory disease remains the leading cause of morbidity and mortality in MPS and is also the most prominent cause of patient-perceived impaired quality of life.[96] Airway obstruction can occur in both the upper and lower airways in MPSs.[13,97,98] The principle cause of the obstruction in MPS I, II, VI, and VII is the multilevel GAG deposition, which in the upper airway leads to nasal mucosal hypertrophy, macroglossia, and adenotonsillar hypertrophy.[99–101] Registry data show that 80% of patients with MPS I demonstrate OSA before the age of 2 years.[102] Despite disease-modifying therapies such as ERT and bone marrow transplantation, 84% of patients with MPS I still undergo adenotonsillectomy.[102] GAG deposition can also result in enlarged and redundant supraglottic tissues, especially in MPS II, where prolapse into the laryngeal inlet can result in severe compromise.[103,104]

Although GAG accumulation leads to overt narrowing of the upper airways, this hypertrophy is often compounded by local inflammation and weakness resulting in laryngopharyngeal malacic changes as well as subglottic laryngotracheomalacia.[105,106] This combination of GAG accumulation and malacial changes leads to multilevel airway obstruction.[107] With the exception of patients with MPS III, these intrinsic upper airway changes are further complicated by limited mouth opening.[107] The impairment of mouth opening is secondary to a combination of temporomandibular joint dysfunction[108] and/or overgrowth of the mandibular coronoid processes.[109]

GAG deposition and inflammation also occur in the lower airway,[110–112] with airway narrowing resulting from malacia seen in all the MPS subtypes.[106,113,114] However, the most severe tracheal abnormalities are seen in MPS IV (tortuosity and "buckling").[115] This exaggerated response is thought to be due to abnormal cartilage metabolism and imbalances between the relatively normal longitudinal growth of the trachea and the severely restricted thoracic cage growth. Indeed, in MPS IV, the tracheal narrowing has been documented as early as 2 years of age. Although the study was cross-sectional, all patients over 15 years of age had a decrease of at least 50% in tracheal caliber, suggesting progression with age.[115]

The combination of chest wall deformities and hepatosplenomegaly[115] does make a significant contribution to the respiratory impact of the MPSs (**Table 3**). Chest wall deformities are part of the general dysostosis multiplex seen in MPS. Particularly the

Table 3
The respiratory impact of the mucopolysaccharidoses

MPS	Name and Enzyme Defect	Main GAGs on Urine Screening	Clinical Symptoms	Respiratory Manifestations: Upper Airway	Respiratory Manifestations: Lower Airway	Restrictive Disease
I	Hurler (H) Hurler-Scheie (HS) Scheie (S) Iduronidase deficiency	DS HS	Coarse facies, otitis media, hepatosplenomegaly, umbilical/inguinal hernias, dysostosis multiplex, cervical spine instability potential neurologic decline (Hurler), corneal clouding, joint stiffness, valvular heart disease	+++	++	++
II	Hunter Iduronate—I-sulphatase deficiency	DS HS	As MPS1 but no corneal clouding	+++	++	+
II	Sanfilippo (A–D) A) Heparan *N*-sulfatase B) Alpha-N-acetylglucosaminidase C) Acetyl-coenzyme A:alpha-glucosaminide acetyltransferase D) *N*-acetylglucosamine-6-sulfate	HS	Stage 1—Initially asymptomatic/mild developmental delay Stage 2—hyperactivity and grossly impaired sleep (mainly neurologic) Stage 3—neurologic decline gastrostomy and bed bound	–/+ Otitis media common	–/+	–/+
III	Morquio (A and B) A) *N*-acetylgalactosamine 6-sulfatase B) Beta-galactosidase	KS, CS	Severe skeletal deformity cervical spine instability genu valgum, pectus carinatum and kyphoscoliosis? short stature, valvular heart disease, corneal clouding, joint hypermobility	++	+++	+++
VI	Maroteaux–Lamy *N*-acetylgalactosamine 4-sulfatase	DS, CS	As per MPS 1, but with a greater chance of cervical spine instability but without/minimal neurologic compromise	+++	++	++
VII	Sly Beta-glucuronidase	DS, HS, CS	Hydrops fetalis and as per MPS I	++	++	++

pectus carinatum, kyphoscoliosis and rib abnormalities—both shape (oar) and angulation (more horizontal)—as well as induration of the costovertebral complex and the elevation of the diaphragms all contribute to the reduction in pulmonary function.[13,115] Chest wall pathology is most closely tied to stature and is thus most prevalent in MPS IV, although it is also seen in the more severe phenotypes of MPS I, II, and VI.[13] Finally, MPS I, IV, and VI are associated with atlantoaxial subluxation and odontoid hypoplasia that may result in spinal cord compression[116] that, if involving the C3 to C5 nerve roots, can decrease diaphragmatic function and ventilation.[13]

A comprehensive evaluation of respiratory function should be attempted in all patients with MPS, with spirometry, PSG, flexible nasoendoscopy, and imaging all contributing to overall management and perioperative safety.[107,117] Although central apnoeas have been noted with progressive neurologic involvement,[117] the commonest form of sleep disordered breathing found on PSG is OSA. The limited published PSG data suggest that OSA is present in 70% to 100% of patients with MPS I, II, and VI, although most prominently in MPS I and II.[118–121] Although nasoendoscopy is a very useful tool to access laryngeal involvement and inspiratory supraglottic collapse, this tool can be challenging in the young and those with neurocognitive impairment.[122] Three-dimensional CT reconstructions of the large airways can help with preoperative planning, with reported alterations in anesthetic decision making in more than 20% of cases.[105]

Disease Associated with Recurrent Respiratory Infections

A number of both endocrine and metabolic disorders are associated with increased risk of respiratory infections. The best example is the autosomal recessive form of pseudohypoaldosteronism owing to defective action of the epithelial sodium channel, whose 3 subunits are encoded by SCNN1A, SCNN1B, and SCNN1G. Alpha subunit variants have been associated chronic disease and are reportedly clinically indistinguishable from cystic fibrosis.[123,124] Impaired neutrophil function in GSD 1B and G6PC3 (severe congenital neutropenia type 4) also predispose to increased respiratory infections. Recurrent infection is also a hallmark of immune dysregulation, polyendocrinopathy, enteropathy, X-linked syndrome and immune dysregulation, polyendocrinopathy, enteropathy, X-linked–like disorders, with up to 30% of affected patients having recurrent pulmonary disease.[125] The most significant metabolic impairment of the immunologic function, however, is seen in patients with adenosine deaminase 1, which in its most severe form causes severe combined immunodeficiency. The recurrent opportunistic infections that arise from decreased T and B cells result from the build-up of adenosine and its derivatives.[126] By the time of diagnosis, these patients often have chronic respiratory insufficiency and autoimmune phenomena, including cytopenias and antithyroid antibodies. Allergies and an elevated serum IgE are often present.[127]

PULMONARY HYPERTENSION

Although in the World Health Organization classification of pulmonary hypertension, metabolic disease falls within category 5, the multifactorial subclassification,[128] the commonest metabolic causes are due to mitochondrial dysfunction. It is seen in both defects predominately affecting mitochondrial energetics such as LIPT1,[129] Tmem70,[130] and NFU1,[131] and in those affecting more diverse mitochondrial functions such as the glycine cleavage system (nonketotic hyperglycinemia),[132] DNA transcription (mitochondrial seryl-tRNA synthetase),[133] or amino acid transport (SLC25A26).[134]

Typically, the disorders predominately affecting energetics present in the neonatal period, are multisystemic in nature and have a prominent neurologic component.

Outside the neonatal period, metabolic disorders resulting in pulmonary hypertension are rare. Historically, Gaucher's disease was the commonest cause with pulmonary hypertension occurring in 5% of splenectomized patients.[54,135] However, the advent of ERT and the resultant reduction in splenectomies, seems to have resolved this.

Intracellular processing defects in cobalamin (vitamin B_{12}), typically cobalamin C has been seen to present with isolated pulmonary hypertension in both children[136] and adults.[137] It has, however, recently also been associated with diffuse lung parenchymal disease.[138] It seems most likely that the microangiopathy associated with the high levels of homocysteine and organic acids is the basis of the pulmonary hypertension. The typical presentation of cobalamin C is with developmental delay and failure to thrive from poor enteral tolerance in the first 6 months of life.[139]

CLINICAL CARE POINTS

- The normal range of biochemical investigations especially those used in the investigation of biochemical disease are not as well established as more classical normal ranges and more prone to sampling errors. Thus, if is there is disparity between the clinical and biochemical phenotype further discussion with the reference laboratory should be sought.
- While next generation sequencing is revolutionising medicine, given the number of VUS (variants of unknown significance) generated in panel testing, functional investigation where possible as outlined above is still the authors first line suggestion currently.

DISCLOSURE

The authors have nothing to disclose.

REFERENCES

1. Tokatli A, Coşkun T, Ozalp I, et al. The major presenting symptom in a biotinidase-deficient patient: laryngeal stridor. J Inherit Metab Dis 1992;15(2):281–2.
2. Dionisi-Vici C, Bachmann C, Graziani MC, et al. Laryngeal stridor as a leading symptom in a biotinidase-deficient patient. J Inherit Metab Dis 1988;11(3):312–3.
3. Baumgartner ER, Suormala TM, Wick H, et al. Biotinidase deficiency: a cause of subacute necrotizing encephalomyelopathy (Leigh syndrome). Report of a case with lethal outcome. Pediatr Res 1989;26(3):260–6.
4. Jaeger B, Bosch AM. Clinical presentation and outcome of riboflavin transporter deficiency: mini review after five years of experience. J Inherit Metab Dis 2016;39(4):559–64.
5. Bosch AM, Stroek K, Abeling NG, et al. The Brown-Vialetto-Van Laere and Fazio Londe syndrome revisited: natural history, genetics, treatment and future perspectives. Orphanet J Rare Dis 2012;7:83.
6. Sperl W, Geiger R, Lehnert W, et al. Stridor as the major presenting symptom in riboflavin-responsive multiple acyl-CoA dehydrogenation deficiency. Eur J Pediatr 1997;156(10):800–2.

7. Xi J, Wen B, Lin J, et al. Clinical features and ETFDH mutation spectrum in a cohort of 90 Chinese patients with late-onset multiple acyl-CoA dehydrogenase deficiency. J Inherit Metab Dis 2013;37(3):399–404.
8. Shoback D. Clinical practice. Hypoparathyroidism. N Engl J Med 2008;359(4): 391–403.
9. Clarke BL, Brown EM, Collins MT, et al. Epidemiology and Diagnosis of Hypoparathyroidism. J Clin Endocrinol Metab 2016;101(6):2284–99.
10. Mannstadt M, Bilezikian JP, Thakker RV, et al. Hypoparathyroidism. Nat Rev Dis Primers 2017;3:17055.
11. Broomfield A, Sweeney MG, Woodward CE, et al. Paediatric single mitochondrial DNA deletion disorders: an overlapping spectrum of disease. J Inherit Metab Dis 2015;38(3):445–57.
12. Labarthe F, Benoist JF, Brivet M, et al. Partial hypoparathyroidism associated with mitochondrial trifunctional protein deficiency. Eur J Pediatr 2006;165(6): 389–91.
13. Muhlebach MS, Wooten W, Muenzer J. Respiratory manifestations in mucopolysaccharidoses. Paediatr Respir Rev 2011;12(2):133–8.
14. Ehlert K, Frosch M, Fehse N, et al. Farber disease: clinical presentation, pathogenesis and a new approach to treatment. Pediatr Rheumatol Online J 2007; 5:15.
15. Pavone L, Moser HW, Mollica F, et al. Farber's lipogranulomatosis: ceramidase deficiency and prolonged survival in three relatives. Johns Hopkins Med J 1980; 147(5):193–6.
16. Haraoka G, Muraoka M, Yoshioka N, et al. First case of surgical treatment of Farber's disease. Ann Plast Surg 1997;39(4):405–10.
17. Ladenson PW, Goldenheim PD, Ridgway EC. Prediction and reversal of blunted ventilatory responsiveness in patients with hypothyroidism. Am J Med 1988; 84(5):877–83.
18. Siafakas NM, Salesiotou V, Filaditaki V, et al. Respiratory muscle strength in hypothyroidism. Chest 1992;102(1):189–94.
19. Sorensen JR, Winther KH, Bonnema SJ, et al. Respiratory manifestations of hypothyroidism: a systematic review. Thyroid 2016;26(11):1519–27.
20. Tan HL, Urquhart DS. Respiratory complications in Children with Prader Willi Syndrome. Paediatr Respir Rev 2017;22:52–9.
21. Davi MV, Dalle Carbonare L, Giustina A, et al. Sleep apnoea syndrome is highly prevalent in acromegaly and only partially reversible after biochemical control of the disease. Eur J Endocrinol 2008;159(5):533–40.
22. Lin HY, Lin SP, Lin CC, et al. Polysomnographic characteristics in patients with Prader-Willi syndrome. Pediatr Pulmonol 2007;42(10):881–7.
23. Paterson WF, Donaldson MD. Growth hormone therapy in the Prader-Willi syndrome. Arch Dis Child 2003;88(4):283–5.
24. Spagnolo P, Bush A. Interstitial lung disease in children younger than 2 years. Pediatrics 2016;137(6):e20152725.
25. Bloom W. Splenomegaly (Type Gaucher) and Lipoid-Histiocytosis (Type Niemann). Am J Pathol 1925;1(6). 595-626.9.
26. Rao AR, Parakininkas D, Hintermeyer M, et al. Bilateral lung transplant in Gauchers type-1 disease. Pediatr Transplant 2005;9(2):239–43.
27. Schneider EL, Epstein CJ, Kaback MJ, et al. Severe pulmonary involvement in adult Gaucher's disease. Report of three cases and review of the literature. Am J Med 1977;63(3):475–80.

28. Guillemot N, Troadec C, de Villemeur TB, et al. Lung disease in Niemann-Pick disease. Pediatr Pulmonol 2007;42(12):1207–14.
29. Lian X, Yan C, Yang L, et al. Lysosomal acid lipase deficiency causes respiratory inflammation and destruction in the lung. Am J Physiol Lung Cell Mol Physiol 2004;286(4):L801–7.
30. Aflaki E, Moaven N, Borger DK, et al. Lysosomal storage and impaired autophagy lead to inflammasome activation in Gaucher macrophages. Aging Cell 2016;15(1):77–88.
31. Allen MJ, Myer BJ, Khokher AM, et al. Pro-inflammatory cytokines and the pathogenesis of Gaucher's disease: increased release of interleukin-6 and interleukin-10. QJM 1997;90(1):19–25.
32. Dhami R, He X, Gordon RE, et al. Analysis of the lung pathology and alveolar macrophage function in the acid sphingomyelinase–deficient mouse model of Niemann-Pick disease. Lab Invest 2001;81(7):987–99.
33. Kurko J, Vähä-Mäkilä M, Tringham M, et al. Dysfunction in macrophage toll-like receptor signaling caused by an inborn error of cationic amino acid transport. Mol Immunol 2015;67(2 Pt B):416–25.
34. Yao P, Fox PL. Aminoacyl-tRNA synthetases in medicine and disease. EMBO Mol Med 2013;5(3):332–43.
35. Valimahamed-Mitha S, Berteloot L, Ducoin H, et al. Lung involvement in children with lysinuric protein intolerance. J Inherit Metab Dis 2015;38(2):257–63.
36. Santamaria F, Parenti G, Guidi G, et al. Early detection of lung involvement in lysinuric protein intolerance: role of high-resolution computed tomography and radioisotopic methods. Am J Respir Crit Care Med 1996;153(2):731–5.
37. Parto K, Svedström E, Majurin ML, et al. Pulmonary manifestations in lysinuric protein intolerance. Chest 1993;104(4):1176–82.
38. Santamaria F, Brancaccio G, Parenti G, et al. Recurrent fatal pulmonary alveolar proteinosis after heart-lung transplantation in a child with lysinuric protein intolerance. J Pediatr 2004;145(2):268–72.
39. Hadchouel A, Wieland T, Griese M, et al. Biallelic mutations of methionyl-tRNA synthetase cause a specific type of pulmonary alveolar proteinosis prevalent on Réunion Island. Am J Hum Genet 2015;96(5):826–31.
40. Sun Y, Hu G, Luo J, et al. Mutations in methionyl-tRNA synthetase gene in a Chinese family with interstitial lung and liver disease, postnatal growth failure and anemia. J Hum Genet 2017;62(6):647–51.
41. Enaud L, Hadchouel A, Coulomb A, et al. Pulmonary alveolar proteinosis in children on La Réunion Island: a new inherited disorder? Orphanet J Rare Dis 2014; 9:85.
42. Cassiman D, Packman S, Bembi B, et al. Cause of death in patients with chronic visceral and chronic neurovisceral acid sphingomyelinase deficiency (Niemann-Pick disease type B and B variant): literature review and report of new cases. Mol Genet Metab 2016;118(3):206–13.
43. Mendelson DS, Wasserstein MP, Desnick RJ, et al. Type B Niemann-pick disease: findings at chest radiography, thin-section CT, and pulmonary function testing. Radiology 2006;238(1):339–45.
44. Frazier AA, Franks TJ, Cooke EO, et al. Pulmonary alveolar proteinosis. Radiographics 2008;28(3):883–99.
45. Baldi BG, Santana AN, Takagaki TY, et al. Lung cyst: an unusual manifestation of Niemann-Pick disease. Respirology 2009;14(1):134–6.

46. Arda IS, Gençoğlu A, Coşkun M, et al. A very unusual presentation of Niemann-Pick disease type B in an infant: similar findings to congenital lobar emphysema. Eur J Pediatr Surg 2005;15(4):283–6.
47. Vanier MT. Complex lipid trafficking in Niemann-Pick disease type C. J Inherit Metab Dis 2014;38(1):187–99.
48. Schofer O, Mischo B, Püschel W, et al. Early-lethal pulmonary form of Niemann-Pick type C disease belonging to a second, rare genetic complementation group. Eur J Pediatr 1998;157(1):45–9.
49. Millat G, Chikh K, Naureckiene S, et al. Niemann-Pick disease type C: spectrum of HE1 mutations and genotype/phenotype correlations in the NPC2 group. Am J Hum Genet 2001;69(5):1013–21.
50. Bjurulf B, Spetalen S, Erichsen A, et al. Niemann-Pick disease type C2 presenting as fatal pulmonary alveolar lipoproteinosis: morphological findings in lung and nervous tissue. Med Sci Monit 2008;14(8):CS71–5.
51. Goitein O, Elstein D, Abrahamov A, et al. Lung involvement and enzyme replacement therapy in Gaucher's disease. QJM 2001;94(8):407–15.
52. Elstein D, Alcalay R, Zimran A. The emergence of Parkinson disease among patients with Gaucher disease. Best Pract Res Clin Endocrinol Metab 2015;29(2): 249–59.
53. Kerem E, Elstein D, Abrahamov A, et al. Pulmonary function abnormalities in type I Gaucher disease. Eur Respir J 1996;9(2):340–5.
54. Weinreb NJ, Barbouth DS, Lee RE. Causes of death in 184 patients with type 1 Gaucher disease from the United States who were never treated with enzyme replacement therapy. Blood Cell Mol Dis 2018;68:211–7.
55. Amir G, Ron N. Pulmonary pathology in Gaucher's disease. Hum Pathol 1999; 30(6):666–70.
56. Lee SY, Mak AW, Huen KF, et al. Gaucher disease with pulmonary involvement in a 6-year-old girl: report of resolution of radiographic abnormalities on increasing dose of imiglucerase. J Pediatr 2001;139(6):862–4.
57. Pelini M, Boice D, O'Neil K, et al. Glucocerebrosidase treatment of type I Gaucher disease with severe pulmonary involvement. Ann Intern Med 1994; 121(3):196–7.
58. Santamaria F, Parenti G, Guidi G, et al. Pulmonary manifestations of Gaucher disease: an increased risk for L444P homozygotes? Am J Respir Crit Care Med 1998;157(3 Pt 1):985–9.
59. Vellodi A, Ashworth M, Finnegan N, et al. Pulmonary hemorrhage in type 3 Gaucher disease: a case report. J Inherit Metab Dis 2010;33(Suppl 3):S329–31.
60. Carson KF, Williams CA, Rosenthal DL, et al. Bronchoalveolar lavage in a girl with Gaucher's disease. A case report. Acta Cytol 1994;38(4):597–600.
61. J D, et al. Pulmonary disease in type III Gaucher disease refractory to conventional enzyme replacement therapy. Mol Genet Metab 2014;111(2):s34–5.
62. de Boer GM, van Dussen L, van den Toorn LM, et al. Lung transplantation in Gaucher disease: a learning lesson in trying to avoid both Scylla and Charybdis. Chest 2016;149(1):e1–5.
63. Jones SA, Valayannopoulos V, Schneider E, et al. Rapid progression and mortality of lysosomal acid lipase deficiency presenting in infants. Genet Med 2015;18(5):452–8.
64. Broomfield A, Kenth J, Bruce IA, et al. Respiratory complications of metabolic disease in the paediatric population: a review of presentation, diagnosis and therapeutic options. Paediatr Respir Rev 2019;32:55–65.

65. Li Y, Qin Y, Li H, et al. Lysosomal acid lipase over-expression disrupts lamellar body genesis and alveolar structure in the lung. Int J Exp Pathol 2007;88(6): 427–36.
66. Bush D, Sremba L, Lomax K, et al. Neonatal onset interstitial lung disease as a primary presenting manifestation of mucopolysaccharidosis type I. JIMD Rep 2019;43:71–7.
67. Smets K, Van Daele S. Neonatal pulmonary interstitial glycogenosis in a patient with Hunter syndrome. Eur J Pediatr 2011;170(8):1083–4.
68. Valayannopoulos V, de Blic J, Mahlaoui N, et al. Laronidase for cardiopulmonary disease in hurler syndrome 12 years after bone marrow transplantation. Pediatrics 2010;126(5):e1242–7.
69. Eisengart JB, Jarnes J, Ahmed A, et al. Long-term cognitive and somatic outcomes of enzyme replacement therapy in untransplanted Hurler syndrome. Mol Genet Metab Rep 2017;13:64–8.
70. Lecube A, Simó R, Pallayova M, et al. Pulmonary function and sleep breathing: two new targets for type 2 diabetes care. Endocr Rev 2017;38(6):550–73.
71. HERS HG. Alpha-glucosidase deficiency in generalized glycogenstorage disease (Pompe's disease). Biochem J 1963;86:11–6.
72. Foley AR, Menezes MP, Pandraud A, et al. Treatable childhood neuronopathy caused by mutations in riboflavin transporter RFVT2. Brain 2014;137(Pt 1): 44–56.
73. van den Hout HM, Hop W, van Diggelen OP, et al. The natural course of infantile Pompe's disease: 20 original cases compared with 133 cases from the literature. Pediatrics 2003;112(2):332–40.
74. Byrne BJ, Kishnani PS, Case LE, et al. Pompe disease: design, methodology, and early findings from the Pompe Registry. Mol Genet Metab 2011; 103(1):1–11.
75. Broomfield A, Fletcher J, Davison J, et al. Response of 33 UK patients with infantile-onset Pompe disease to enzyme replacement therapy. J Inherit Metab Dis 2016;39(2):261–71.
76. Hahn A, Praetorius S, Karabul N, et al. Outcome of patients with classical infantile Pompe disease receiving enzyme replacement therapy in Germany. JIMD Rep 2015;20:65–75.
77. Leung EC, Mhanni AA, Reed M, et al. Outcome of perinatal hypophosphatasia in Manitoba Mennonites: a retrospective cohort analysis. JIMD Rep 2013;11:73–8.
78. Padidela R. Asfotase alfa treatment in perinatal and infantile hypophosphatasia: safe and sustained efficacy. Lancet Diabetes Endocrinol 2019;7(2):76–8.
79. Whyte MP, Simmons JH, Moseley S, et al. Asfotase alfa for infants and young children with hypophosphatasia: 7 year outcomes of a single-arm, open-label, phase 2 extension trial. Lancet Diabetes Endocrinol 2019;7(2):93–105.
80. Chinoy A, Mughal MZ, Padidela R. Current status in therapeutic interventions of neonatal bone mineral metabolic disorders. Semin Fetal Neonatal Med 2020; 25(1):101075.
81. Forlino A, Marini JC. Osteogenesis imperfecta. Lancet 2016;387(10028): 1657–71.
82. McAllion SJ, Paterson CR. Causes of death in osteogenesis imperfecta. J Clin Pathol 1996;49(8):627–30.
83. Shapiro JR, Burn VE, Chipman SD, et al. Pulmonary hypoplasia and osteogenesis imperfecta type II with defective synthesis of alpha I(1) procollagen. Bone 1989;10(3):165–71.

84. Tam A, Chen S, Schauer E, et al. A multicenter study to evaluate pulmonary function in osteogenesis imperfecta. Clin Genet 2018;94(6):502–11.
85. Wang TG, Yang GF, Alba A. Chronic ventilator use in osteogenesis imperfecta congenita with basilar impression: a case report. Arch Phys Med Rehabil 1994;75(6):699–702.
86. Coman D, Irving M, Kannu P, et al. The skeletal manifestations of the congenital disorders of glycosylation. Clin Genet 2008;73(6):507–15.
87. Grünewald S. The clinical spectrum of phosphomannomutase 2 deficiency (CDG-Ia). Biochim Biophys Acta 2009;1792(9):827–34.
88. Maquet E, Costagliola S, Parma J, et al. Lethal respiratory failure and mild primary hypothyroidism in a term girl with a de novo heterozygous mutation in the TITF1/NKX2.1 gene. J Clin Endocrinol Metab 2009;94(1):197–203.
89. Berger KI, Fagondes SC, Giugliani R, et al. Respiratory and sleep disorders in mucopolysaccharidosis. J Inherit Metab Dis 2012;36(2):201–10.
90. Muenzer J. Early initiation of enzyme replacement therapy for the mucopolysaccharidoses. Mol Genet Metab 2014;111(2):63–72.
91. Pal AR, Mercer J, Jones SA, et al. Substrate accumulation and extracellular matrix remodelling promote persistent upper airway disease in mucopolysaccharidosis patients on enzyme replacement therapy. PLoS One 2018;13(9):e0203216.
92. Bigger BW, Begley DJ, Virgintino D, et al. Anatomical changes and pathophysiology of the brain in mucopolysaccharidosis disorders. Mol Genet Metab 2018;125(4):322–31.
93. Simonaro CM, Ge Y, Eliyahu E, et al. Involvement of the Toll-like receptor 4 pathway and use of TNF-alpha antagonists for treatment of the mucopolysaccharidoses. Proc Natl Acad Sci U S A 2010;107(1):222–7.
94. Simonaro CM, D'Angelo M, He X, et al. Mechanism of glycosaminoglycan-mediated bone and joint disease: implications for the mucopolysaccharidoses and other connective tissue diseases. Am J Pathol 2008;172(1):112–22.
95. Khan S, Alméciga-Díaz CJ, Sawamoto K, et al. Mucopolysaccharidosis IVA and glycosaminoglycans. Mol Genet Metab 2017;120(1–2):78–95.
96. Soni-Jaiswal A, Mercer J, Jones SA, et al. Mucopolysaccharidosis I; Parental beliefs about the impact of disease on the quality of life of their children. Orphanet J Rare Dis 2016;11(1):96.
97. Pal AR, Langereis EJ, Saif MA, et al. Sleep disordered breathing in mucopolysaccharidosis I: a multivariate analysis of patient, therapeutic and metabolic correlators modifying long term clinical outcome. Orphanet J Rare Dis 2015;10:42.
98. Jones SA, Wynn R. Mucopolysaccharidoses: clinical features and diagnosis. UpToDate; 2017. Available at: https://www.uptodate.com/contents/mucopolysaccharidoses-clinical-features-and-diagnosis?search=MPS%20IV&source=search_result&selectedTitle=1~15&usage_type=default&display_rank=1#H10.
99. Myer CM. Airway obstruction in Hurler's syndrome–radiographic features. Int J Pediatr Otorhinolaryngol 1991;22(1):91–6.
100. Morimoto N, Kitamura M, Kosuga M, et al. CT and endoscopic evaluation of larynx and trachea in mucopolysaccharidoses. Mol Genet Metab 2014;112(2):154–9.
101. Gönüldaş B, Yılmaz T, Serap Sivri H, et al. Mucopolysaccharidosis: otolaryngologic findings, obstructive sleep apnea and accumulation of glucosaminoglycans in lymphatic tissue of the upper airway. Int J Pediatr Otorhinolaryngol 2014;78(6):944–9.

102. Arn P, Bruce IA, Wraith JE, et al. Airway-related symptoms and surgeries in patients with mucopolysaccharidosis I. Ann Otol Rhinol Laryngol 2015;124(3):198–205.
103. Shapiro J, Strome M, Crocker AC. Airway obstruction and sleep apnea in Hurler and Hunter syndromes. Ann Otol Rhinol Laryngol 1985;94(5 Pt 1):458–61.
104. Yoskovitch A, Tewfik TL, Brouillette RT, et al. Acute airway obstruction in Hunter syndrome. Int J Pediatr Otorhinolaryngol 1998;44(3):273–8.
105. Ingelmo PM, Parini R, Grimaldi M, et al. Multidetector computed tomography (MDCT) for preoperative airway assessment in children with mucopolysaccharidoses. Minerva Anestesiol 2011;77(8):774–80.
106. Shih SL, Lee YJ, Lin SP, et al. Airway changes in children with mucopolysaccharidoses. Acta Radiol 2002;43(1):40–3.
107. Walker R, Belani KG, Braunlin EA, et al. Anaesthesia and airway management in mucopolysaccharidosis. J Inherit Metab Dis 2013;36(2):211–9.
108. de Almeida-Barros RQ, de Medeiros PFV, de Almeida Azevedo MQ, et al. Evaluation of oral manifestations of patients with mucopolysaccharidosis IV and VI: clinical and imaging study. Clin Oral Investig 2018;22(1):201–8.
109. Coleman M, De Kruijf M, Jones SA, et al. Coronoid process hyperplasia as a cause of reduced mouth opening capacity in children with mucopolysaccharidoses. Br J Oral Maxillofac Surg 2018;56(10):e15–6.
110. Peters ME, Arya S, Langer LO, et al. Narrow trachea in mucopolysaccharidoses. Pediatr Radiol 1985;15(4):225–8.
111. Yasuda E, Fushimi K, Suzuki Y, et al. Pathogenesis of Morquio A syndrome: an autopsied case reveals systemic storage disorder. Mol Genet Metab 2013;109(3):301–11.
112. Tomatsu S, Alméciga-Díaz CJ, Barbosa H, et al. Therapies of mucopolysaccharidosis IVA (Morquio A syndrome). Expert Opin Orphan Drugs 2013;1(10):805–18.
113. Tomatsu S, Averill LW, Sawamoto K, et al. Obstructive airway in Morquio A syndrome, the past, the present and the future. Mol Genet Metab 2016;117(2):150–6.
114. Rutten M, Ciet P, van den Biggelaar R, et al. Severe tracheal and bronchial collapse in adults with type II mucopolysaccharidosis. Orphanet J Rare Dis 2016;11:50.
115. Walker PP, Rose E, Williams JG. Upper airways abnormalities and tracheal problems in Morquio's disease. Thorax 2003;58(5):458–9.
116. Broomfield A, Zuberi K, Mercer J, et al. Outcomes from 18 years of cervical spine surgery in MPS IVA: a single centre's experience. Childs Nerv Syst 2018;34(9):1705–16.
117. Muenzer J, Beck M, Eng CM, et al. Multidisciplinary management of Hunter syndrome. Pediatrics 2009;124(6):e1228–39.
118. Moreira GA, Kyosen SO, Patti CL, et al. Prevalence of obstructive sleep apnea in patients with mucopolysaccharidosis types I, II, and VI in a reference center. Sleep Breath 2014;18(4):791–7.
119. Leighton SE, Papsin B, Vellodi A, et al. Disordered breathing during sleep in patients with mucopolysaccharidoses. Int J Pediatr Otorhinolaryngol 2001;58(2):127–38.
120. Nashed A, Al-Saleh S, Gibbons J, et al. Sleep-related breathing in children with mucopolysaccharidosis. J Inherit Metab Dis 2009;32(4):544–50.
121. Wooten WI, Muenzer J, Vaughn BV, et al. Relationship of sleep to pulmonary function in mucopolysaccharidosis II. J Pediatr 2013;162(6):1210–5.

122. Kamin W. Diagnosis and management of respiratory involvement in Hunter syndrome. Acta Paediatr 2008;97(457):57–60.
123. Schaedel C, Marthinsen L, Kristoffersson AC, et al. Lung symptoms in pseudohypoaldosteronism type 1 are associated with deficiency of the alpha-subunit of the epithelial sodium channel. J Pediatr 1999;135(6):739–45.
124. Hanukoglu A, Bistritzer T, Rakover Y, et al. Pseudohypoaldosteronism with increased sweat and saliva electrolyte values and frequent lower respiratory tract infections mimicking cystic fibrosis. J Pediatr 1994;125(5 Pt 1):752–5.
125. Gambineri E, Ciullini Mannurita S, Hagin D, et al. Clinical, immunological, and molecular heterogeneity of 173 patients with the phenotype of immune dysregulation, polyendocrinopathy, enteropathy, X-Linked (IPEX) Syndrome. Front Immunol 2018;9:2411.
126. Hershfield MS, Arredondo-Vega FX, Santisteban I. Clinical expression, genetics and therapy of adenosine deaminase (ADA) deficiency. J Inherit Metab Dis 1997;20(2):179–85.
127. Lawrence MG, Barber JS, Sokolic RA, et al. Elevated IgE and atopy in patients treated for early-onset ADA-SCID. J Allergy Clin Immunol 2013;132(6):1444–6.
128. Simonneau G, Robbins IM, Beghetti M, et al. Updated clinical classification of pulmonary hypertension. J Am Coll Cardiol 2009;54(1 Suppl):S43–54.
129. Tort F, Ferrer-Cortès X, Thió M, et al. Mutations in the lipoyltransferase LIPT1 gene cause a fatal disease associated with a specific lipoylation defect of the 2-ketoacid dehydrogenase complexes. Hum Mol Genet 2014;23(7):1907–15.
130. Catteruccia M, Verrigni D, Martinelli D, et al. Persistent pulmonary arterial hypertension in the newborn (PPHN): a frequent manifestation of TMEM70 defective patients. Mol Genet Metab 2014;111(3):353–9.
131. Ahting U, Mayr JA, Vanlander AV, et al. Clinical, biochemical, and genetic spectrum of seven patients with NFU1 deficiency. Front Genet 2015;6:123.
132. Cataltepe S, van Marter LJ, Kozakewich H, et al. Pulmonary hypertension associated with nonketotic hyperglycinaemia. J Inherit Metab Dis 2000;23(2):137–44.
133. Belostotsky R, Ben-Shalom E, Rinat C, et al. Mutations in the mitochondrial seryl-tRNA synthetase cause hyperuricemia, pulmonary hypertension, renal failure in infancy and alkalosis, HUPRA syndrome. Am J Hum Genet 2011;88(2):193–200.
134. Kishita Y, Pajak A, Bolar NA, et al. Intra-mitochondrial methylation deficiency due to mutations in SLC25A26. Am J Hum Genet 2015;97(5):761–8.
135. Lo SM, Liu J, Chen F, et al. Pulmonary vascular disease in Gaucher disease: clinical spectrum, determinants of phenotype and long-term outcomes of therapy. J Inherit Metab Dis 2011;34(3):643–50.
136. Iodice FG, Di Chiara L, Boenzi S, et al. Cobalamin C defect presenting with isolated pulmonary hypertension. Pediatrics 2013;132(1):e248–51.
137. Grange S, Bekri S, Artaud-Macari E, et al. Adult-onset renal thrombotic microangiopathy and pulmonary arterial hypertension in cobalamin C deficiency. Lancet 2015;386(9997):1011–2.
138. Liu J, Peng Y, Zhou N, et al. Combined methylmalonic acidemia and homocysteinemia presenting predominantly with late-onset diffuse lung disease: a case series of four patients. Orphanet J Rare Dis 2017;12(1):58.
139. Morel CF, Lerner-Ellis JP, Rosenblatt DS. Combined methylmalonic aciduria and homocystinuria (cblC): phenotype-genotype correlations and ethnic-specific observations. Mol Genet Metab 2006;88(4):315–21.

Pulmonary Manifestations of Immunodeficiency and Immunosuppressive Diseases Other than Human Immunodeficiency Virus

Susan E. Pacheco, MD, James M. Stark, MD, PhD*

KEYWORDS

- Primary immunodeficiency • Secondary immunodeficiency • Immunosuppression
- Pulmonary infection • Humoral immunity • Cell-mediated immunity
- Innate immunity • Chemotherapy

KEY POINTS

- The upper and lower respiratory tracts are frequently involved in patients with primary or secondary immunodeficiencies.
- Primary and secondary immunodeficiencies may predispose to recurrent bacterial and viral respiratory infections, or infections by unusual or opportunistic organisms (eg, viruses, fungi, mycobacteria).
- Oncologic diseases and their treatment may predispose to respiratory abnormalities as a result of the underlying malignancy, treatment regime, and the resulting immunosuppression (like the primary immunodeficiencies).
- Organ transplant may result in pulmonary abnormalities related to problems with the transplanted organ function (rejection) and from immunosuppression.
- Pulmonary complications resulting from primary and secondary immunodeficiency require a systematic approach for appropriate diagnosis and treatment.

INTRODUCTION

Clinicians are often faced with children with too many respiratory infections or unusual pneumonias. The difficulty becomes not only diagnosing the cause (infectious or noninfectious) but also determining whether there is an underlying immune disorder that predisposes to repeated or atypical pneumonias. This article begins with a

Department of Pediatrics, Division of Pulmonary Medicine, Allergy-Immunology, and Sleep, McGovern Medical School at UTHealth, 6431 Fannin Street MSB 3.228, Houston, TX 77030, USA
* Corresponding author.
E-mail address: James.M.Stark@uth.tmc.edu

Pediatr Clin N Am 68 (2021) 103–130
https://doi.org/10.1016/j.pcl.2020.09.004
pediatric.theclinics.com

discussion of lung immunity. Then it focuses on defects in cellular or humoral immunity associated with primary immunodeficiency disorders (PIDs) that contribute to respiratory diseases. This article cannot provide an exhaustive review of PID but focuses on the major classes and common PIDs as examples of alterations in the immune system that predispose to pulmonary infectious and to noninfectious processes. The focus of the article then changes to a discussion of immunodeficiency resulting from chemotherapy or immunosuppression following organ transplant. The article concludes with a discussion of infectious agents and diagnostic tools available to define these pulmonary complications in these patients.

IMMUNOLOGY OF THE RESPIRATORY TRACT

The respiratory tract is an open gate from the outside world, continuously exposing the lung and host defenses to external pathogens, allergens, and toxicants. The large surface area of the conducting airways and alveolar surfaces (>70 m^2 in adults) poses a great challenge for the lung defenses in immunocompetent hosts. Innate (physical, chemical, and cellular defenses) and adaptive immune responses have evolved in the entire respiratory tract to prevent airway injury and contain infection. Beyond their role in mucociliary clearance, the ciliated epithelium of the conducting airways produces a series of secreted products (eg, lysozyme, lactoferrin, immunoglobulin [Ig] A secretory component, phospholipase-A2, proteases, antioxidants, and cationic peptides) that serve to neutralize pathogens or enhance the immune response. Admixed in the glycoprotein mucin layer produced by goblet cells and facilitated by secretory IgA (SIgA) and IgM, the ciliary epithelium propels entrapped particles or neutralized microorganisms out from the lung toward the pharynx. Nonciliated club cells, the major secretory cells in the bronchial epithelium of the respiratory zone, produce an array of compounds that facilitate airway defense and repair. Microorganisms not expelled by these physical barriers or those reaching the respiratory units are phagocytized by alveolar macrophages or detected by sensor cells such as airways epithelial cells and dendritic cells.[1]

Alveolar macrophages are the first line of defense against organisms reaching the lower airway, mediating their effects by phagocytosis, secretion of bactericidal compounds such as lysozyme, cationic proteins, reactive oxygen species, complement components and C1q inhibitor, and IgG-mediated opsonization in the alveolar space. Epithelial cells may recognize microorganisms by their recognition receptors, such as toll-like receptors. The ensuing immune activation conduces to expression of type I and type III interferons, chemokines, and cytokines that, in turn, activate tissue-resident lymphoid cells. This process leads to amplification of the immune response by activation and recruitment of effector cells for pathogen clearing, and macrophage differentiation and dendritic cell maturation into antigen-presenting cells. Once activated, these dendritic cells migrate to the draining lymph nodes where they initiate the adaptive immune response by presenting antigen to T cells and B cells, resulting in antibody production and generation of antigen-specific effector T cells. Moreover, the local inflammatory responses in the airway increase expression of adhesion molecules and release of chemokines (eg, interleukin [IL] 8) and other soluble factors that facilitate neutrophil recruitment into the airway and subsequent activation.[1]

The primary antibodies in the respiratory tract are secretory IgA and IgG. Secretory IgA, a dimer of IgA2, is bound to the secretory component (SC), a remnant of the polymeric Ig receptor, produced by epithelial cells. SIgA is the most abundant immunoglobulin in the upper and conductive airway's fluid, and serves several functions, including neutralization of viruses and toxins, enhancement of lactoferrin and lactoperoxidase activities, and inhibition of microbial growth. Because SIgA is able to bind 2 antigens simultaneously, it may form large antigen-antibody complexes that may be removed by mucociliary clearance. SIgA and multimeric IgM at the bronchial surface are primarily derived from the mucosa-associated lymphatic tissue.[2] Bronchus-associated lymphoid tissue in humans is not normally present in the lower respiratory tract but may be induced in response to respiratory infections.[3] IgG is the primary antibody found in lower respiratory secretions and alveoli, where it constitutes about 5% of the total protein content found in bronchoalveolar lavage (BAL).[4] In contrast with SIgA, which is actively transported into the airway, IgG reaches the airway largely by transudation through the mucosa, although local secretion by intraluminal lymphocytes contributes to the presence IgG in the airways and alveolar space.[5] IgG functions by opsonizing microbes for phagocytosis and killing, activating the complement cascade, and neutralizing many bacterial endotoxins and viruses. The IgG subclasses IgG1 and IgG3 are of particular importance in lung defenses because they may facilitate complement fixation. IgG2 functions as type-specific antibody against pathogens such as pneumococci or *Haemophilus influenzae*.[6]

Several types of T (thymus derived) lymphocytes (T cells) contribute to both lung immunity and lung injury. All mature T cells express a unique T-cell receptor (TCR) consisting of α and β chains ($\alpha\beta$) in most T cells, whereas a smaller population has TCR composed of γ and δ chains. Almost all $\alpha\beta$ T cells are cluster of differentiation (CD) 4(+) or CD8(+). CD4(+) T cells are called T-helper (Th) cells, whereas CD8(+) T cells are termed cytotoxic/suppressor cells.[1] B-cell and T-cell deficiencies play significant roles in immunodeficiency and in pulmonary dysfunction.

PRIMARY IMMUNODEFICIENCIES

There are now more than 400 PIDs characterized clinically and/or at the molecular level.[7,8] Although once considered rare, it is estimated that 1 in 1200 people worldwide are potentially living with a form of PID.[7,9] Patients with PID may present with symptoms involving the upper and/or lower airways, including recurrent infections of the respiratory tract, immune dysregulation (eg, chronic inflammation, autoimmunity, allergy, lymphoproliferation), structural abnormalities (eg, hilar or mediastinal adenopathy, bronchiectasis, obstructive and restrictive lung disease), or malignancy.[10] The kind of infectious organism involved may suggest the type of immune defect, although there is considerable overlap between PIDs. Likewise, noninfectious manifestations (hilar or mediastinal adenopathy, obstructive and restrictive lung diseases, autoimmune and interstitial lung diseases, or malignancy) may be seen in several subgroups of PID.[10] The following discussion of pulmonary manifestations of primary immunodeficiencies follows the classification of the International Union of Immunological Societies (IUIS), focusing on the subgroups that may have a significant pulmonary component[7,8] (**Fig. 1**).

Immunodeficiencies Affecting Cellular and Humoral Immunity

Combined immunodeficiencies (immunodeficiencies affecting cellular and humoral immunity) result from defects involving both T-cell and B-cell lineages, or from altered T cell–dependent signaling that leads to impaired B-cell function. The availability of genetic testing along with newborn screening (NBS) for severe combined immunodeficiency (SCID) has allowed early diagnosis and better understanding of the prevalence, morbidity, and mortality of many of these diseases. Early detection has improved prompt preventive interventions as well as lifesaving treatment

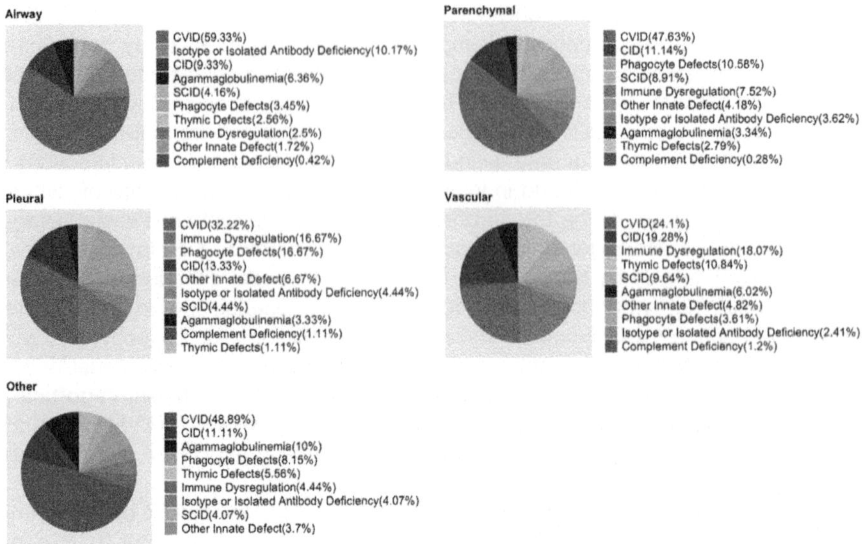

Fig. 1. Prevalence of PIDs by pulmonary location and disorder type. The prevalence of disease caused by the major classes of primary immunodeficiency disorders by location within the respiratory system. CID, combined immunodeficiency; CVID, common variable immunodeficiency; SCID, severe combined immunodeficiency. (*From* Patrawala M, Cui Y, Peng L, et al. Pulmonary disease burden in primary immune deficiency disorders. J of Clinical Immunology 2020; 40: 340; with permission.)

options, such as enzyme replacement therapy and hematopoietic stem cell transplant (HSCT).

Severe combined immunodeficiency

SCID is the most profound immunodeficiency, characterized by a severe reduction in the number and function of CD3-expressing T-cells, lymphopenia, and extreme susceptibility to infections. The lack of CD3 cells creates an intense immune impairment with severe T-cell dysfunction and impaired antibody production. Mutations in at least 17 different genes have been associated with SCID.[7] Besides the CD3 impairment, different mutations are associated with distinct cellular immune phenotypes characterized by presence or absence of CD19 B cells or natural killer (NK) (CD16/56) cells. X-linked SCID, the most common form of SCID, is caused by mutation in IL2 receptor γ chain. Most of the remaining defects have an autosomal recessive (AR) pattern of inheritance.[7] Before the NBS for SCID, a common clinical presentation was diarrhea and failure to thrive in the first months of life, and/or persistent infections with opportunistic or common pathogens. Implementation of the NBS for SCID in the United States, Puerto Rico, and in at least 20 countries[11] has allowed early detection of this disease, clinical intervention before severe infections occur, and definition of its prevalence at about 1 in 58,000.[12] Patients with SCID may develop pneumonia and/or disseminated infections with opportunistic organisms and other pathogens such as *Pneumocystis jiroveci*, *Candida* spp, adenovirus, respiratory syncytial virus (RSV), parainfluenza virus type 3, Epstein-Barr virus (EBV), and cytomegalovirus (CMV). Moreover, they are at risk of severe disseminated infection when immunized with live virus vaccines such as polio, measles-mumps-rubella vaccine, varicella, or bacillus Calmette-Guérin.

Adenosine deaminase - severe combined immunodeficiency syndrome

Mutations in the adenosine deaminase (ADA) gene result in autosomal recessive (AR) ADA-SCID syndrome (SCIDS), which makes up about 15% of all SCID cases. Although susceptible to opportunistic infections, infectious agents are not always behind the pulmonary manifestations of ADA-SCIDS, despite clinical and radiographic similarities to the other types of SCID.[13] In the analysis of a small cohort of patients, *P jiroveci* was isolated from 11 of 19 patients with X-linked SCID, but not from 19 patients with ADA-SCIDS. A similar pattern was observed for RSV and parainfluenza. ADA is a key enzyme in the purine salvage pathway, and its deficiency results in the accumulation of toxic metabolites that alter T-cell, B-cell, and NK-cell function, leading to the SCID phenotype. The resulting pulmonary abnormalities are reversible by enzyme (ADA) replacement therapy and HSCT.[14] Pulmonary alveolar proteinosis (PAP) is a frequent finding in patients with ADA-SCIDS, even in the absence of infection. Up to 20% of patients with ADA-SCIDS may have delayed-onset disease[15]; therefore, ADA-SCIDS must be suspected in any infant or child with PAP, because it may be missed by NBS for SCIDS.[16]

The hyper–immunoglobulin M syndromes

Hyper-IgM (HIGM) syndrome is characterized by normal or increased levels of IgM and absent or markedly decreased levels of IgG (<2 standard deviations [SD] for age) and IgA, that result from defects in T cell–driven immunoglobulin class switch recombination (CSR).[17] The most common form (>70% of cases) is the X-linked recessive HIGM syndrome type I caused by mutation in the CD40 ligand (CD40L, CD154), expressed in activated CD4+ lymphocytes. These mutations impede interaction with CD40 on B cells and CSR.[18] HIGM type III, involving mutation of CD40, is rare, but the clinical phenotype, including susceptibility to opportunistic infections early in life, is similar to that of X-linked HIGM. The most common complications in children with HIGM syndrome are pneumonia and upper airway infections caused by bacterial, viral, and fungal organisms. *P jiroveci* pneumonia is a common manifestation of HIGM types I and III, although pneumonia by viral pathogens, *Histoplasma*, and encapsulated organisms may also occur.[19] Patients may present with cryptococcus infections, hilar and mediastinal lymphadenopathies, and PAP[17] (see **Fig. 1**). HIGM types II and IV may present with recurrent respiratory tract infections, but not caused by *P jiroveci*. These types of HIGM and other conditions having pulmonary manifestations have been described.[20]

Other forms of combined immunodeficiency

Recurrent sinopulmonary infection may be one of the manifestations of patients with mutations in the major histocompatibility complex (ie, MHCI, MHCII), and IL21 deficiency. Pneumocystis infections are also seen in patients with IKAROS, CARD11, and IL21R deficiency.[7]

Combined Immunodeficiencies with Associated Syndromic Features

These immunodeficiencies include a diverse group of diseases with various immunologic and nonimmunologic abnormalities. These disorders are characterized by defects of lymphocyte function and/or number, cytokine production, or immune activation, in association with characteristic clinical phenotypes or congenital anomalies.

22q11.2 microdeletion (DiGeorge syndrome)

The presentation of this condition is often multisystemic, but cardiac and immune abnormalities are seen in more than 70% of patients.[21] The immunologic defects are mainly related to variable thymic hypoplasia with lower than normal T-cell numbers, although normal T-cell proliferation is present in most patients. Less than 1% of patients present with complete DiGeorge syndrome, with absent thymic tissue and T cells, and a severe combined immunodeficiency picture. Despite of their T-cell abnormalities, patients with DiGeorge syndrome do not experience opportunistic or severe infections. Functional humoral immune defects have recently been described. These patients may present with recurrent sinopulmonary infections and poor response to polysaccharide antigens.[21,22] Patients without humoral immunodeficiency may still have recurrent upper and lower airway infections, because of airway structure and associated anatomic abnormalities. Laryngomalacia, tracheomalacia, bronchomalacia, subglottic stenosis, and other abnormalities are common, and some patients require tracheostomy[23] (see **Fig. 1**).

Classic X-linked Wiskott-Aldrich syndrome

These patients present with eczema, thrombocytopenia with small platelets, and recurrent infections, as a result of mutations in the Wiskott-Aldrich syndrome (WAS) protein (WASp). The classic or severe form of WAS has complete absence of WASp, presenting with an early, severe deficient innate immunity, T-cell and B-cell defects, and increased susceptibility to fungal, viral, bacterial and opportunistic infections.[24] Recurrent otosinopulmonary infections develop in the first year of life. Pulmonary infections may be caused by encapsulated bacteria (*Streptococcus pneumoniae*), viruses (herpes simplex virus), or opportunistic organisms (*Aspergillus* and *P jiroveci*)[24] (see **Fig. 1**). Death usually results from infection, vasculitis, autoimmune cytopenias, hemorrhages, or lymphoreticular malignancy.

Ataxia-telangiectasia

Ataxia-telangiectasia (AT) is an AR disorder caused by mutation in the ATM (AT mutated) gene, which codes for a protein required for DNA repair. During childhood, patients develop progressive loss of motor function and oculocutaneous telangiectasias, and have malignant predisposition.[25] The immune defect results from abnormal T-cell and B-cell numbers and function, which makes these patients susceptible to recurrent upper and lower respiratory infections with organisms such *Pseudomonas aeruginosa* and *Staphylococcus aureus* or encapsulated bacteria[25] (see **Fig. 1**). Infections with opportunistic organisms are uncommon. Up to 25% of patients with AT develop a distinct form of interstitial lung disease (ILD) of unknown cause unrelated to the chemotherapy-associated pulmonary fibrosis or parenchymal malignant disease.[25] Because of increased radiosensitivity, imaging that exposes these patients to ionizing radiation should be minimized, because repeated exposure to x-rays places them at risk for lymphoreticular cancers and adenocarcinoma[25] (see **Fig. 1**).

Coloboma, heart abnormalities, choanal atresia, retardation of growth, genital and ear anomalies syndrome

Besides their well-described congenital defects, patients with CHARGE (coloboma, heart abnormalities, choanal atresia, retardation of growth, genital and ear anomalies) syndrome may experience combined humoral and cellular immunodeficiency with an SCID phenotype.[26] They may develop viral and bacterial respiratory tract infections and, rarely, opportunistic infections. Swallowing problems and gastroesophageal reflux disease are common and may lead to recurrent, potentially fatal aspiration[27] (see **Fig. 1**).

Jacobsen syndrome

Patients with Jacobsen syndrome, or chromosome 11q deletion syndrome, may experience recurrent sinopulmonary infections caused by impaired T cells, B cells and NK cells.[28]

Lung disease immunodeficiency and chromosomal breakage syndrome

Lung disease immunodeficiency and chromosomal breakage syndrome is an AR chromosome breakage syndrome that alters the function of T and B cells. Patients with this recently described condition develop severe acute respiratory distress syndrome (ARDS) following viral pneumonia.[29]

Hyper–immunoglobulin E syndromes

The hyper-IgE syndromes (HIESs) should be considered once the possibility of increased IgE level stemming from atopic disorders, parasitic diseases, allergic bronchopulmonary aspergillosis, and some autoimmune conditions is excluded. In general, the HIESs present with eczema, recurrent lung and skin infections, and increased IgE level.[30] There are several monogenic mutations associated with these conditions but the 2 most common forms are autosomal dominant (AD)-HIES or Job syndrome (caused by a heterozygous mutation in the STAT-3 gene) and the AR-HIES (caused by a biallelic mutation in the DOCK8 gene).[31] Besides their syndromic features, skeletal (frequent fractures) and dental abnormalities, patients with AD-HIES, present early in life with recurrent skin infections, mucocutaneous candidiasis, deep abscesses, and pyogenic pneumonias. Pneumonias are frequently caused by *S aureus*, encapsulated organisms, and *Aspergillus* sp. Absence of systemic inflammation may delay diagnosis and treatment and lead to pulmonary complications such as pneumatoceles, empyema, and bronchiectasis in up to 70% of patients.[30,31] Once the parenchyma is damaged, these patients may be more susceptible to infection or colonization with other pathogens, such as nontuberculous mycobacteria (NTM), molds, and *Pseudomonas*.[30,31] Patients with AR-HIES share similar clinical features with AD-HIES. However, they do not have skeletal and dental abnormalities but impaired response to polysaccharide antigens (see **Fig. 1**).

Anhidrotic ectodermal dysplasias

Anhidrotic ectodermal dysplasias (EDAs) are characterized by deficient differentiation of ectoderm tissues: skin, hair, teeth, and sweat glands. Mutations in the IKBKG gene cause X-linked recessive EDA with immune deficiency (EDA-ID), and mutations in the NFKBIA gene cause autosomal dominant EDA-ID. These patients experience recurrent airway infections with opportunistic organisms such as *P jiroveci*[32] and with organisms such as pneumococci, *S aureus*, *Pseudomonas* spp., *H influenzae*, *Klebsiella pneumoniae*, *Serratia marcescens*, viruses, and mycobacteria. The paucity of secretory glands in the airways may lead to atrophic rhinitis and ciliary dysfunction, making these patients more susceptible to chronic airway problems and infectious complications[32] (see **Fig. 1**).

Primary Immunodeficiency Disorder with Predominantly Antibody Deficiencies

Antibody deficiencies or humoral immunodeficiencies are the most common forms of PID, accounting for more than 50% of cases.[33] They may include milder forms, such as transient hypogammaglobulinemia of infancy, asymptomatic (selective IgA deficiency), IgG subclasses deficiency, and specific antibody deficiency, and more severe forms of common variable immunodeficiency (CVID) and agammaglobulinemia. The onset and severity of sinopulmonary infections, autoimmunity, and malignancy depend on the underlying defect.[33] Infections are caused by encapsulated organisms such as *H influenzae*, pneumococci, and *Moraxella catarrhalis*, although infections with nontypeable or nonencapsulated organism also occur. Noninfectious manifestations of antibody deficiencies include ILDs such as granulomatous-lymphocytic ILD (GLILD), cryptogenic organizing pneumonia (COP), follicular bronchiolitis, lymphoid hyperplasia, and lymphocytic interstitial pneumonitis (LIP)[2] (see **Fig. 1**).

Selective immunoglobulin A deficiency

Immunoglobulin A deficiency (IgAD), the most common PID, is characterized by absent levels of serum IgA (<7 mg/dL) in the presence of normal serum levels of IgG and IgM, in a patient older than 4 years of age, in whom other causes of hypogammaglobulinemia have been excluded.[34] It has an incidence of about 1 in 600 described in the Western world,[35] but its frequency varies with ethnic background. There is a maturational defect in IgA-bearing B cells that impedes progression to IgA-secreting plasma cells, although a definite genetic abnormality has not been identified. Symptomatic patients frequently have associated IgG2 subclass deficiency. Recurrent sinopulmonary infections are the most common manifestations associated with symptomatic IgAD,[36] usually with organisms such as *H influenzae* and *S pneumoniae*. Rarely, some patients develop bronchiectasis or CVID over time. Many patients with IgAD have respiratory allergies and atopic dermatitis, as well as gastrointestinal infections, malabsorption, and autoimmunity[36,37] (see **Fig. 1**).

The congenital agammaglobulinemias

Congenital agammaglobulinemias are manifested by impaired production of IgG, immunoglobulin, and IgM; severely decreased or absent circulating CD19 or B cells; and increased susceptibility to infections. X-linked agammaglobulinemia (XLA), the first PID to be recognized,[38] results from mutations in the Bruton tyrosine kinase (BTK) that lead to arrested development at the pre–B-cell level, with preservation of T-cell numbers and function. XLA constitutes about 85% of cases of congenital agammaglobulinemia, with an incidence between 1 in 100,000 and 1 in 200,000 depending on ethnicity.[39] The AR forms of agammaglobulinemia have a similar, severe reduction of all immunoglobulin classes and absence of peripheral B cells, in the absence of BTK mutations.[39] Mu heavy chain locus mutations are the most common in AR agammaglobulinemia, involving up 50% of patients without BTK mutation in some series.[40] The clinical presentation of AR agammaglobulinemia is similar to BTK, but the symptoms may be more severe. All children with agammaglobulinemia present with severe bacterial infections after 3 to 6 months of life, when in utero–acquired maternal IgG antibodies decline. Many patients develop bronchiectasis early despite adequate replacement treatment with gamma globulin. Patients frequently experience recurrent bouts of otitis media (OM) and sinusitis.[39,41] Recurrent OM and absent tonsils should alert clinicians to the possibility of this disorder.[41] Infections with pneumococci, *H influenzae*, *Mycoplasma*, and occasionally *P jiroveci* occur.[42] Other manifestations of congenital agammaglobulinemia include pseudomonas sepsis and increased susceptibility to chronic enteroviral infections (see **Fig. 1**).

Common variable immunodeficiency

CVID is a group of antibody deficiencies characterized by decreased production of IgG (usually <0.4 g/L) in combination with decreased IgA and/or IgM level, weak or absent antibody response to vaccines, and absence of any other immunodeficiency condition.[43] This group is almost always associated with pulmonary complications with onset in childhood, or midadolescence to young adulthood. CVID is the most common symptomatic humoral immunodeficiency in adults, ranging between 1 in 10,000 and 1 in 100,000 cases. Children may account for up to 30% of patients with CVID.[7,43,44]

Unlike XLA, patients with CVID have circulating CD19 B cells (although in variable numbers) and T-cell abnormalities (reduced numbers of naive CD4+ cells and occasional impairment of lymphoproliferative responses).

CVID likely represents several different genetic disorders whose causes remain elusive in most patients. Most cases are sporadic, although 5% to 25% are familial with an autosomal dominant pattern of inheritance. There are several mutations associated with disease in patients that fulfill criteria for CVID, but they only account for about 2% of patients with CVID.[44] Patients with CVID have recurrent sinopulmonary infections, including otitis, sinusitis, bronchitis, and pneumonia (see **Fig. 1**).

Pulmonary infection is the most serious complication. Infecting pathogens are those that require antibody for opsonization and phagocytosis, such as pneumococci, *H influenzae*, *Mycoplasma*, and nontypeable *H influenzae*. Immune dysregulation may be responsible for the autoimmune and inflammatory manifestations of CVID. Chronic lung disease has been reported in 30% to 60% of patients, and bronchiectasis in more than 50%.[45] Noninfectious pulmonary disease becomes common in adolescence and early adulthood.

CVID shows 2 very different clinical phenotypes: (1) recurrent airway infections, which may lead to bronchiectasis; and (2) ILD or CVID-ILD, observed in up to 20% of these patients. The often-used term GLILD (Granulomatous-Lymphocytic Interstitial Lung Disease) is misleading because granulomas are not always present in tissue biopsy.[46,47] Lung biopsies in these patients show the presence of mainly CD4+ T lymphocytes, CD8+ T cells, B cells, and absence of FOXP3-positive T-regulatory cells.[47] The differential diagnosis of GLILD is broad, including infection, lymphoid interstitial pneumonia, and malignancy. GLILD is frequently considered a systemic disease because it is often accompanied by conditions such as idiopathic thrombocytopenic purpura, splenomegaly, hepatitis, arthritis, inflammatory bowel disease, or hemolytic anemia. The multisystemic nature of GLILD, including sarcoidlike noncaseating granulomas on histology, often leads to confusion with sarcoidosis. Progressive ILD in patients with CVID has been associated with lower IgG level, higher IgM level, and severe thrombocytopenia.[45] Although characteristic of CVID, GLILD has been described in other primary immunodeficiencies, such as the 22q11 deletion syndrome, Kabuki syndrome, Good syndrome, LRBA (lipopolysaccharide [LPS]-responsive and beige-like anchor protein) mutations, cytotoxic T lymphocyte–associated protein 4 mutations, and recombination-activating genes (RAG) mutations.[48] Immunoglobulin replacement has led to major improvement in the management of infections in CVID, preventing acute infections, and slowing progression of chronic infections.

Selective IgM deficiency

IgM deficiency is a disorder of unknown inheritance pattern and poorly defined mechanism, characterized by serum IgM (<2 SD of the mean), normal IgG and IgG subclasses, IgA and T-cell function. Vaccine response may be normal to both protein and polysaccharide antigens,[49] although impaired response to unconjugated polysaccharide antigens may be found in up to 45% of patients.[50] Recurrent infections are common, including otosinusitis, bronchitis, and pneumonia, and other systemic infections usually caused by organisms such as *Pseudomonas*, pneumococci, *H influenzae*, *Neisseria meningitidis*, and *Aspergillus fumigatus*[50] (see **Fig. 1**).

Specific antibody deficiency

Patients with specific antibody deficiency have normal immunoglobulin classes, normal protein antigen vaccine responses, but impaired antibody responses to pure polysaccharide antigens such as those from pneumococci.[51,52] This condition is one of the most common presentations of immunodeficient pediatric patients with recurrent sinopulmonary infections. The diagnosis of this disease is debated because there is no clear definition of the magnitude or number of pneumococcal serotypes that define a normal response.[52] Neither an inheritance pattern nor a mechanism for this condition has been identified, but decreased numbers of switched memory B cells, known to be key elements in protection from polysaccharide-encapsulated bacteria, occur in this patient population.[52]

Diseases of Immune Dysregulation

This group of diseases is composed of disorders in immune regulatory pathways that result in alteration of normal immune cell function leading to lung disease. Although this article does not provide an exhaustive review of these disorders, it reviews some conditions that have significant pulmonary manifestations.[7,8]

Lysinuric protein intolerance

The SLCA7 gene encodes a protein that is a component of the lysine amino acid transporter at the basolateral plasma membrane of epithelial cells (discussed in Alexander A. Broomfield and colleagues' article, "Pulmonary Manifestations of Endocrine and Metabolic Diseases in Children," elsewhere in this issue). Most of the symptoms of lysinuric protein intolerance are linked to urea cycle abnormality caused by impaired transport of cationic amino acids. However, lung involvement may be severe, resulting in PAP, interstitial fibrosis, and lipid deposition in the interstitium and alveolar spaces that leads to respiratory failure[53] (see **Fig. 1**).

Hermansky-Pudlak syndrome

Hermansky-Pudlak syndrome (HPS) is a group of AR disorders characterized by varying degrees of oculocutaneous albinism, visual impairment, susceptibility to skin cancer, and excessive bleeding and bruising. It results from abnormal regulation of lysosome-related organelles derived from the endosomal system, resulting in loss of function in diverse physiologic systems. Patients with the most common HPS subtypes (HPS1 and HPS4) have progressive pulmonary fibrosis that is lethal in the fourth to fifth decade of life without lung transplant. The primary cause seems to be defective biogenesis of lamellar bodies in the alveolar type 2 cells resulting in reduced surfactant synthesis and secretion, which leads to inflammation and ultimately to lung fibrosis[54] (see **Fig. 1**; discussed in Bernard A. Cohen and Nelson L. Turcios' article, "Pulmonary Manifestations of Skin Disorders in Children," elsewhere in this issue).

Itchy E3 ubiquitin protein ligase deficiency

Itchy E3 ubiquitin protein ligase (ITCH) is a ubiquitin ligase that plays a prominent role in preventing autoinflammation in humans and mice. ITCH exists in an autoinhibited state at baseline that becomes activated by phosphorylation leading to ubiquitination, which marks specific proteins for degradation by the lysosome or proteasome. In humans, ITCH deficiency is rare, but in 1 study 9 out of 10 patients with ITCH deficiency had chronic lung disease with baseline lung inflammation (mixed lymphocytic infiltrate without fibrosis on lung pathology) and recurrent pneumonia (see **Fig. 1**). The second most common presentation was autoimmunity.[55]

Congenital Defects of Phagocyte Numbers or Function

Congenital defects of phagocyte number or function consist primarily of defects involving the function of neutrophil and monocyte/macrophages. In general, these conditions involve deficiencies in movement (eg, chemotaxis), cell recruitment or activation, and intracellular killing.

Chronic granulomatous disease

Chronic granulomatous disease (CGD) is caused by defects in the reduced nicotinamide adenine dinucleotide phosphate oxidase complex responsible for the production of superoxide. X-linked CGD is the most common form, with severe phenotype and early presentation, compared with the AR form described in female patients. The hallmark of this disease is the occurrence of purulent inflammation caused by catalase-positive, low-grade pyogenic bacteria. This syndrome should be considered in any individual with recurrent catalase-positive bacterial or fungal infections. Pulmonary infections are the most frequent presentation. *Aspergillus*, *Burkholderia*, and *S aureus* are the most commonly reported pathogens in patients with CGD[56] (see **Fig. 1**). Other complications thought to be related to immune dysregulation include ILD, pleural effusions, chronic obstructive pulmonary disease, and noninfectious granulomas.[57]

Leukocyte adhesion deficiencies

Leukocyte adhesion deficiencies (LADs) are rare conditions with 3 major types, involving defects in leukocyte migration and adhesion: (1) defects in β2 integrins (LAD-I), (2) impaired fucosylation and function of selectin ligands (LAD-II), and (3) impaired activation of β integrins (LAD-III).[1,58] LAD-1, the most common, presents early in life, usually with delayed detachment of the umbilical cord. Patients with the severe phenotype (CD18 expression <2%) have recurrent pneumonia, OM, and sepsis.[59] Nonhealing, chronic ulcers are frequent complications. The prognosis is poor without allogeneic HSCT. Recently, cystic fibrosis (CF) has been added to the list of human inborn error of immunity as a cell-type selective LAD disease.[7] CFTR (the major protein defect in CF) has been suggested to play a regulatory role in β-integrin activation and chemotaxis of mononuclear cells in these patients[60] (see **Fig. 1**).

Hereditary pulmonary alveolar proteinosis

Hereditary pulmonary alveolar proteinosis (PAP) is caused by X-linked mutations (CSF2RA) or AR mutations (CSF2RB), encoding granulocyte-macrophage colony-stimulating factor receptor subunits.[61] These mutations alter the recycling of pulmonary surfactant components, resulting in accumulation of surfactant proteins in the airspace. The clinical presentation of these patients varies, ranging from asymptomatic to respiratory failure.

Defects in Intrinsic and Innate Immunity

Many of the defects that alter intrinsic and innate immunity result from changes that affect cytokine production, cytokine receptors, or participation in the intracellular signaling cascades that activate immune cell function. Loss of intracellular signaling pathways results in increased susceptibility to bacterial, viral, fungal, or mycobacterial infections[7,8] (see **Fig. 1**).

CARD9 and MYD88 deficiencies

Innate pattern recognition receptors and Toll-like receptors provide surveillance against invading extracellular organisms. These receptors mediate their signaling through intracellular signaling adaptors, including Caspase recruitment domain-containing protein 9 (CARD9) and Myeloid differentiation primary response protein (MYD88). Defective CARD9 manifests extreme susceptibility to fungal infection but not to bacterial, viral, or parasitic infection.[62] MYD88 deficiency results in development of life-threatening pyogenic bacterial infection without increased susceptibility to fungal disease.[63]

MDA5 viral immunity and autoimmune disease

Melanoma differentiation-associated protein 5 (MDA5) is a member of the RLR (RIG1-like receptor) family of cytosolic receptors that recognizes long intracellular double-stranded RNA (dsRNA) molecules. Activation of MDA5 by dsRNA binding results in interactions with other adaptors, leading to transcription of genes encoding type I interferons, which coordinate cellular immune responses to virus infection.[1,64] In addition, mutations in the IFIH1 gene (encoding MDA5) may lead to interferon-driven autoinflammatory disease.[64,65]

Complement Deficiencies

Complement defects are among the rarest immunodeficiencies. Complement defects are associated with increased susceptibility to infections, systemic or local inflammatory conditions (including systemic lupus erythematosus [SLE]), and thrombotic disorders.[66,67] These patients are at increased risk of developing pyogenic infections with organisms such as pneumococci, *H influenzae*, and *Neisseria* spp. Early SLE and pneumonia complicated by empyema and pneumatoceles has been reported in C1r deficiency.[66,67]

C3 deficiency presents the most severe phenotype, including recurrent OM, pneumonia, sepsis, meningitis, and osteomyelitis, most commonly caused by pneumococci, *N meningitidis*, *Klebsiella* spp, *Escherichia coli*, and *Streptococcus pyogenes*.[66,67] Complement components interact with Toll-like receptors and modify B cell–mediated and T cell–mediated immunity; alterations in this signaling may contribute to the development of autoimmune disorders.

Hereditary angioedema (HAE) is an autosomal dominant disease resulting from a mutation in the C1-esterase inhibitor gene leading to low serum C4 levels. It is characterized by potentially life-threatening attacks of cutaneous and submucosal swelling.[68] Angioedema is the manifestation of transient increases in vascular permeability. Bradykinin has been identified as the mediator of swelling in HAE with C1 inhibitor deficiency. Recurrent attacks in a school-aged child of cutaneous angioedema (asymmetric, nonpruritic, and nonpitting) without urticaria associated with severe abdominal pain should alert the clinician to consider HAE. Treatments for acute attacks and prophylaxis are available[7,69] (see **Fig. 1**).

Diagnosis of Primary Immunodeficiencies

The early diagnosis of patients with a PID is critical for the implementation of treatment modalities that help decrease the morbidity and mortality of this fragile population. Once considered rare, it is estimated that about 1 in 1200 people are potentially living with a PID.[7,9] Despite the available resources, including access to a vast amount of electronic medical information, and evaluation resources, more than half of the individuals with a PID are not diagnosed until they are 30 years of age or older, with an average time of 12.4 years between onset of symptoms and diagnosis. A third of these patients developed permanent impairment of lung function at the time of diagnosis, and family history of PID was absent in up to 80% of the population (https://primaryimmune.org/wp-content/uploads/2011/04/Primary-Immunodeficiency-Diseases-in-America-2007The-Third-National-Survey-of-Patients.pdf). If a PID is suspected, screening tests should be performed and/or appropriate referral made. The importance of working with or referring the patient to an immunologist cannot be overemphasized, because more advanced testing, specialized treatments, as well as long-term follow-up is required. Likewise, the interpretation of some immunologic tests is not always straightforward.

In general, the immune evaluation of a child with a suspected PID is guided by the age, clinical presentation, organ system involvement, and specific pathogens if available. The diagnosis is often suggested by the clinical presentation or type of infectious microorganisms, but significant overlap may occur. A series of basic screening tests are available that facilitate ruling out or ruling in some of the previously discussed PIDs (**Table 1**). When indicated, both quantitative and qualitative tests are performed, because conducting only a quantitative evaluation may lead to underdiagnosis or overdiagnosis. For example, the presence of normal IgG levels does not always translate to a functional or protective immune response, and decreased IgG levels do not always translate to immunodeficiency.

Genetic testing using chromosomal microarray, gene panels, or whole-exome sequencing is being used with increased frequency in this patient population.[70] These tests are useful in confirming the diagnosis and outlining management in at least 40% of cases.[71]

SECONDARY IMMUNODEFICIENCIES

Overview

The malignancy, chemotherapy, or pretransplant and posttransplant drug regimens may alter the number and function of immune cells. Thrombocytopenia, mucositis, and injury to progenitor cells may delay healing and compromise the protective pulmonary epithelial barriers (**Box 1**). Moreover, alteration of normal pulmonary or extrapulmonary organ function may further impair host immune defenses and pulmonary function. These changes may result in immunodeficiency states functionally similar to the primary immunodeficiencies discussed earlier.

Pulmonary Complications of Pediatric Oncology and Cancer Therapy

Pulmonary complications of childhood cancers and cancer therapy may arise because of the primary malignancy itself, immunosuppression with secondary infections, or as complications of the cancer regimen (**Table 2**). These complications are discussed in detail in Lama Elbahlawan and colleagues' article, "Pulmonary Manifestations of Hematologic and Oncologic Diseases in Children," elsewhere in this issue.

Malignancies may have a myriad of effects on lung function. Space-occupying tumors may cause obstruction or compression of the superior vena cava (SVC), airways, or other mediastinal structures causing SVC or superior mediastinum syndromes resulting in respiratory distress. Likewise, SVC syndrome may also develop from thrombosis secondary to central lines, causing cough, hoarseness, dyspnea, orthopnea, chest pain, or syncope. Airway decompression may require surgery, radiation therapy, steroids, or use of alternate chemotherapeutic agents.[72]

Hyperleukocytosis syndrome (>100,000 cells/μL) may occur in 10% of nonlymphoblastic leukemias or CML generating hyperviscosity, which may damage the pulmonary microcirculation, causing pulmonary vascular injury, hypoxemia, and pulmonary hemorrhage.[73] Tumors within the thoracic or abdominal cavities or tumors involving the chest wall may impair the normal diaphragmatic excursion and chest wall motion, or decrease lung volume. Lung tumors may manifest as hemoptysis or postobstructive pneumonia. Extrinsic compression of an airway may occur because of tumor or adenopathy, causing stridor, wheezing, or postobstructive pneumonia. Secondary invasive solid tumors on either side of the diaphragm may lead to

Table 1
Laboratory evaluation for immunodeficiency

Quantitative	Functional	Comments
Humoral Evaluation		
Serum IgG, IgA, IgM	Vaccine titers to protein and polysaccharide antigens	May help exclude diseases such as IgAD, HIGM syndrome, CVID, XLA IgA level may be increased in the severe form of WAS, and decreased in AT
CD19 (B cells) by flow cytometry	—	CD19 cells absent in XLA and low or absent in CVID
Cellular Evaluation		
CBC with differential	—	Lymphopenia in SCIDS Decreased mean platelet volume in the severe form of WAS
NBS TCR excision circle	—	Diagnosis of SCIDS
PBL phenotyping by flow cytometry (eg, CD3, CD34CD8, CD19, CD16/56, CD45RA, CD45RO, HLADR)	Delayed hypersensitivity skin test (DHST) (eg, *Candida*, tetanus, PPD) or in vitro LP to mitogens and antigens	PBL phenotyping is used for the diagnosis of various PIDs based on the presence or absence of different cell subsets Both DHST and in vitro LP assays measure cell-mediated immunity DHST has variable sensitivity, not useful for infants or if negative In vitro LP lymphocytes with mitogens is useful in the diagnosis of SCIDS
Complement Defects Evaluation		
Individual components (eg, C2, C3, C4) C1 esterase inhibitor levels	Classic complement pathway hemolytic activity measuring 50% (CH50) or 100% RBC lysis (CH100) Alternative complement pathway hemolytic activity measuring 50% (AP50) or 100% RBC lysis (AP100) C1 esterase inhibitor functional assay	C2 deficiency is the most common complement defect C4 is always decreased in type I and II hereditary angioedema (C1-esterase inhibitor deficiency)

(*continued on next page*)

Table 1
(*continued*)

Quantitative	Functional	Comments
Phagocyte Defects Evaluation		
—	Dihydrorhodamine test or NBT	Abnormal in CGD
Cell surface expression of β2 integrin (CD18) by flow cytometry	—	Absent in leukocyte adhesion deficiency

Abbreviations: CBC, complete blood count; DHST, delayed hypersensitivity skin testing; LP, lymphoproliferation; PBL, peripheral blood lymphocytes; RBC, red blood cell; CH50, complement hemolytic activity causing 50% lysis of treated sheep red blood cells; CH100, complement hemolytic activity causing 100% lysis of treated sheep red blood cells; AP50, alternative complement pathway hemolytic activity causing lysis of 50% treated sheep red blood cells; AP100, alternative complement pathway hemolytic activity causing lysis of 50% treated sheep red blood cells; NBT, nitroblue tetrazolium- a measure of cells ability to produce reactive oxygen species; PPD, purified protein deriviaive of mycobacterium tuberculosis.

pulmonary impairment and restrictive lung disease. In addition, altered control of ventilation may result from intracranial tumors, manifesting as central apnea or hypoventilation.[74,75]

Chemotherapeutic agents and/or radiation therapy may lead to both infectious (caused by immunosuppression) and noninfectious pulmonary complications.[74,76,77] Radiation therapy, cancer chemotherapy, and immunosuppressive agents may directly damage the lung by disrupting the epithelial barriers or altering the host primary defenses.[1] Moreover, they may lead to secondary organ dysfunction (kidney, liver, heart), which may alter normal pulmonary function or predispose to pneumonia (see **Box 1**, **Table 2**).

Complications of chemotherapy and radiation therapy may occur early or late in the course of treatment. Early-onset consequences include bronchospasm, hypersensitivity reactions, and pulmonary edema. With improved survival from malignancies, more children are presenting with late pulmonary complications of their therapies. Pulmonary injury may express as diffuse alveolar damage, interstitial disease, and obliterative bronchiolitis (bronchiolitis obliterans syndrome [BOS]) with resultant obstructive or restrictive lung disease, decreased exercise tolerance, and need for supplemental O_2 therapy. In addition, radiation therapy to the lungs, mediastinal structures, and vertebrae may cause abnormal growth of the chest cavity.[75]

Pulmonary infections are common complications of cancer therapies. The magnitude and duration of the neutropenia determine the risk of infection (see **Table 2**). Moreover, chemotherapy may alter neutrophil function or cause breakdown of mucosal barriers that allows microbial invasion[78] (see **Box 1**). Alkylating agents, purine analogues, and newer monoclonal antibody regimens may cause prolonged, severe, multilineage cytopenias that weaken immunity.[79] Infections often arise from normal skin or mucosal bacterial flora. Opportunistic infections may occur secondary to reduced cellular defenses.

Transplant-Related Pulmonary Complications

Transplant has become the curative treatment of organ failure and for several malignancies, hematologic conditions, and immunodeficiency diseases.

Box 1

Factors predisposing to infection and pulmonary complications following treatment of cancer, organ transplant and subsequent immunosuppression

Underlying disease
- Alteration in cellular immunity, or phagocytic cell number, or function secondary to the underlying disease, malignancy, or autoimmune state

Change in physical barriers
- Breakdown in the physical barriers caused by mucositis, defective healing
- Effects of chemotherapy
- Graft-versus-host disease
- New routes of entry (intravenous catheters, shunts, drains)

Prolonged or recurrent use of broad-spectrum antibiotic, antifungal, or antiviral therapies for acute infections or prophylaxis
- Alteration of resident normal microbiota that allows secondary bacterial or fungal overgrowth
- Selection for drug-resistant pathogens
- Environmental effects (selection of resistant organisms in the hospital unit/home environment)

Quantitative defects in normal circulating or resident immune cells caused by underlying disease or suppressive therapy
- Neutropenia
- Lymphopenia
- Thrombocytopenia
- Macrophage deficiency

Qualitative defects and functional abnormalities in immune cells
- Neutrophil and macrophage migration defects or abnormal phagocytosis/cell killing
- Lymphocytes: defective antibody production and dysfunction of cytotoxic cells

Defective function of respiratory muscles or thoracic cage, or development of scoliosis caused by space-occupying tumors, radiation therapy, or surgery impairing cough and airway clearance

Surgery and complications
- Strictures or denervation
- Drains and catheters
- Wound dehiscence

Extrapulmonary organ dysfunction
- Liver, heart, or renal failure caused by primary disease or secondary to toxicities of medications

Other underlying disease
- Diabetes, chronic obstructive pulmonary disease

Nutritional defects caused by inability to feed or absorb feeding: mucositis, feeding intolerance
- Deficiencies in vitamins, iron, essential fatty acids
- Synthetic defects caused by liver or renal dysfunction
- Catabolic state/defective wound healing

Infectious risks
- Colonization of skin or mucosal surfaces
- Persistent or latent viral infections in the recipient (EBV, CMV, herpes simplex virus, herpesvirus 6)
- Latent infection in transplanted organs or blood products
- Infected blood products
- Extent of preexisting immunity caused by immunization or prior infection of the patient
- Acute infections acquired from donor organs or blood products
- Risk of exposure to community-acquired infections

Table 2
Pulmonary complications of primary immunodeficiency, malignancy, transplant, and immune-suppressive therapies

Complications of the Underlying Disease or Immunosuppressive Therapy	Infectious Complications	Noninfectious Complications
Complications of immunodeficiency state Immunosuppression (related to primary neoplasm or secondary to chemotherapy or radiation therapy) Pulmonary invasion by tumor Airway obstruction Leukemia and lymphomatous involvement with: Leukostasis Leukemic cell lysis Hyperleukocytic reaction Pulmonary hemorrhage Altered ventilation, apnea or hypoventilation Hypoxemia, hypercapnia Poor airway clearance (inefficient cough)	Bacterial infection: Encapsulated organisms Sometimes unusual infections (*Burkholderia cepacia, P aeruginosa*) Viruses: Community-acquired viruses Latent or persistent viruses Fungi: Invasive: (*Aspergillus, Candida, Nocardia*) Environmental: (*Histoplasma, Blastomyces, Coccidioides*) *Pneumocystis jiroveci* Mycobacteria: (*Mycobacterium tuberculosis* and atypical mycobacteria)	Alveolar hemorrhage Superior vena cava syndrome or superior mediastinal syndrome Drug reactions Secondary neoplasms Pulmonary embolism Pulmonary edema (primary pulmonary or caused by heart, renal, or liver dysfunction) Airway obstruction caused by mucositis, lymphadenopathy, or infection ARDS, acute lung injury ILD Interstitial pneumonitis (drug or radiation induced) Obliterative bronchiolitis Graft-vs-host disease Bronchiectasis Transplant rejection

Immunosuppression requires a balance between the need to prevent allograft rejection and preserve organ function, and the cost of leaving the organ recipient susceptible to infection or organ dysfunction[79] (see **Box 1**). Comorbid conditions (preexisting or secondary to the transplant or immunosuppressive agents) may further increase susceptibility to infectious or noninfectious complications (see **Table 2**). It is often difficult to differentiate noninfectious from the infectious complications in immunosuppressed patients without careful investigation.

Transplant rejection is mediated primarily by T cells, although B cell–mediated antibody production plays a role in hyperacute rejection. The immunosuppressive agents are frequently used in combination with different specificities for target cell types or subtypes, or cellular signaling pathways.[79] In addition to their immunosuppressive effects, cyclosporin and tacrolimus may have significant renal side effects that may result in fluid retention and pulmonary edema. Mycophenolate mofetil has fewer renal complications but may cause bone marrow suppression that increases the risk of infection. Monoclonal antibodies such as basiliximab or daclizumab may allow decreased doses of cyclosporine or tacrolimus and thus decrease potential renal toxicity.

Solid organ transplants

Infectious complications of solid organ transplant typically occur in a predictable temporal pattern.[80] Prophylactic regimens have been developed to prevent infections based on these patterns[78] (eg, use of prophylaxis for *P jiroveci* and CMV). Latent viral or fungal infections (latent in the host or in the donated organ) occur early following transplant. Portopulmonary hypertension, pulmonary hypertension, and hepatopulmonary syndrome may occur in children with liver failure and should be considered in children with otherwise unexplained hypoxemia after transplant.[79]

Lung transplant

Lung transplant presents a unique set of problems for immunosuppression in the transplanted organ (prevention of rejection vs risk of infection) in part because the transplanted lung is an interface between the outside environment and the host defenses.[1] A defect in pulmonary host defenses may result in an increased susceptibility to infection or increased propensity to inflammation that may lead to rejection manifested as graft-versus-host disease (GvHD), or development of obliterative bronchiolitis.[81] Local damage to the lung defenses further contributes to propensity to infection: denervation of the transplanted organ results in decreased cough reflexes; ischemic injury to the mucosa disrupts the mucociliary transport; the anastomosis site may develop strictures, impaired airway clearance, and airway obstruction.[82] Infectious agents may be passively transferred from the donor to the recipient. Early deaths following transplant result from graft failure, infection, technical issues, and multiorgan dysfunction. Infectious complications result in significant morbidity and mortality, accounting for almost 50% of the deaths.[83] Beyond 1 year posttransplant, obliterative bronchiolitis, chronic rejection,[84] and posttransplant lymphoproliferative disease (PTLD) are the main causes of morbidity and mortality. Allograft rejection is less common in children than in adults; however, surveillance and timely and accurate diagnosis of rejection may be both more important and more difficult in children because of the frequency of viral respiratory infections in this age group.

Hematopoietic stem cell transplant

HSCT presents an even greater challenge to lung defenses (see **Box 1**, **Table 2**). Several factors may contribute to the severe and sustained immunocompromise in HSCT recipients (discussed in Lama Elbahlawan and colleagues' article, "Pulmonary Manifestations of Hematologic and Oncologic Diseases in Children," elsewhere in this issue). Immune deficits result in the high frequency of life-threatening bacterial, viral, and opportunistic infections in HSCT recipients.[85] Noninfectious complications may also cause significant morbidity and mortality in these patients[86] (see **Box 1**, **Table 2**).

Post-HSCT complications occur in predictable temporal patterns.[85,86] This sequence of the immunologic recovery and immunosuppressive therapy results in the susceptibility to infectious and noninfectious complications that occur in HSCT recipients.[85,86] During the preengraftment phase, patients are most susceptible to bacterial and viral infections. After neutrophil recovery (postengraftment phase), T-cell and B-cell immunity remains abnormal, predisposing the patient to infections with fungi, viruses, mycobacteria, and parasites. Patients remain susceptible to encapsulated organisms because of inability to generate specific antibody responses. The development of GvHD further increases the risk of infection, in part because of treatment with corticosteroids and other immunosuppressive agents, and disruption of mucosal barriers.[1,87]

Noninfectious complications following HSCT include airway obstruction by mucositis, pulmonary edema, diffuse alveolar hemorrhage, and pulmonary embolism. Chronic obstructive pulmonary disease may be detected in up to 20% of long-term survivors of HSCT, usually resulting from GvHD, preparative regimen, and infection.[85]

Late-onset pulmonary disease includes BOS, COP,[86] diffuse alveolar damage, and interstitial pneumonia.[86] BOS is diagnosed in lung biopsy specimens by the characteristic histopathologic changes: peribronchiolar fibrosis and varying degrees of intraluminal fibrous obliteration with circumferential narrowing of the terminal bronchioles.[88] In the absence of lung biopsy, BOS may be diagnosed clinically based on the 2014 NIH chronic GvHD consensus scoring.[89] These criteria include decrease in forced expiratory volume in 1 second, increase in residual Volume (RV) and RV/Total Lung Capacity (TLC) (evidence of obstructive airway changes), reduction in distance walked in 6-minute walk test, air trapping or bronchiectasis on computed tomography (CT), and worsening in symptom severity score.[89,90] In children, these pulmonary function changes may not always indicate BOS requiring biopsy for definitive diagnosis.[91] The patterns of histopathology and abnormal airway physiology are similar in BOS associated with HSCT and lung transplant recipients.[88]

PTLD is often associated with T-cell dysfunction in the presence of EBV-infected B cells.[92] The mean interval to its development is 5 to 6 months posttransplant, with a cumulative incidence of 1% to 20% at 10 years. Several factors contribute to the risk of PTLD, including the age of the recipient, type of transplant and preparative regimen, and the ongoing immunosuppressive therapy.[92] PTLD is one of the most severe complications of solid organ transplant and HSCT.[92] Treatment includes a reduction in immunosuppression and the use of rituximab (anti-CD20 monoclonal antibody).

INFECTIONS IN IMMUNODEFICIENCY STATES

Immunodeficiency states (primary or secondary) may increase the susceptibility of the child to respiratory infections. Specific pathogens of concern in this population are discussed next.

Viral Infections

Respiratory viral infections pose a particular challenge to immunodeficient and immunocompromised patients and cause significant morbidity and mortality[93] (**Table 3**). Vaccines and effective antiviral agents are available for few of these viruses. Common childhood infections (eg, RSV, varicella) may be life threatening in immunodeficient or immunocompromised children.[79,80] Early diagnosis is essential for limiting the morbidity and mortality caused by influenza and RSV. Because patients with viral infections shed virus longer and have higher viral titers than immunocompetent hosts, prolonged courses of treatment may be necessary. Multiplex real-time polymerase chain reaction (PCR) or enzyme immunoassays (enzyme-linked immunosorbent assay) are frequently used to detect respiratory viruses.[89] Quantitative PCR is used to identify and quantify CMV and EBV infections[94] (see **Table 3**).

Fungal Infections

Invasive fungal disease is associated with significant morbidity and mortality in immunocompromised or immunosuppressed patients.[65,95] Invasive infections (eg, *Aspergillus*, *Candida*, *Mucor*) often occur in hospitalized patients; however, environmental fungi may cause significant respiratory disease[65,95–97] (see **Table 3**). Early detection of invasive fungal disease is critical because outcomes depend on early and appropriate antifungal therapy (see **Table 3**). Despite the development of potent antifungal agents, mortality associated with fungal infections remains high. *P jiroveci* pneumonia is discussed in Lama Elbahlawan and colleagues' article, "Pulmonary Manifestations of Hematologic and Oncologic Diseases in Children," elsewhere in this issue.

Table 3
Viral and fungal disease in immunocompromised or immunodeficient children

	Clinical Picture	Diagnosis
Viruses		
AV, BV, CV, IV, hMPV, hPIV, RSV, RV	Pneumonia, bronchitis, bronchiolitis Upper respiratory infection	PCR, culture, EIA
CMV	Pneumonia, disseminated disease	PCR, cytology, culture
EBV	Range of disease: reactive interstitial disease to lymphoma	PCR, EBV cytotoxic T cell, EBV PCR (quantitative)
Fungus		
A fumigatus	Colonization tracheobronchitis Pulmonary aspergillosis	Culture, histopathology, serum galactomannan, BAL galactomannan Blood or sputum PCR
Candida albicans	Sepsis, disseminated disease, reticulonodular disease or ground-glass opacities on CXR	Blood, respiratory cultures β (1→3) D-glucan (nonspecific)
Mucor	Rhinopulmonary disease, angioinvasive Parenchymal abscess or nodules Upper lobes	Histopathology
P jiroveci	Hypoxemia, interstitial pneumonia Ground-glass opacities on CT	Microscopic evaluation BAL with staining, indirect immunofluorescence, PCR
Endemic Fungi		
Histoplasma	Disseminated disease Multiorgan involvement	Histoplasma antigen urine or serum Histoplasma serology
Coccidioides	Dyspnea, CXR similar to bacterial pneumonia	Culture, cytology Antigen detection blood, BAL
Blastomyces	Diffuse pneumonia	Culture, cytology, serum antibody Urine testing for blastomyces adhesion-1 antigen

Abbreviations: AV, adenovirus; BV, bocavirus; CV, coronavirus; CXR, chest radiograph; EIA, enzyme immunoassay; hMPV, human metapneumovirus; hPIV, human parainfluenza virus; IV, influenza virus; PCR, polymerase chain reaction.

Mycobacterial Infections

Immunodeficiency or immunosuppressive therapies may alter T-cell number or function, predisposing to infection by intracellular pathogens, including mycobacteria. The gold standard for identification of *Mycobacterium tuberculosis* (MTB) and the nontuberculous mycobacteria (NTM) remains the culture of clinical specimens. In immunocompromised patients, interferon-γ blood tests (interferon-γ release assays) have greater sensitivity and specificity than tuberculin skin testing, but may have false-negative results in nearly 40% of patients, particularly in patients with low CD4 T-cell counts.[98] However, neither can distinguish infection from disease.

PCR-based molecular methods such as Xpert MTB/RIF (Xpert Ultra, endorsed by the World Health Organization since 2010) have improved the tuberculosis diagnostic time and detection of rifampicin resistance using a combination of specimens (induced sputum with 3%–5% hypertonic saline, even in young infants, and nasopharyngeal samples), with almost 90% sensitivity against a gold standard of culture-confirmed disease with high specificity.[99,100]

Published guidelines for the identification and treatment of *M tuberculosis* and NTM primarily focus on infection in immunocompetent patients.[101] There are few evidence-based recommendations to guide the treatment of immunocompromised patients.[102,103]

DIAGNOSIS AND TREATMENT OF RESPIRATORY ABNORMALITIES IN IMMUNOINCOMPETENT OR IMMUNOSUPPRESSED CHILDREN

In children with suspected immune defects, the medical history, physical examination, and routine microbial surveillance are important first steps to identify the source of complications. Timing of the symptoms relative to drug therapies or changes in immunosuppressive agents could point to the infection or noninfectious complications. There is an improved likelihood of patient recovery if the cause is identified early so the lung findings and aggressive diagnostic studies are warranted.

Diagnostic Imaging and Pulmonary Function Testing

Pulmonary changes on chest radiographs may be delayed or modified in immunocompromised patients because of the inability to generate a local inflammatory response. They remain valuable to detect pulmonary disorder.[76,77,96] Changes in pulmonary function tests that suggest developing restrictive or obstructive lung disease or diffusion defects may indicate the development of acute or chronic rejection. CT scans are helpful in assessing for changes associated with rejection. However, lung biopsy remains the most accurate diagnostic tool for acute and chronic rejection.[91] Chest CT is particularly useful when the chest radiograph is negative or when findings on chest radiographs are nonspecific. Moreover, it is useful in defining areas of lung involvement to target invasive studies (biopsy, BAL). Spiral CT angiograms and ventilation/perfusion studies may be diagnostic if pulmonary thromboembolism is a consideration. High-resolution CT showing a mosaic pattern of patchy hyperinflation and hypoattenuation may be suggestive of BOS.[76,77,96]

Culture and Special Stains for Pulmonary Pathogens

Spontaneous or induced sputum samples may provide valuable information to diagnose bacterial and fungal causes of pulmonary infiltrates. In addition, nasal aspirates are studied by rapid and specific PCR techniques to identify common viral respiratory pathogens[93] (see **Table 3**).

Serum and Urine Studies

Blood cultures may identify disseminated bacterial and fungal infections. Detection of galactomannan in blood or BAL is highly suggestive of invasive *Aspergillus*. Measurement of (1-3)-β-D-glucan is a nonspecific test that may suggest several invasive organisms, including *Aspergillus* and *Candida*. Urine antigen studies for *Histoplasma* and *Blastomyces* may suggest active infection by endemic fungi.

Flexible Bronchoscopy with Bronchoalveolar Lavage

Flexible fiberoptic bronchoscopy with BAL or with transbronchial biopsy are useful tools for diagnosing pulmonary complications in immunocompromised patients.[104] BAL may provide specimens for culture, cytology, PCR, and immunohistochemistry. Bronchoscopy may identify endobronchial obstruction caused by infection or tumor. Protected brush specimens may decrease contamination of the lower respiratory samples from upper airway bacteria or fungi acquired passing the scope through the nasopharynx. Cytologic stains or PCR may detect pathogens such as *P jiroveci* and mycobacteria. Invasive pathogens (*Aspergillus*, *Mucor*) may be detectable only by biopsy; however, analysis of BAL samples for fungal antigens [galactomannan or (1-3)-β-D-glucan] may increase the detection of potential infection by *A fumigatus* and *Candida albicans*, respectively (see **Table 3**). The presence of blood in BAL fluid may suggest pulmonary hemorrhage, possibly related to diffuse alveolar hemorrhage, or mucormycosis[85,86] (see **Table 3**). Several novel methods have been developed to improve the BAL diagnostic yield (eg, multiplex PCR and metagenomic next-generation sequencing assays).

Lung Biopsy

Transbronchial lung biopsies may be diagnostic of lung disorders,[104] but may be difficult to perform in young children because of the bronchoscope size, the airway size, and the lack of biopsy instruments that can pass through the small suction channel (1.2 mm) of the pediatric bronchoscope. Small adult bronchoscopes are used in older/larger children because the larger suction channel (2 mm) allows passage of biopsy instruments. Biopsy samples may help identify invasive pathogens undetectable by BAL (eg, invasive *Aspergillus* or *Mucor*),[105] in addition to detecting ILD, acute rejection (lung transplant), GvHD, and BOS in HSCT and lung transplant patients.[104] However, because of the small sample size and sampling error, open lung biopsy (OLB) may be necessary to identify the cause of the lung disorder.

Needle lung biopsy under CT or fluoroscopic guidance may have high yield for peripheral lung lesions (particularly suspected fungal lesions) that cannot be reached with flexible fiberoptic bronchoscopy. The major risks associated with transthoracic biopsy are pneumothorax and bleeding. In addition, because of the small needle size, sampling error may occur with this procedure.

OLB remains the gold standard for diagnosis of pulmonary abnormalities in immunocompromised patient. It allows the surgeon to visualize and select optimal sites for biopsy and to obtain adequate quantities of lung tissue for analysis. The use of mini-thoracotomy or video-assisted thoracoscopic surgery allows a smaller incision and faster recovery. Although OLB provides the most definitive information in immunocompromised patients, timing of the biopsies and the potential need for repeated biopsies (particularly if lung rejection, GvHD, or obliterative bronchiolitis are considerations) limit the use of repeated open biopsy.

SUMMARY

Pulmonary symptoms and pulmonary complications in immunodeficient or immunocompromised patients may be diagnostic challenges for clinicians. The immunologic defects resulting from primary immunodeficiencies or immunosuppression may predispose to lung infection in patients with primary or secondary T-cell defects, or immunosuppressed patients following transplant. Infectious and noninfectious complications may be difficult to differentiate. Clinicians caring for these patients must maintain a high index of suspicion for both infectious and noninfectious pulmonary complications and have a thorough approach in the evaluation of these complex patients. Input from pulmonology and immunology specialists is essential for the diagnosis and care of these complex patients.

CLINICAL CARE POINTS

- Primary immunodeficiencies are relatively common (estimated 1/1200 worldwide) and must be considered in children with unusual or unexplained pulmonary infections, inflammatory processes, structural abnormalities or malignancies.
- More than half of individuals with primary immunodeficiencies are not diagnosed until they are 30 years of age or older- one third of these have developed permanent impairment of lung function at the time of diagnosis.
- Malignancy, chemotherapy, or pre-transplant and post-transplant drug regimens can result in alterations in pulmonary function and predispose to secondary immunodeficiencies.
- Primary and secondary immunodeficiencies can predispose to both infectious and noninfectious pulmonary complications that require thorough investigation and may be difficult to distinguish.
- PCR based diagnostic studies improve the time to diagnosis and the diagnostic accuracy for many primary immunodeficiencies and many infectious agents found in patients with primary and secondary immunodeficiencies.

DISCLOSURE

The authors have nothing to disclose.

REFERENCES

1. Smith KG, Kamdar AA, Stark JM. Lung Defenses: Intrinsic, Innate, and Adaptive. In: Wilmott R, Deterding R, Li A, et al, editors. Kendig's disorders of the respiratory tract in children. 9 edition. Philadelphia: Elsevier; 2019. p. 120–33.
2. Baumann U, Routes JM, Soler-Palacin P, et al. The Lung in Primary Immunodeficiencies: New Concepts in Infection and Inflammation. Front Immunol 2018;9: 1837.
3. Sato S, Kiyono H. The mucosal immune system of the respiratory tract. Curr Opin Virol 2012;2(3):225–32.
4. Reynolds HY, Newball HH. Analysis of proteins and respiratory cells obtained from human lungs by bronchial lavage. J Lab Clin Med 1974;84(4):559–73.
5. Reynolds HY. Immunoglobulin G and its function in the human respiratory tract. Mayo Clin Proc 1988;63(2):161–74.
6. Siber GR, Schur PH, Aisenberg AC, et al. Correlation between serum IgG-2 concentrations and the antibody response to bacterial polysaccharide antigens. N Engl J Med 1980;303(4):178–82.
7. Tangye SG, Al-Herz W, Bousfiha A, et al. Human Inborn Errors of Immunity: 2019 Update on the Classification from the International Union of Immunological Societies Expert Committee. J Clin Immunol 2020;40(1):24–64.
8. Patrawala M, Cui Y, Peng L, et al. Pulmonary Disease Burden in Primary Immune Deficiency Disorders: Data from USIDNET Registry. J Clin Immunol 2020;40(2): 340–9.

9. Bousfiha AA, Jeddane L, Ailal F, et al. A phenotypic approach for IUIS PID classification and diagnosis: guidelines for clinicians at the bedside. J Clin Immunol 2013;33(6):1078–87.
10. Yazdani R, Abolhassani H, Asgardoon MH, et al. Infectious and Noninfectious Pulmonary Complications in Patients With Primary Immunodeficiency Disorders. J Investig Allergol Clin Immunol 2017;27(4):213–24.
11. Quinn J, Orange JS, Modell V, et al. The case for severe combined immunodeficiency (SCID) and T cell lymphopenia newborn screening: saving lives...one at a time. Immunol Res 2020;68(1):48–53.
12. Kwan A, Puck JM. History and current status of newborn screening for severe combined immunodeficiency. Semin Perinatol 2015;39(3):194–205.
13. Booth C, Algar VE, Xu-Bayford J, et al. Non-infectious lung disease in patients with adenosine deaminase deficient severe combined immunodeficiency. J Clin Immunol 2012;32(3):449–53.
14. Grunebaum E, Cutz E, Roifman CM. Pulmonary alveolar proteinosis in patients with adenosine deaminase deficiency. J Allergy Clin Immunol 2012;129(6): 1588–93.
15. Flinn AM, Gennery AR. Adenosine deaminase deficiency: a review. Orphanet J Rare Dis 2018;13(1):65.
16. Speckmann C, Neumann C, Borte S, et al. Delayed-onset adenosine deaminase deficiency: strategies for an early diagnosis. J Allergy Clin Immunol 2012; 130(4):991–4.
17. Leven EA, Maffucci P, Ochs HD, et al. Hyper IgM Syndrome: a Report from the USIDNET Registry. J Clin Immunol 2016;36(5):490–501.
18. Nicolaides RE, de la Morena MT. Inherited and acquired clinical phenotypes associated with neuroendocrine tumors. Curr Opin Allergy Clin Immunol 2017; 17(6):431–42.
19. Winkelstein JA, Marino MC, Ochs H, et al. The X-linked hyper-IgM syndrome: clinical and immunologic features of 79 patients. Medicine (Baltimore) 2003; 82(6):373–84.
20. de la Morena MT. Clinical Phenotypes of Hyper-IgM Syndromes. J Allergy Clin Immunol Pract 2016;4(6):1023–36.
21. Maggadottir SM, Sullivan KE. The diverse clinical features of chromosome 22q11.2 deletion syndrome (DiGeorge syndrome). J Allergy Clin Immunol Pract 2013;1(6):589–94.
22. Gennery AR. Immunological aspects of 22q11.2 deletion syndrome. Cell Mol Life Sci 2012;69(1):17–27.
23. Jones JW, Tracy M, Perryman M, et al. Airway Anomalies in Patients With 22q11.2 Deletion Syndrome: A 5-Year Review. Ann Otol Rhinol Laryngol 2018; 127(6):384–9.
24. Candotti F. Clinical Manifestations and Pathophysiological Mechanisms of the Wiskott-Aldrich Syndrome. J Clin Immunol 2018;38(1):13–27.
25. Bhatt JM, Bush A, van Gerven M, et al. ERS statement on the multidisciplinary respiratory management of ataxia telangiectasia. Eur Respir Rev 2015;24(138): 565–81.
26. Wong MT, Schölvinck EH, Lambeck AJ, et al. CHARGE syndrome: a review of the immunological aspects. Eur J Hum Genet 2015;23(11):1451–9.
27. Blake KD, Prasad C. CHARGE syndrome. Orphanet J Rare Dis 2006;1:34.
28. Dalm VASH, Driessen GJA, Barendregt BH, et al. The 11q Terminal Deletion Disorder Jacobsen Syndrome is a Syndromic Primary Immunodeficiency. J Clin Immunol 2015;35(8):761–8.

29. van der Crabben SN, Hennus MP, McGregor GA, et al. Destabilized SMC5/6 complex leads to chromosome breakage syndrome with severe lung disease. J Clin Invest 2016;126(8):2881–92.
30. Freeman AF, Olivier KN. Hyper-IgE Syndromes and the Lung. Clin Chest Med 2016;37(3):557–67.
31. Al-Shaikhly T, Ochs HD. Hyper IgE syndromes: clinical and molecular characteristics. Immunol Cell Biol 2019;97(4):368–79.
32. Fete T. Respiratory problems in patients with ectodermal dysplasia syndromes. Am J Med Genet A 2014;164a(10):2478–81.
33. Bonilla FA, Khan DA, Ballas ZK, et al. Practice parameter for the diagnosis and management of primary immunodeficiency. J Allergy Clin Immunol 2015;136(5): 1186–205.e1-8.
34. Geha RS, Notarangelo LD, Casanova JL, et al. Primary immunodeficiency diseases: an update from the International Union of Immunological Societies Primary Immunodeficiency Diseases Classification Committee. J Allergy Clin Immunol 2007;120(4):776–94.
35. Janzi M, Kull I, Sjoberg R, et al. Selective IgA deficiency in early life: association to infections and allergic diseases during childhood. Clin Immunol 2009;133(1): 78–85.
36. Cunningham-Rundles C. Physiology of IgA and IgA deficiency. J Clin Immunol 2001;21(5):303–9.
37. Yel L. Selective IgA deficiency. J Clin Immunol 2010;30(1):10–6.
38. Bruton OC. Agammaglobulinemia. Pediatrics 1952;9(6):722–8.
39. Plebani A, Lougaris V. Agammaglobulinemia. In: Sullivan K, Striehm ER, editors. Stiehm's immune deficiencies. First Edition. Cambridge (MA): Academic Press; 2014. p. 329–46. Chapter 13.
40. Plebani A, Soresina A, Rondelli R, et al. Clinical, immunological, and molecular analysis in a large cohort of patients with X-linked agammaglobulinemia: an Italian multicenter study. Clin Immunol 2002;104(3):221–30.
41. Conley ME, Howard V. Clinical findings leading to the diagnosis of X-linked agammaglobulinemia. J Pediatr 2002;141(4):566–71.
42. Jongco AM, Gough JD, Sarnataro K, et al. X-linked agammaglobulinemia presenting as polymicrobial pneumonia, including Pneumocystis jirovecii. Ann Allergy Asthma Immunol 2014;112(1):74–5.e2.
43. Cunningham-Rundles C. The many faces of common variable immunodeficiency. Hematol Am Soc Hematol Educ Program 2012;2012:301–5.
44. Bonilla FA, Barlan I, Chapel H, et al. International Consensus Document (ICON): Common Variable Immunodeficiency Disorders. J Allergy Clin Immunol Pract 2016;4(1):38–59.
45. Maglione PJ, Overbey JR, Cunningham-Rundles C. Progression of Common Variable Immunodeficiency Interstitial Lung Disease Accompanies Distinct Pulmonary and Laboratory Findings. J Allergy Clin Immunol Pract 2015;3(6): 941–50.
46. Hurst JR, Warnatz K. Interstitial lung disease in primary immunodeficiency: towards a brighter future. Eur Respir J 2020;55(4):2000089.
47. Rao N, Mackinnon AC, Routes JM. Granulomatous and lymphocytic interstitial lung disease: a spectrum of pulmonary histopathologic lesions in common variable immunodeficiency–histologic and immunohistochemical analyses of 16 cases. Hum Pathol 2015;46(9):1306–14.

48. Sood AK, Funkhouser W, Handly B, et al. Granulomatous-Lymphocytic Interstitial Lung Disease in 22q11.2 Deletion Syndrome: a Case Report and Literature Review. Curr Allergy Asthma Rep 2018;18(3):14.
49. Janssen LMA, Macken T, Creemers MCW, et al. Truly selective primary IgM deficiency is probably very rare. Clin Exp Immunol 2018;191(2):203–11.
50. Gupta S, Gupta A. Selective IgM Deficiency-An Underestimated Primary Immunodeficiency. Front Immunol 2017;8:1056.
51. Sorensen RU, Edgar D. Specific Antibody Deficiencies in Clinical Practice. J Allergy Clin Immunol Pract 2019;7(3):801–8.
52. Perez E, Bonilla FA, Orange JS, et al. Specific Antibody Deficiency: Controversies in Diagnosis and Management. Front Immunol 2017;8:586.
53. Ogier de Baulny H, Schiff M, Dionisi-Vici C. Lysinuric protein intolerance (LPI): a multi organ disease by far more complex than a classic urea cycle disorder. Mol Genet Metab 2012;106(1):12–7.
54. Bowman SL, Bi-Karchin J, Le L, et al. The road to lysosome-related organelles: Insights from Hermansky-Pudlak syndrome and other rare diseases. Traffic 2019;20(6):404–35.
55. Field NS, Moser EK, Oliver PM. Itch regulation of innate and adaptive immune responses in mice and humans. J Leukoc Biol 2020;108(1):353–62.
56. Marciano BE, Spalding C, Fitzgerald A, et al. Common severe infections in chronic granulomatous disease. Clin Infect Dis 2015;60(8):1176–83.
57. Henrickson SE, Jongco AM, Thomsen KF, et al. Noninfectious Manifestations and Complications of Chronic Granulomatous Disease. J Pediatr Infect Dis Soc 2018;7(suppl_1):S18–24.
58. Harris ES, Weyrich AS, Zimmerman GA. Lessons from rare maladies: leukocyte adhesion deficiency syndromes. Curr Opin Hematol 2013;20(1):16–25.
59. Almarza Novoa E, Kasbekar S, Thrasher AJ, et al. Leukocyte adhesion deficiency-I: A comprehensive review of all published cases. J Allergy Clin Immunol Pract 2018;6(4):1418–20.e10.
60. Sorio C, Montresor A, Bolomini-Vittori M, et al. Mutations of Cystic Fibrosis Transmembrane Conductance Regulator Gene Cause a Monocyte-Selective Adhesion Deficiency. Am J Respir Crit Care Med 2016;193(10):1123–33.
61. Trapnell BC, Nakata K, Bonella F, et al. Pulmonary alveolar proteinosis. Nat Rev Dis Primers 2019;5(1):16.
62. Drummond RA, Franco LM, Lionakis MS. Human CARD9: A Critical Molecule of Fungal Immune Surveillance. Front Immunol 2018;9:1836.
63. von Bernuth H, Picard C, Puel A, et al. Experimental and natural infections in MyD88- and IRAK-4-deficient mice and humans. Eur J Immunol 2012;42(12):3126–35.
64. Dias Junior AG, Sampaio NG, Rehwinkel J. A Balancing Act: MDA5 in Antiviral Immunity and Autoinflammation. Trends Microbiol 2019;27(1):75–85.
65. Tissot F, Agrawal S, Pagano L, et al. ECIL-6 guidelines for the treatment of invasive candidiasis, aspergillosis and mucormycosis in leukemia and hematopoietic stem cell transplant patients. Haematologica 2017;102(3):433–44.
66. Ricklin D, Hajishengallis G, Yang K, et al. Complement: a key system for immune surveillance and homeostasis. Nat Immunol 2010;11(9):785–97.
67. Schröder-Braunstein J, Kirschfink M. Complement deficiencies and dysregulation: Pathophysiological consequences, modern analysis, and clinical management. Mol Immunol 2019;114:299–311.

68. Maurer M, Magerl M, Ansotegui I, et al. The international WAO/EAACI guideline for the management of hereditary angioedema-The 2017 revision and update. Allergy 2018;73(8):1575–96.
69. Tangye SG, Al-Herz W, Bousfiha A, et al. Correction to: Human Inborn Errors of Immunity: 2019 Update on the Classification from the International Union of Immunological Societies Expert Committee. J Clin Immunol 2020;40(1):65.
70. Heimall JR, Hagin D, Hajjar J, et al. Use of Genetic Testing for Primary Immunodeficiency Patients. J Clin Immunol 2018;38(3):320–9.
71. Quinn J, Modell V, Holle J, et al. Jeffrey's insights: Jeffrey Modell Foundation's global genetic sequencing pilot program to identify specific primary immunodeficiency defects to optimize disease management and treatment. Immunol Res 2020;68(3):126–34.
72. Nossair F, Schoettler P, Starr J, et al. Pediatric superior vena cava syndrome: An evidence-based systematic review of the literature. Pediatr Blood Cancer 2018; 65(9):e27225.
73. Ruggiero A, Rizzo D, Amato M, et al. Management of Hyperleukocytosis. Curr Treat Options Oncol 2016;17(2):7.
74. Josephson MB, Goldfarb SB. Pulmonary complications of childhood cancers. Expert Rev Respir Med 2014;8(5):561–71.
75. Versluys AB, Bresters D. Pulmonary Complications of Childhood Cancer Treatment. Paediatr Respir Rev 2016;17:63–70.
76. Chavhan GB, Babyn PS, Nathan PC, et al. Imaging of acute and subacute toxicities of cancer therapy in children. Pediatr Radiol 2016;46(1):9–20 [quiz: 26–8].
77. Shelmerdine SC, Chavhan GB, Babyn PS, et al. Imaging of late complications of cancer therapy in children. Pediatr Radiol 2017;47(3):254–66.
78. Knackstedt ED, Danziger-Isakov L. Infections in pediatric solid-organ transplant recipients. Semin Pediatr Surg 2017;26(4):199–205.
79. Blondet NM, Healey PJ, Hsu E. Immunosuppression in the pediatric transplant recipient. Semin Pediatr Surg 2017;26(4):193–8.
80. Duncan MD, Wilkes DS. Transplant-related immunosuppression: a review of immunosuppression and pulmonary infections. Proc Am Thorac Soc 2005; 2(5):449–55.
81. Gadre S, Turowski J, Budev M. Overview of Lung Transplantation, Heart-Lung Transplantation, Liver-Lung Transplantation, and Combined Hematopoietic Stem Cell Transplantation and Lung Transplantation. Clin Chest Med 2017; 38(4):623–40.
82. Porteous MK, Lee JC. Primary Graft Dysfunction After Lung Transplantation. Clin Chest Med 2017;38(4):641–54.
83. Benden C. Pediatric lung transplantation. J Thorac Dis 2017;9(8):2675–83.
84. Bryant R 3rd, Morales D, Schecter M. Pediatric lung transplantation. Semin Pediatr Surg 2017;26(4):213–6.
85. Collaco JM, Gower WA, Mogayzel PJ Jr. Pulmonary dysfunction in pediatric hematopoietic stem cell transplant patients: overview, diagnostic considerations, and infectious complications. Pediatr Blood Cancer 2007;49(2):117–26.
86. Ahya VN. Noninfectious Acute Lung Injury Syndromes Early After Hematopoietic Stem Cell Transplantation. Clin Chest Med 2017;38(4):595–606.
87. Singh N, Loren AW. Overview of Hematopoietic Cell Transplantation for the Treatment of Hematologic Malignancies. Clin Chest Med 2017;38(4):575–93.
88. Bergeron A, Cheng GS. Bronchiolitis Obliterans Syndrome and Other Late Pulmonary Complications After Allogeneic Hematopoietic Stem Cell Transplantation. Clin Chest Med 2017;38(4):607–21.

89. Hakim A, Cooke KR, Pavletic SZ, et al. Diagnosis and treatment of bronchiolitis obliterans syndrome accessible universally. Bone Marrow Transpl 2019;54(3): 383–92.
90. Jagasia MH, Greinix HT, Arora M, et al. National Institutes of Health Consensus Development Project on Criteria for Clinical Trials in Chronic Graft-versus-Host Disease I. The 2014 Diagnosis and Staging Working Group Report. Biol Blood Marrow Transpl 2015;21(3):389–401.e1.
91. Towe C, Chester OA, Ferkol T, et al. Bronchiolitis obliterans syndrome is not specific for bronchiolitis obliterans in pediatric lung transplant. J Heart Lung Transplant 2015;34(4):516–21.
92. Petrara MR, Giunco S, Serraino D, et al. Post-transplant lymphoproliferative disorders: from epidemiology to pathogenesis-driven treatment. Cancer Lett 2015; 369(1):37–44.
93. Pochon C, Voigt S. Respiratory Virus Infections in Hematopoietic Cell Transplant Recipients. Front Microbiol 2018;9:3294.
94. Cho SY, Lee DG, Kim HJ. Cytomegalovirus Infections after Hematopoietic Stem Cell Transplantation: Current Status and Future Immunotherapy. Int J Mol Sci 2019;20(11):2666.
95. Hage CA, Carmona EM, Evans SE, et al. Summary for Clinicians: Microbiological Laboratory Testing in the Diagnosis of Fungal Infections in Pulmonary and Critical Care Practice. Ann Am Thorac Soc 2019;16(12):1473–7.
96. Katragkou A, Fisher BT, Groll AH, et al. Diagnostic Imaging and Invasive Fungal Diseases in Children. J Pediatr Infect Dis Soc 2017;6(suppl_1):S22–31.
97. Ma L, Cisse OH, Kovacs JA. A Molecular Window into the Biology and Epidemiology of Pneumocystis spp. Clin Microbiol Rev 2018;31(3). e00009-18.
98. Ndzi EN, Nkenfou CN, Gwom LC, et al. The pros and cons of the QuantiFERON test for the diagnosis of tuberculosis, prediction of disease progression, and treatment monitoring. Int J Mycobacteriol 2016;5(2):177–84.
99. Eddabra R, Ait Benhassou H. Rapid molecular assays for detection of tuberculosis. Pneumonia (Nathan) 2018;10:4.
100. Pena T, Klesney-Tait J. Mycobacterial Infections in Solid Organ and Hematopoietic Stem Cell Transplantation. Clin Chest Med 2017;38(4):761–70.
101. Lange C, Dheda K, Chesov D, et al. Management of drug-resistant tuberculosis. Lancet 2019;394(10202):953–66.
102. Longworth SA, Daly JS. Management of infections due to nontuberculous mycobacteria in solid organ transplant recipients-Guidelines from the American Society of Transplantation Infectious Diseases Community of Practice. Clin Transplant 2019;33(9):e13588.
103. WHO. WHO guidelines on tuberculosis infection and control 2019 update. In. Vol WHO/CDS/TB/2019.1 License CC By-NC-SA 3.0 IGO. Geneva (Switzerland): World Health Organization; 2019.
104. Wong JY, Westall GP, Snell GI. Bronchoscopic procedures and lung biopsies in pediatric lung transplant recipients. Pediatr pulmonology 2015;50(12):1406–19.
105. De La Cruz O, Silveira FP. Respiratory Fungal Infections in Solid Organ and Hematopoietic Stem Cell Transplantation. Clin Chest Med 2017;38(4):727–39.

Respiratory Complications in Children and Adolescents with Human Immunodeficiency Virus

Leah Githinji, MD, PhD, Heather J. Zar, MD, PhD*

KEYWORDS

• HIV • Children • Lower respiratory tract infection • Chronic lung disease

KEY POINTS

- Respiratory disease represents the major burden of mortality and morbidity in children with human immunodeficiency virus (HIV).
- Substantial decrease in acute and opportunistic respiratory infections has occurred as a result of antiretroviral therapy (ART).
- Pulmonary tuberculosis (TB) presenting as acute or chronic disease is common in TB-endemic areas and is more prevalent in children with HIV than in children who are not infected, even with use of ART.
- Chronic lung disease is common with improved survival of children infected with HIV perinatally.
- Chronic lung disease ranges from asymptomatic mild lung function impairment to bronchiectasis or bronchiolitis obliterans, the commonest manifestation.

INTRODUCTION

Respiratory disease is a major cause of morbidity and mortality among children with human immunodeficiency virus (HIV) globally.[1,2] Early diagnosis of HIV in infants and availability of antiretroviral therapy (ART) have resulted in improved survival with less acute diseases.[3] However, in some areas where children have suboptimal access to ART, acute lower respiratory tract infections (LRTIs) are common.[4] With improved survival, chronic respiratory disease has increasingly emerged, ranging from asymptomatic mildy impaired lung function to bronchiectasis or bronchiolitis obliterans.

EPIDEMIOLOGY

In 2018, 2.8 million children and adolescents were infected with HIV, 90% living in sub-Saharan Africa, with 190,000 new infections reported.[5] Although there has

Department of Paediatrics and Child Health, South Africa MRC Unit on Child & Adolescent Health, University of Cape Town, Red Cross War Memorial Children's Hospital, ICH Building, Klipfontein Road, Rondebosch 7700, South Africa
* Corresponding author.
E-mail address: Heather.Zar@uct.ac.za

Pediatr Clin N Am 68 (2021) 131–145
https://doi.org/10.1016/j.pcl.2020.09.016 pediatric.theclinics.com

been much progress in ART availability, 790,000 (46%) children with HIV were not receiving ART in 2018.[5] Prevention of mother-to-child transmission programs have nearly doubled since 2010, leading to decreases in vertical HIV transmission and an increase in HIV-exposed uninfected (HEU) children (who are HIV negative but born to an infected mother) who have an increased risk of LRTI in the first 6 months of life.[6] Globally, about 1.4 million HEU children are born annually, with approximately 14.8 million HEU children worldwide.[7] The scope of the respiratory involvement in patients with HIV ranges from acute lung infection to chronic lung disease (**Box 1**).

ACUTE LOWER RESPIRATORY TRACT INFECTION

Early diagnosis of HIV and use of ART and trimethoprim (TMP)-sulfamethoxazole (SMX) (cotrimoxazole) prophylaxis have reduced the incidence and mortality from LRTI,[8,9] but this continues to be a leading cause of hospitalization and death in children with HIV.[10] Risk factors for LRTI may be general (overcrowding, poverty, adverse environmental exposure, malnutrition, and lack of vaccination) or HIV specific (immunosuppression, impaired response to vaccines, or immune dysregulation). LRTI is frequently caused by several coinfections; multiple pathogens may be associated with more severe disease.[11]

BACTERIAL LOWER RESPIRATORY TRACT INFECTION

The use of ART[8] and pneumococcal conjugate vaccine (PCV) and *Haemophilus influenzae* type b (Hib) vaccines has reduced the incidence and severity of bacterial LRTI in children with HIV.[12] Other pathogens include *Staphylococcus aureus*, *H influenzae*, *Escherichia coli*, *Salmonella* spp, and *Klebsiella* spp.[13] The incidence of pneumonia caused by *Bordetella pertussis* is higher in HIV-positive and HEU children compared with unexposed children.[14] The clinical manifestations and radiographic findings of bacterial pneumonia are similar to those in HIV-negative children.

PULMONARY TUBERCULOSIS

Children with HIV are at increased risk for developing pulmonary tuberculosis (PTB) compared with uninfected children, although ART has reduced its incidence.[15] Although ART decreases the risk of tuberculosis (TB) infection, its full protective potential is only evident 1 to 2 years after starting ART.[16] TB incidence is estimated to

Box 1
Spectrum of human immunodeficiency virus–associated lung disease

Acute LRTI
- Infections: Viral, bacterial, *Pneumocystis jiroveci* pneumonia (PCP), *Mycobacterium tuberculosis*, nontuberculous mycobacteria, fungal

Chronic disease
- Asymptomatic impairment in lung function
- Bronchiolitis obliterans/chronic obstructive pulmonary disease
- Bronchiectasis
- Interstitial lung disease
- Asthma
- Immune reconstitution inflammatory syndrome
- Pulmonary hypertension
- Malignancy

range from 0.3 to 25.3 per 100 person-years in children with HIV; estimates are that 15% of children starting ART in sub-Saharan Africa will develop TB disease.[16]

HIV-TB coinfection is associated with worse clinical and radiological outcomes and higher mortality compared with children without HIV infection.[17] HIV-TB coinfection also poses several challenges, including drug-drug interactions, overlapping drug toxicities, and potential for immune reconstitution inflammatory syndrome (IRIS; a paradoxical clinical and radiological worsening following initiation of ART). Because of the association of HIV and TB, children presenting with TB disease should be tested for HIV infection and screening for TB should be done in children with HIV.

PTB in children with HIV may present as acute pneumonia or with chronic cough, fever, weight loss, or failure to thrive.[18] Extrapulmonary TB may occur more frequently. Chest radiographic findings include lobar consolidation with airway compression (**Fig. 1**), pleural effusion, fibrosis, miliary TB, hilar lymphadenopathy (**Fig. 2**), and rarely bronchoesophageal fistula.

Annual screening of children with HIV for TB infection is recommended using the tuberculin skin test in children who have a negative test. A reaction greater than 5 mm is considered positive. However, the sensitivity of skin testing is reduced in children with HIV compared with uninfected children; a blood interferon gamma assay has a higher sensitivity and specificity for diagnosis of TB infection in children with HIV. However, neither can distinguish infection from disease.

Diagnosis of PTB may be challenging.[19] The availability of the polymerase chain reaction (PCR)–based molecular method Xpert MTB/rifampin (RIF) (Xpert Ultra) has improved the rapid diagnosis of TB and detection of rifampicin resistance; using a combination of specimens (induced sputum and nasopharyngeal samples), sensitivity was almost 90% against a gold standard of culture-confirmed disease, with high specificity.[20] Xpert on stool is promising in children with HIV.[21] Testing of urine for *Mycobacterium*-specific lipoarabinomannan (LAM) reduces mortality in adults with advanced HIV,[22] but accuracy in children is variable, with sensitivity ranging from 43% to 65% and low or moderate specificity.[23,24] A more sensitive version, Fuji-LAM, has a sensitivity of 87% in adults with HIV, with CD4 counts less than or equal

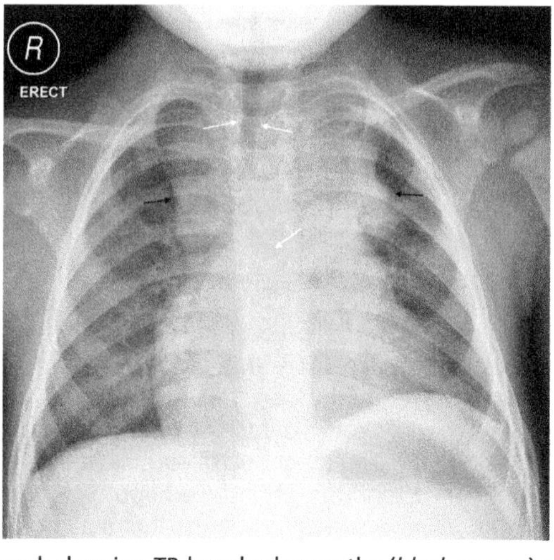

Fig. 1. Chest radiograph showing TB lymphadenopathy (*black arrows*) with compression of left main bronchus and trachea (*white arrows*). (*Courtesy of* A.-M. Du Plessis, MBChB, MMed, FCRad(SA), Cape Town, South Africa.)

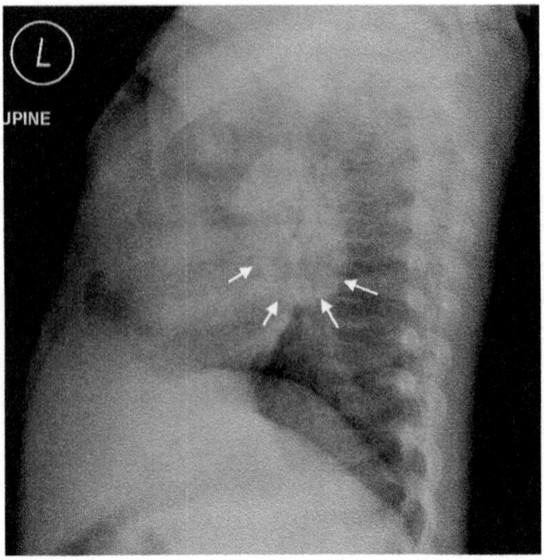

Fig. 2. Lateral chest radiograph showing hilar lymphadenopathy (*arrows*) caused by TB (doughnut sign). (*Courtesy of* A.-M. Du Plessis, MBChB, MMed, FCRad(SA), Cape Town, South Africa.)

to 100 cells/mm.[3,25] Nontuberculous mycobacteria (NTM) may cause disease in immunosuppressed children but is uncommon with ART use.[26] Isolated pulmonary disease with *Mycobacterium avium* complex (MAC) is rare.[26]

VIRAL LOWER RESPIRATORY TRACT INFECTION

Viral LRTI is common from respiratory syncytial virus (RSV), influenza, parainfluenza, human metapneumovirus, or adenovirus.[27] Children who are not on ART are more likely to develop severe RSV pneumonia,[28] requiring hospitalization, oxygen, or mechanical ventilation.[29] Outcomes from influenza LRTIs were similar in children with and without HIV.[30] Measles and varicella virus may cause severe pneumonia in severely immunosuppressed children with CD4 counts less than 200 cells/mm^3.[3,31]

Cytomegalovirus (CMV) may cause pneumonitis, but this is less common with the use of ART.[32] CMV pneumonitis presents with dry cough and radiological features of interstitial disease. Definitive diagnosis of CMV lung disease requires lung biopsy, but CMV viral load on bronchoalveolar lavage (BAL) or blood may be a useful indicator.[33]

FUNGAL LOWER RESPIRATORY TRACT INFECTION

Pneumocystis jiroveci is the most common opportunistic pathogen in infants with HIV with pneumonia who are not receiving TMP-SMX prophylaxis or ART. Clinical manifestations include acute cough fever, tachypnea, and hypoxemia. Common chest radiographic changes are hyperinflation, diffuse bilateral opacities, and perihilar reticulonodular infiltrates (**Fig. 3**). The diagnosis is established by PCR on respiratory specimens, with a higher yield reported on induced sputum or BAL compared with nasopharyngeal aspirates.[34] Other fungal infections that may occur in the context of severe immunosuppression include aspergillosis, histoplasmosis, candidiasis, and cryptococcosis. Cultures of bone marrow, cerebrospinal fluid, and lymph node or lung biopsy may be diagnostic.

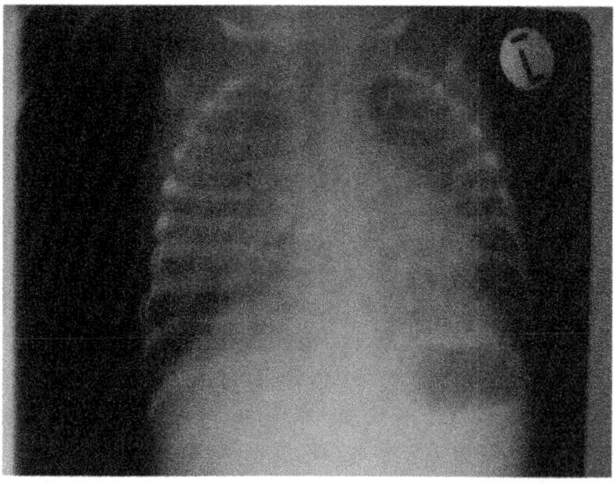

Fig. 3. Chest radiograph with bilateral opacification caused by *P jiroveci* pneumonia. (*Courtesy of* A.-M. Du Plessis, MBChB, MMed, FCRad(SA), Cape Town, South Africa.)

CHRONIC RESPIRATORY ILLNESS

Clinical Spectrum

Chronic lung disease has increasingly emerged in children with HIV as they survive longer. The clinical presentation includes chronic cough, dyspnea, digital clubbing, hypoxemia at rest, and exercise intolerance.[3,35] In Zimbabwean adolescents with HIV (n = 385, <2% on ART), almost 60% had chronic cough[35]; in a second cohort (n = 116, 69% on ART), 35% had resting hypoxemia and 10% had digital clubbing.[36] Exercise intolerance has been reported more commonly in adolescents with than those without HIV.[37] However, the spectrum of chronic disease in adolescents with HIV well established on ART is mild, with few reporting chronic cough (15%, n = 515) and normal oxygen saturation on exertion.[38]

Chronic lung disease includes bronchiolitis obliterans, bronchiectasis, chronic reactive airways disease or interstitial lung disease (see **Box 1**). Bronchiolitis obliterans predominates. Predisposing factors include delayed access to ART, immune dysregulation, recurrent or chronic infection, pulmonary aspiration because of esophagitis caused by *Candida*, herpes simplex virus or CMV (uncommon with ART use), adverse environmental exposures, malnutrition, or.[8] Rarely, bronchoesophageal fistula, a complication of PTB, may contribute to chronic aspiration and lung disease.

A higher incidence of asthma has been reported in children with HIV on ART compared with ART-naive children (35% vs 11%),[39] or compared with HEU children (34% vs 25%),[40] attributed to IRIS.[39] However, asthma medication as a marker for asthma was used in these studies. A lower rate of bronchodilator responsiveness has been reported in youth with HIV compared with HEU youth (9% vs 17%).[41]

Malignancies such as Kaposi sarcoma or non-Hodgkin lymphoma are rare in patients receiving ART. Pulmonary hypertension may occur as a sequela of chronic lung disease leading to *cor pulmonale*.[42] Primary pulmonary hypertension has also been reported in adolescents with HIV.[43]

Lung Function

Adolescents with HIV, well established on ART, had mildly reduced lung function, with increased airway resistance and lung clearance index compared with controls not infected with HIV.[38] Lung function impairment was less severe in children on ART for longer duration.[44] Lung function abnormalities include irreversible airway obstructive changes[35,38,45] and abnormal exercise testing.[45] Diffusion capacity abnormalities are rare in adolescents with HIV[38] compared with adults.[46] Longitudinal changes in spirometry indicate that lung function tracks through adolescence with persistence of impairment despite ART.[47,48] Prior LRTI or TB was associated with reduced lung function.[47] Irreversible airway obstruction suggests bronchiolitis obliterans as the predominant chronic disease.[49,50]

Chest Radiology

In the pre-ART era, nodular opacities indicative of lymphocytic interstitial pneumonia dominated chronic chest radiographic changes; this has disappeared with ART.[51] Two studies of chest computed tomography (CT) of perinatally infected adolescents on ART for at least 5 years in Zimbabwe (n = 84) and in South Africa (n = 100) showed decreased attenuation identified on expiratory films[49,50] as the predominant finding, a feature of bronchiolitis obliterans (**Fig. 4**). The extent of mosaic attenuation correlated with lung function impairment.[50] Tramlines and ring shadows are common radiological findings in children on ART and are features of bronchiectasis[50] (**Fig. 5**).

Chest ultrasound may be useful for the diagnosis of disseminated TB to show focal splenic lesions or abdominal lymphadenopathy.[52] and for identifying pneumonia or mediastinal adenopathy, suggesting PTB.[53,54]

Human Immunodeficiency Virus–Exposed Uninfected Children

HEU children have an increased risk of LRTI, especially in the first 6 months of life,[27,55] compared with infants not exposed to HIV. Lung function may be impaired in HEU infants shortly after birth[56] but is similar to that in unexposed children at 2 years, except for HEU children whose mothers had uncontrolled HIV disease during pregnancy.[57] Several mechanisms for increased susceptibility to LRTI in HEU infants may be relevant, including in utero HIV or ART exposure, lack of transfer of sufficient functional maternal antibodies, lack of breastfeeding, higher exposure to infectious agents, or immune dysregulation.[58]

MANAGEMENT OF HUMAN IMMUNODEFICIENCY VIRUS–ASSOCIATED LUNG DISEASE

Treatment

For LRTI, empiric antibiotics should be given and oxygen as well as other supportive care.[26] If intravenous (IV) antibiotics are needed, beta-lactam antibiotics (with or

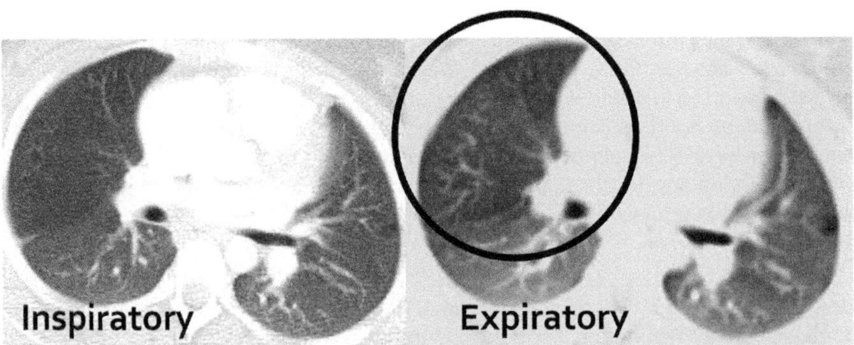

Fig. 4. Bronchiolitis obliterans in a child with HIV on ART showing air trapping (*circle*) on expiratory views of the CT scan. (*Courtesy of* A.-M. Du Plessis, MBChB, MMed, FCRad(SA), Cape Town, South Africa.)

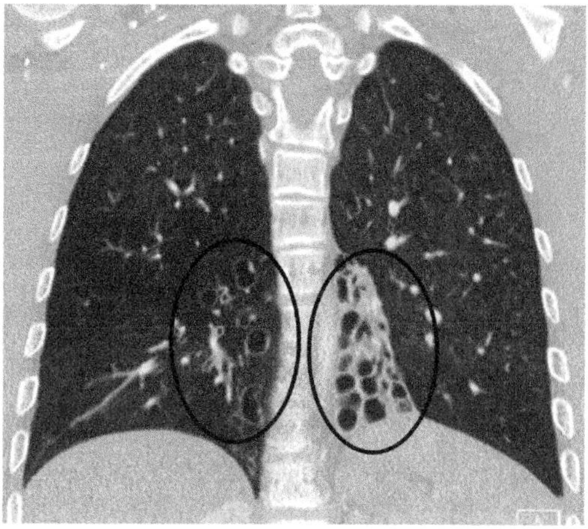

Fig. 5. Bilateral lower lobe bronchiectasis (*circles*) in an adolescent with HIV on ART. (*Courtesy of* A.-M. Du Plessis, MBChB, MMed, FCRad(SA), Cape Town, South Africa.)

without an aminoglycoside) or amoxicillin-clavulanic acid or a cephalosporin may be used.[13,26] The recommended treatment of LRTI in children with HIV is outlined in **Table 1**. If *S aureus* is suspected, cloxacillin should be given; for methicillin-resistant *S aureus*, vancomycin or clindamycin are indicated.[13]

Oral therapy is preferable; empiric treatment with high-dose oral amoxicillin is recommended. Addition of azithromycin or another macrolide should be considered if pertussis, *Mycoplasma*, or *Chlamydia* are suspected.[26] High-dose oral or IV cotrimoxazole for 21 days should be given for suspected or confirmed *P jirovecii* pneumonia (PCP), with corticosteroids in those with hypoxemia.[59] For CMV pneumonitis, ganciclovir intravenously or oral valganciclovir should be given[13] (**Table 2**). Neuraminidase inhibitors (eg, oseltamivir) may be effective for influenza if given early in the disease.[26]

Three or 4 drugs are recommended for PTB, with isoniazid (INH), RIF, pyrazinamide, and ethambutol for 2 months and 4 months of continuation phase with INH and rifampicin[60] (see **Table 1**). US guidelines recommend a 2-month initiation phase with 4 drugs and a longer continuation phase of 7 months with rifampin and INH, although 4 months may be used in those with minimal disease.[26] Doses of drugs are similar for children with and without HIV,[13] but drug interactions with ART must be considered, especially with the use of rifampin. In young children on a protease inhibitor with lopinavir/ritonavir, superboosting with additional ritonavir (ratio 1:1) is needed.[26] No adjustments are needed for those on an efavirenz-based regimen.[26] Recent WHO recommendations are to transition to 2 non-nucleoside reverse transcriptase inhibitors and dolutegravir, but the dosage to overcome drug interactions with rifampin has not been established. Rifabutin may be used rather than rifampin, but its use is limited because of lack of pediatric formulations, high cost, and lack of availability. ART should be started within 2 to 8 weeks of TB treatment in ART-naive children, to minimize potential development of IRIS. Prednisone should be used for airway obstruction or when IRIS occurs (see **Table 1**). Treatment of NTM involves at least 12 months of azithromycin or clarithromycin, ethambutol with or without rifampin, and amikacin.[61]

The management of chronic lung disease aims to preserve lung function by improving airway clearance, promoting growth, and preventing or treating intercurrent

Table 1
Treatment of lower respiratory tract infection in children with human immunodeficiency virus

Infection	Regimen
Pneumonia	Empiric antibiotic therapy with broad-spectrum antibiotics either IV or oral. Oral is preferable if possible First-line IV treatment options: Ampicillin (or penicillin) 50 mg/kg/dose 6 hourly plus gentamicin 7.5 mg/kg once daily or amoxicillin-clavulanate 30 mg/kg/dose (of amoxicillin component) 8 hourly IV for 5 days or ceftriaxone 50 mg/kg twice daily alone as second-line treatment First line oral treatment: Amoxicillin 45 mg/kg/dose 12 hourly for 5 d Add azithromycin (or other macrolide): 10 mg/kg orally daily for 5 d if pertussis, *Mycoplasma pneumoniae*, *Chlamydia pneumoniae*, or *Chlamydia trachomatis* suspected
S aureus pneumonia	Oral or IV cloxacillin (50 mg/kg 6 hourly) for 1–4 wk Add vancomycin 10–20 mg/kg/dose 6 hourly or clindamycin for methicillin-resistant *S aureus*
P jirovecii pneumonia suspected	Cotrimoxazole (TMP/SMX) oral or IV (5 mg/kg/dose TMP and 25 mg/kg/dose SMX) 6 hourly for 21 d Prednisone 1–2 mg/kg/d tapered over 21 d. Continue prophylaxis thereafter
CMV	Ganciclovir 5 mg/kg/dose 12 hourly; switch to oral valganciclovir (16 mg/kg/dose 12 hourly) with clinical improvement) for up to 6 wk
Influenza	Oseltamivir for 5 d
Pulmonary tuberculosis	INH (10–15 mg/kg, maximum dose 300 mg/d) RIF (10–20 mg/kg, max. dose 600 mg/d) PZA (30–40 mg/kg, maximum 2 g/d) ETA (15–25 mg/kg; maximum 2.5 g/d) 2-mo initiation phase: INH, RIF, PZA, and ETA, then continuation phase of 4–7 mo: INH and RIF Add prednisone 1–2 mg/kg/d tapered over 4–6 wk for airway compression or IRIS

Abbreviations: INH, isoniazid; PZA, pyrazinamide; RIF, rifampicin; ETA, ethambutol.
Data from Nuttall JJ. Current antimicrobial management of community-acquired pneumonia in HIV-infected children. Expert Opinion on Pharmacotherapy. 2019;20(5):595-608 and Panel on Antiretroviral Guidelines for Adults and Adolescents. Guidelines for the Use of Antiretroviral Agents in Adults and Adolescents with HIV. Department of Health and Human Services. Available at http://www.aidsinfo.nih.gov/ContentFiles/AdultandAdolescentGL.pdf. Accessed May 2020.

infections. Prophylactic azithromycin in children with HIV with bronchiectasis has not been well studied, although preliminary results of a randomized controlled trial showed a decrease in hospitalizations or acute exacerbations.[62]

Prevention

Preventive strategies for lung disease in children with HIV are summarized in **Table 2**.

1 Early initiation of ART. ART should be initiated as soon as the diagnosis of HIV is established, to optimize lung health and function.
2. Optimize nutrition. Good nutrition is essential to ensure adequate lung growth, protect against LRTI and PCP, and optimize lung function.

Table 2
Prevention strategies for lung disease in children with human immunodeficiency virus

Intervention	Strategy
Immunization	Regular immunization schedule including: Diphtheria, pertussis, tetanus; measles; pneumococcal conjugate; and *H influenzae* type b vaccination Annual influenza vaccine
Nutrition	Exclusive breastfeeding for 6 mo Optimize nutritional intake
Tobacco smoke and air pollution exposure	Avoid maternal and household tobacco smoking Minimize exposure to indoor and outdoor pollution Prevent adolescent smoking
TMP-SMX (cotrimoxazole) prophylaxis	1. All infants with HIV, regardless clinical stage or immunologic status 2. Children with HIV 1–6 y old if CD4 count <500 cells/mm^3 or CD4 <15% 3. Children with HIV >6 y old with CD4 counts ≤200 cells/μL, or WHO stage 2, 3 or 4 disease
INH prophylaxis	6–9 mo of INH prophylaxis in children exposed to a household contact or person with TB infection 36 mo of INH prophylaxis in adolescents with HIV
HIV prevention	Prevention of mother-to-child transmission Strategies to prevent horizontal transmission in adolescents
HIV treatment	Early use of effective combination ART as soon as HIV is diagnosed

Data from Panel on Antiretroviral Guidelines for Adults and Adolescents. Guidelines for the Use of Antiretroviral Agents in Adults and Adolescents with HIV. Department of Health and Human Services. Available at http://www.aidsinfo.nih.gov/ContentFiles/AdultandAdolescentGL.pdf. Accessed May 2020.

3. Immunization. All children should receive standard immunizations, including diphtheria, pertussis, tetanus; measles; pneumococcal conjugate; and Hib. The nature and degree of immunosuppression in children with HIV may affect the efficacy and duration of vaccine-induced protection.[63] Children with HIV treated with ART from early infancy and responsive to therapy have similar immunogenicity and immune responses to most childhood vaccines compared with infants not exposed to HIV.[64] HEU infants may have lower concentrations of transplacental acquired antibodies for some vaccine-preventable diseases[65]; however, their immune responses to vaccines are not impaired.[65] Furthermore, there is similar persistence of protective antibody concentrations and memory responses in HEU children compared with children unexposed to HIV.[66] The need for further booster doses of PCV in older children with HIV is unclear, particularly with the use of ART. WHO currently recommends that a booster dose of PCV be considered in the second year of life in children with HIV who received their 3-dose primary PCV series in infancy.[67] Influenza vaccine should be given annually.
4. Prevent exposure to tobacco smoke and pollution. Minimizing exposure to tobacco smoke or pollution antenatally and postnatally reduces the risk of LRTI, wheezing, and impaired lung function.
5. Chemoprophylaxis
   5.1 Cotrimoxazole

Cotrimoxazole is highly effective for prevention of PCP and may also offer protection against bacterial pneumonia. WHO recommends providing life-long cotrimoxazole prophylaxis, regardless of CD4 counts, in areas with a high prevalence of malaria or bacterial infections.[68] However, in other regions, PCP prophylaxis may be discontinued in children with HIV on ART.[26]

US guidelines[26] recommend cotrimoxazole prophylaxis for:

1. All infants with HIV, irrespective of clinical stage or immunologic status
2. Children with HIV 1 to 6 years of age if their CD4 counts are less than 500 cells/mm^3 or CD4 percentage is less than 15%
3. Children with HIV more than 6 years of age with CD4 counts less than or equal to 200 cells/μL

WHO guidelines recommend PCP prophylaxis for HEU infants from 4 to 6 weeks of age until HIV infection has been excluded after cessation of breastfeeding.[69] However, a recently randomized controlled trial showed that cotrimoxazole prophylaxis conferred no survival advantage in HEU children.[70]

5.2 Isoniazid

INH prophylaxis is highly effective to prevent TB disease.[71] However, under-use, especially in high-burden TB settings, is a challenge. At least 6 months of INH should be given to all children with HIV who have a close contact with TB or who have a positive tuberculin skin test, once TB disease has been excluded.[72] US guidelines recommend 9 months of INH (10–15 mg/kg/d) to treat latent TB infection in children with HIV provided that TB disease has been excluded.[26] Shorter regimens have also been recommended to improve adherence. WHO recommends at least 36 months of INH prophylaxis in adolescents with HIV where TB disease has been excluded, in high TB endemic areas, regardless of ART use or immune reconstitution.[60]

5.3 Valganciclovir

Prophylaxis with valganciclovir may be considered for children with HIV greater than or equal to 6 years of age who have CD4 cell counts less than 50 cells/mm^3 or less than 6 years old with CD4 less than 5%. Primary prophylaxis may be discontinued when the CD4 cell count is greater than 100 cells/mm^3 for children greater than or equal to 6 years of age, or greater than 10% in children less than 6 years of age.[26]

5.4 Azithromycin

Azithromycin is used to prevent MAC in children with advanced immunosuppression, defined as CD4 <1 year: <750 cells/mm, 1 to <2 years: <500 cells/mm, 2 to <6 years: <75 cells/mm3, ≥6 years: <50 cells/mm.[3,26]

6. Maternal health. Enhancing maternal health, including optimal control of HIV disease and avoiding smoking before and during pregnancy, is a critical strategy to attain lung health in children. Children born to mothers who had poorly controlled HIV disease during pregnancy had impaired lung function at 2 years of age.[57]

SUMMARY AND FUTURE RECOMMENDATIONS

Although acute LRTI was a major cause of morbidity and mortality pre-ART, the incidence has reduced substantially with early HIV diagnosis, use of ART, and better vaccines. Tuberculosis, viral or bacterial pneumonia, PCP, or CMV pneumonitis remain prevalent in children with HIV in settings of suboptimal ART use or with late HIV diagnosis. HEU infants have an increased risk of LRTI in the first 6 months of life. With improved survival and control of HIV, chronic lung disease has become common, ranging from asymptomatic mild lung function impairment to bronchiolitis obliterans and bronchiectasis. Chronic lung disease is associated with prior LRTI or PTB. Delayed initiation of ART is a key factor. General and HIV-specific measures to promote lung health should be strengthened. More research is needed to understand the progression and spectrum of HIV-associated chronic lung disease and develop new preventive strategies.

CLINICS CARE POINTS

- Early diagnosis of HIV and prompt initiation of ART is key to preserve lung health.
- LRTI is the commonest acute infection and may be caused by bacteria, viruses, M tuberculosis or fungi. The incidence of LRTI has reduced substantially with use of ART, cotrimoxazole prophylaxis and immunisation.
- HIV-exposed uninfected infants have a higher risk of LRTI than unexposed infants.
- Chronic lung disease, most commonly bronchiolitis obliterans or bronchiectasis, is increasingly prevalent due to longer survival of HIV-infected children.
- Empiric treatment with broad spectrum antibiotics should be used for LRTI; for children with suspected PCP, cotrimoxazole should be added with corticosteroids (in hypoxic children).
- General preventive strategies including optimising nutrition, avoidance of smoke exposure and immunisation are important to reduce lung disease in HIV-infected children.
- Specific preventive interventions such as cotrimoxazole or INH prophylaxis are highly effective for reducing respiratory infections or TB.

ACKNOWLEDGMENTS

The authors thank Dr Anne-Marie Du Plessis for providing images.

DISCLOSURE

The authors have nothing to disclose.

REFERENCES

1. Ferrand RA, Bandason T, Musvaire P, et al. Causes of acute hospitalization in adolescence: burden and spectrum of HIV-related morbidity in a country with an early-onset and severe HIV epidemic: a prospective survey. PLoS Med 2010;7(2):e1000178.
2. McHugh G, Rylance J, Mujuru H, et al. Chronic morbidity among older children and adolescents at diagnosis of HIV infection. J Acquir Immune Defic Syndr 2016;73(3):275–81.
3. Frigati LJ, Ameyan W, Cotton MF, et al. Chronic comorbidities in children and adolescents with perinatally acquired HIV infection in sub-Saharan Africa in the era of antiretroviral therapy. Lancet Child Adolesc Health 2020;4(9):688–98.
4. Bates M, Mudenda V, Mwaba P, et al. Deaths due to respiratory tract infections in Africa: a review of autopsy studies. Curr Opin Pulm Med 2013;19(3):229–37.
5. UNAIDS. 2019. Available at: https://www.unaids.org/en/resources/documents/2019/2019-UNAIDS-data. Accessed March 27, 2020.

6. Le Roux DM, Myer L, Nicol MP, et al. Incidence and severity of childhood pneumonia in the first year of life in a South African birth cohort: the Drakenstein Child Health Study. Lancet Glob Health 2015;3(2):e95–103.
7. Slogrove AL, Powis KM, Johnson LF, et al. Estimates of the global population of children who are HIV-exposed and uninfected, 2000–18: a modelling study. Lancet Glob Health 2020;8(1):e67–75.
8. B-Lajoie M-R, Drouin O, Bartlett G, et al. Incidence and prevalence of opportunistic and other infections and the impact of antiretroviral therapy among HIV-infected children in low-and middle-income countries: a systematic review and meta-analysis. Clin Infect Dis 2016;62(12):1586–94.
9. Violari A, Cotton MF, Gibb DM, et al. Early antiretroviral therapy and mortality among HIV-infected infants. N Engl J Med 2008;359(21):2233–44.
10. Theodoratou E, McAllister DA, Reed C, et al. Global, regional, and national estimates of pneumonia burden in HIV-infected children in 2010: a meta-analysis and modelling study. Lancet Infect Dis 2014;14(12):1250–8.
11. McNally LM, Jeena PM, Gajee K, et al. Effect of age, polymicrobial disease, and maternal HIV status on treatment response and cause of severe pneumonia in South African children: a prospective descriptive study. Lancet 2007; 369(9571):1440–51.
12. Bliss SJ, O'Brien KL, Janoff EN, et al. The evidence for using conjugate vaccines to protect HIV-infected children against pneumococcal disease. Lancet Infect Dis 2008;8(1):67–80.
13. Nuttall JJ. Current antimicrobial management of community-acquired pneumonia in HIV-infected children. Expert Opin Pharmacother 2019;20(5):595–608.
14. Muloiwa R, Dube FS, Nicol MP, et al. Incidence and diagnosis of pertussis in South African children hospitalized with lower respiratory tract infection. Pediatr Infect Dis J 2016;35(6):611–6.
15. Walters E, Cotton MF, Rabie H, et al. Clinical presentation and outcome of tuberculosis in human immunodeficiency virus infected children on anti-retroviral therapy. BMC Pediatr 2008;8(1):1.
16. Dodd PJ, Prendergast AJ, Beecroft C, et al. The impact of HIV and antiretroviral therapy on TB risk in children: a systematic review and meta-analysis. Thorax 2017;72(6):559.
17. Salvadori N, Ngo-Giang-Huong N, Duclercq C, et al. Incidence of tuberculosis and associated mortality in a cohort of human immunodeficiency virus-infected children initiating antiretroviral therapy. J Pediatr Infect Dis Soc 2017;6(2):161–7.
18. Oliwa JN, Karumbi JM, Marais BJ, et al. Tuberculosis as a cause or comorbidity of childhood pneumonia in tuberculosis-endemic areas: a systematic review. Lancet Respir Med 2015;3(3):235–43.
19. Nicol MP, Zar HJ. New specimens and laboratory diagnostics for childhood pulmonary TB: progress and prospects. Paediatr Respir Rev 2011;12(1):16–21.
20. Zar HJ, Workman L, Isaacs W, et al. Rapid diagnosis of pulmonary tuberculosis in African children in a primary care setting by use of Xpert MTB/RIF on respiratory specimens: a prospective study. Lancet Glob Health 2013;1(2):e97–104.
21. MacLean E, Sulis G, Denkinger CM, et al. Diagnostic Accuracy of Stool Xpert MTB/RIF for detection of pulmonary tuberculosis in children: a systematic review and meta-analysis. J Clin Microbiol 2019;57(6):e02057.
22. Peter JG, Zijenah LS, Chanda D, et al. Effect on mortality of point-of-care, urine-based lipoarabinomannan testing to guide tuberculosis treatment initiation in HIV-positive hospital inpatients: a pragmatic, parallel-group, multicountry, open-label, randomised controlled trial. Lancet 2016;387(10024):1187–97.

23. LaCourse SM, Pavlinac PB, Cranmer LM, et al. Stool Xpert MTB/RIF and urine lipoarabinomannan for the diagnosis of tuberculosis in hospitalized HIV-infected children. AIDS 2018;32(1):69–78.
24. Nicol MP, Allen V, Workman L, et al. Urine lipoarabinomannan testing for diagnosis of pulmonary tuberculosis in children: a prospective study. Lancet Glob Health 2014;2(5):e278–84.
25. Broger T, Nicol MP, Székely R, et al. Diagnostic accuracy of a novel tuberculosis point-of-care urine lipoarabinomannan assay for people living with HIV: A meta-analysis of individual in-and outpatient data. PLoS Med 2020;17(5):e1003113.
26. Panel on Antiretroviral Guidelines for Adults and Adolescents. Guidelines for the Use of Antiretroviral Agents in Adults and Adolescents with HIV. Department of Health and Human Services. Available at: http://www.aidsinfo.nih.gov/ContentFiles/AdultandAdolescentGL.pdf. Accessed May 2,2020.
27. Cohen C, Moyes J, Tempia S, et al. Epidemiology of acute lower respiratory tract infection in HIV-exposed uninfected infants. Pediatrics 2016;137(4):e20153272.
28. Shi T, Balsells E, Wastnedge E, et al. Risk factors for respiratory syncytial virus associated with acute lower respiratory infection in children under five years: Systematic review and meta-analysis. J Glob Health 2015;5(2):020416.
29. Cohen C, Walaza S, Moyes J, et al. Epidemiology of viral-associated acute lower respiratory tract infection among children< 5 years of age in a high HIV prevalence setting, South Africa, 2009–2012. Pediatr Infect Dis J 2015;34(1):66.
30. Madhi SA, Ramasamy N, Bessellar TG, et al. Lower respiratory tract infections associated with influenza A and B viruses in an area with a high prevalence of pediatric human immunodeficiency type 1 infection. Pediatr Infect Dis J 2002; 21(4):291–7.
31. Payne H, Judd A, Donegan K, et al. Incidence of pneumococcal and varicella disease in HIV-infected children and adolescents in the United Kingdom and Ireland, 1996–2011. Pediatr Infect Dis J 2015;34(2):149–54.
32. Yindom L-M, Simms V, Majonga ED, et al. Unexpectedly High Prevalence of Cytomegalovirus DNAemia in older children and adolescents with perinatally acquired human immunodeficiency virus infection. Clin Infect Dis 2019;69(4):580–7.
33. Hsiao N-Y, Zampoli M, Morrow B, et al. Cytomegalovirus viraemia in HIV exposed and infected infants: prevalence and clinical utility for diagnosing CMV pneumonia. J Clin Virol 2013;58(1):74–8.
34. Morrow BM, Samuel CM, Zampoli M, et al. Pneumocystis pneumonia in South African children diagnosed by molecular methods. BMC Res Notes 2014;7(1):26.
35. Ferrand RA, Desai SR, Hopkins C, et al. Chronic lung disease in adolescents with delayed diagnosis of vertically acquired HIV infection. Clin Infect Dis 2012;55(1): 145–52.
36. McHugh G, Simms V, Dauya E, et al. Clinical outcomes in children and adolescents initiating antiretroviral therapy in decentralized healthcare settings in Zimbabwe. J Int AIDS Soc 2017;20(1):21843.
37. Chisati EM, Vasseljen O. Aerobic endurance in HIV-positive young adults and HIV-negative controls in Malawi. Malawi Med J 2015;27(1):5.
38. Githinji LN, Gray DM, Hlengwa S, et al. Lung Function in South African Adolescents Infected Perinatally with HIV and Treated Long-Term with Antiretroviral Therapy. Ann Am Thorac Soc 2017;14(5):722–9.
39. Foster SB, McIntosh K, Thompson B, et al. Increased incidence of asthma in HIV-infected children treated with highly active antiretroviral therapy in the National Institutes of Health Women and Infants Transmission Study. J Allergy Clin Immunol 2008;122(1):159–65.

40. Siberry GK, Leister E, Jacobson DL, et al. Increased risk of asthma and atopic dermatitis in perinatally HIV-infected children and adolescents. Clin Immunol 2012;142(2):201–8.
41. Shearer WT, Jacobson DL, Yu W, et al. Long-term pulmonary complications in perinatally HIV-infected youth. J Allergy Clin Immunol 2017;140(4):1101–11.e7.
42. Kolb TM, Hassoun PM. Right ventricular dysfunction in chronic lung disease. Cardiol Clin 2012;30(2):243–56.
43. Stepffer C, Gaynor E, Lopez M, et al. Pulmonary hypertension associated with the human immunodeficiency virus in children: treatment with sildenafil. A case report. Arch Argent Pediatr 2018;116(3):e437–41.
44. Githinji LN, Gray DM, Zar HJ. Lung function in HIV-infected children and adolescents. Pneumonia 2018;10(1).
45. Rylance J, McHugh G, Metcalfe J, et al. Chronic lung disease in HIV-infected children established on antiretroviral therapy. AIDS 2016;30(18):2795–803.
46. Gingo MR, George MP, Kessinger CJ, et al. Pulmonary function abnormalities in HIV-infected patients during the current antiretroviral therapy era. Am J Respir Crit Care Med 2010;182(6):790–6.
47. Githinji LN, Gray DM, Hlengwa S, et al. Longitudinal Changes in Spirometry in South African Adolescents Perinatally Infected With Human Immunodeficiency Virus Who Are Receiving Antiretroviral Therapy. Clin Infect Dis 2020;70(3):483–90.
48. Rylance S, Rylance J, McHugh G, et al. Effect of antiretroviral therapy on longitudinal lung function trends in older children and adolescents with HIV-infection. PLoS One 2019;14(3):e0213556.
49. du Plessis AM, Andronikou S, Machemedze T, et al. High-resolution computed tomography features of lung disease in perinatally HIV-infected adolescents on combined antiretroviral therapy. Pediatr Pulmonol 2019;54(11):1765–73.
50. Desai SR, Nair A, Rylance J, et al. Human immunodeficiency virus-associated chronic lung disease in children and adolescents in zimbabwe: chest radiographic and high-resolution computed tomographic findings. Clin Infect Dis 2018;66(2):274–81.
51. Pitcher RD, Lombard CJ, Cotton MF, et al. Chest radiographic abnormalities in HIV-infected African children: a longitudinal study. Thorax 2015;70(9):840–6.
52. Belard S, Heuvelings CC, Banderker E, et al. Utility of point-of-care ultrasound in children with pulmonary tuberculosis. Pediatr Infect Dis J 2018;37(7):637–42.
53. Pool K-L, Heuvelings CC, Bélard S, et al. Technical aspects of mediastinal ultrasound for pediatric pulmonary tuberculosis. Pediatr Radiol 2017;47(13):1839–48.
54. Pereda MA, Chavez MA, Hooper-Miele CC, et al. Lung ultrasound for the diagnosis of pneumonia in children: a meta-analysis. Pediatrics 2015;135(4):714.
55. Slogrove AL, Goetghebuer T, Cotton MF, et al. Pattern of infectious morbidity in HIV-exposed uninfected infants and children. Front Immunol 2016;7:164.
56. Gray D, Willemse L, Visagie A, et al. Determinants of early-life lung function in African infants. Thorax 2017;72(5):445–50.
57. Gray DM, Wedderburn CJ, MacGinty RP, et al. Impact of HIV and antiretroviral drug exposure on lung growth and function over 2 years in an African Birth Cohort. AIDS 2020;34(4):549–58.
58. Evans C, Jones CE, Prendergast AJ. HIV-exposed, uninfected infants: new global challenges in the era of paediatric HIV elimination. Lancet Infect Dis 2016;16(6):e92–107.
59. Newberry L, O'Hare B, Kennedy N, et al. Early use of corticosteroids in infants with a clinical diagnosis of Pneumocystis jiroveci pneumonia in Malawi: a

double-blind, randomised clinical trial. Paediatr Int Child Health 2017;37(2): 121–8.
60. World Health Organization. Guidance for national tuberculosis programmes on the management of tuberculosis in children. Geneva (Switzerland): World Health Organization; 2014. www.who.int.
61. Haworth CS, Banks J, Capstick T, et al. British Thoracic Society guidelines for the management of non-tuberculous mycobacterial pulmonary disease (NTM-PD). Thorax 2017;72(Suppl 2):ii1–64.
62. R. F. Azithromycin for treatment of HIV-related chronic lung disease in African children. Conference on Retroviruses and Opportunistic Infections, abstract 86, Boston, MA, March 11, 2020.
63. Madhi SA, Adrian P, Cotton MF, et al. Effect of HIV infection status and antiretroviral treatment on quantitative and qualitative antibody responses to pneumococcal conjugate vaccine in infants. J Infect Dis 2010;202(3):355–61.
64. Simani OE, Izu A, Violari A, et al. Effect of HIV-1 exposure and antiretroviral treatment strategies in HIV-infected children on immunogenicity of vaccines during infancy. AIDS 2014;28(4):531–41.
65. Jallow S, Madhi SA. Pneumococcal conjugate vaccine in HIV-infected and HIV-exposed, uninfected children. Expert Rev Vaccines 2017;16(5):453–65.
66. Simani OE, Izu A, Nunes MC, et al. Effect of HIV exposure and timing of antiretroviral therapy initiation on immune memory responses to diphtheria, tetanus, whole cell pertussis and hepatitis B vaccines. Expert Rev Vaccines 2019;18(1):95–104.
67. World Health Organization. 23-valent pneumococcal polysaccharide vaccine: WHO position paper. Wkly Epidemiol Rec 2008;83(42):373–84. Available at: https://www.who.int/wer/2008/wer8342.pdf.
68. World Health Organization. Guidelines for managing advanced HIV disease and rapid initiation of antiretroviral therapy. 2017. Available at: https://www.who.int/hiv/pub/guidelines/advanced-HIV-disease/en. Accessed April 1, 2020.
69. World Health Organization. Guidelines on post-exposure prophylaxis for HIV and the use of cotrimoxazole prophylaxis for HIV-related infections among adults, adolescents and children: recommendations for a public health approach: December 2014 supplement to the 2013 consolidated guidelines on the use of antiretroviral drugs for treating and preventing HIV infection. In: Vol Accessed April 2020.2014.
70. Daniels B, Coutsoudis A, Moodley-Govender E, et al. Effect of co-trimoxazole prophylaxis on morbidity and mortality of HIV-exposed, HIV-uninfected infants in South Africa: a randomised controlled, non-inferiority trial. Lancet Glob Health 2019;7(12):e1717–27.
71. Zar HJ, Cotton MF, Strauss S, et al. Effect of isoniazid prophylaxis on mortality and incidence of tuberculosis in children with HIV: randomised controlled trial. BMJ 2007;334(7585):136.
72. World Health Organization. Chapter 4: Childhood contact screening and management. Int J Tuberc Lung Dis 2007;11(1):12–5.

Pulmonary Manifestations of Rheumatic Diseases in Children

Mary M. Buckley, MD, C. Egla Rabinovich, MD, MPH*

KEYWORDS

• SLE • JDMS • JIA • jSSc • Sarcoid • PFTs • HRCT

KEY POINTS

- Children with rheumatic disease have rare pulmonary manifestations that may cause significant morbidity and mortality.
- Children with rheumatic disease and lung manifestations are often clinically asymptomatic until disease has significantly progressed, so those at risk should be screened for pulmonary involvement with pulmonary function tests (PFTs).
- BAL and HRCT are important diagnostic modalities for lung disease.
- There has been recent recognition of high mortality-related lung disease in systemic-onset juvenile idiopathic arthritis.
- Early recognition and treatment of lung disease in children with rheumatic diseases may improve outcomes.

INTRODUCTION

Pulmonary manifestations occur in nearly all childhood rheumatic diseases, either secondary to the underlying disease, and/or as adverse effects of drug treatments. Albeit rare, lung disease may be a major cause of morbidity and mortality in these diseases. Symptoms in children may initially be absent or subtle. Those at elevated risk should therefore be screened for pulmonary involvement. Knowledge of the rheumatic diseases in children, along with the disease-specific presentations of pulmonary manifestations, aids in diagnosis and management of lung complications. Each rheumatic disease with relevant pulmonary manifestations is reviewed.

SYSTEMIC LUPUS ERYTHEMATOSUS

Childhood systemic lupus erythematosus (cSLE) is an autoimmune disease, characterized by the presence of autoantibodies in virtually all patients. The activation of

Department of Pediatrics, Division of Rheumatology, Duke University Medical Center, Box 3212 DUMC, Durham, NC 27710, USA
* Corresponding author.
E-mail address: egla.rabinovich@duke.edu

Pediatr Clin N Am 68 (2021) 147–166
https://doi.org/10.1016/j.pcl.2020.09.005 pediatric.theclinics.com
0031-3955/21/

the immune system amplified by lupus autoantibodies together with cytokines and chemokines results in multisystem inflammation and tissue damage. The most common presenting features of cSLE include arthritis, malar rash, nephritis, and central nervous system disease. Prevalence is similar in prepubescent boys and girls, with female predominance increasing after puberty.[1]

The pediatric literature suggests similar arrays of pulmonary manifestations to that of adult systemic lupus erythematosus (SLE) (**Table 1**).[1] The clinical approach to children with cSLE and pulmonary complaints should always include a thorough evaluation for infection. Children have been found to have fewer pulmonary manifestations than adults, including less pleural disease, although pulmonary function test (PFT) abnormalities have been described in up to 48% of a pediatric cohort.[2,3] Mortality has been described to be higher in those children with pulmonary, cardiac, and liver involvement.[4]

Pleuritis, often with pleural effusion, is the most common pulmonary manifestation of cSLE.[1,2,5] Pleural effusions are typically serous or serosanguinous exudates. Hemorrhagic effusions may occur with pulmonary infarcts and infection. Interstitial lung disease (ILD) in cSLE is similar to that seen in mixed connective tissue disease (MCTD), but is less common, with a prevalence of 6%.

Acute lupus pneumonitis is a rare and serious complication of SLE, presenting with acute onset of chest pain, dyspnea, dry cough, and fever with associated significant loss of respiratory function.[6] Coexisting infection is a common observation, suggesting potential trigger. Chest radiographs demonstrate a lower lobe diffuse or patchy acinar infiltrate. Many patients require mechanical ventilation. Histopathologic features of acute lupus pneumonitis include inflammatory cellular infiltrates involving the interstitium and alveolar wall.[7] Complement and immunoglobulin deposition may be seen on direct immunofluorescent staining, but vasculitic lesions are uncommon. Chronic ILD may follow acute lupus pneumonitis.

Pulmonary arterial hypertension (PAH) is characterized by a progressive increase in pulmonary vascular resistance leading to right-sided heart failure and death. PAH develops in up to 14% of cSLE, is often unrecognized in early stages, and carries a poor prognosis.[6,8] In one cohort of cSLE, PAH was seen in 2% of children, with most presenting in the first 2 years of disease onset.[9] Often by the time symptoms are overt, many have progressed to right heart failure. Careful clinical evaluation increases the sensitivity for detecting early PAH. Children are often asymptomatic but may have dyspnea on exertion and cough. Chronic venous thromboembolic disease should be evaluated, because this would mandate anticoagulation. A subset of patients improves or reverses PAH with aggressive immunosuppressive therapy incorporating corticosteroids and cyclophosphamide (CYC).[10]

Diffuse alveolar hemorrhage is an uncommon, but serious manifestation of cSLE with mortality of 40% to 90%.[6,11] It is associated with high anti-dsDNA titers and coexisting renal disease. Hemoptysis with a substantial drop in hematocrit is a typical manifestation accompanied by diffuse, bilateral acinar infiltrates on chest radiograph that might progress rapidly over hours and in some cases just as rapidly resolve. The respiratory compromise seen is often rapid and profound. Treatment recommendations are based on anecdotal evidence and case series, but therapy is generally aggressive with intravenous corticosteroid dosing and consideration of CYC, rituximab, and/or plasmapheresis.[12]

Venous thrombosis and thromboembolism are the most common thrombotic complications of antiphospholipid antibody syndrome that may be associated with SLE, and may lead to development of PAH.[13] Therefore, patients with cSLE presenting with acute dyspnea should undergo evaluation for pulmonary embolism. Catastrophic

Table 1
Noninfectious pulmonary complications of adult SLE and MCTD

Pulmonary Manifestation	Estimated Prevalence in SLE	Estimated Prevalence in MCTD	Onset	Presenting Signs and Symptoms	Radiographic Findings	Prognosis	Treatment	Differential Diagnosis
Pleuritis	50%–80%	≤20%	Acute	Pleurisy, dyspnea, orthopnea, pleural rub	Pleural effusion	Good	NSAIDs, CS	Infection, PE, ALP, AH, PTX, drug toxicity
ALP	≤10%	N/A	Acute	Dyspnea, cough, fever, chest pain, pleurisy, hemoptysis; often preceded/associated with infection, hypoxemia	Patchy acinar infiltrates with bibasilar predominance	Poor; mortality up to 50%	CS, PPh, CYC, AZA	Infection, PE, AH, pleuritis, Goodpasture syndrome
AH	Up to 2%	Rare	Acute	Dyspnea, cough, chest pain, drop in hemoglobin, pleurisy, hypoxemia	Patchy acinar infiltrates with bibasilar predominance	Mortality up to 50%	CS, PPh, CYC, AZA	Infection, ALP, PE, vasculitis, Goodpasture syndrome, IPH
Acute reversible hypoxemia	<1%		Acute/chronic	Dyspnea, low FVC, low DLCO	Normal	Good	CS	Infection, PE, early ALP or AH, SLS
Chronic interstitial pneumonitis	3%	20%–50%	Chronic, may be long-term complication of ALP	Dyspnea, cough, low FVC low DLCO, fibrosis	CXR: reticular interstitial infiltrates: ground glass, honeycombing	Poor to good	CS, CYC, AZA	Infection, LIP, drug toxicity, chronic aspiration, PA/h

(*continued on next page*)

Table 1
(continued)

Pulmonary Manifestation	Estimated Prevalence in: SLE	Estimated Prevalence in: MCTD	Onset	Presenting Signs and Symptoms	Radiographic Findings	Prognosis	Treatment	Differential Diagnosis
Shrinking lung disease	<1%		Chronic	Dyspnea, orthopnea, low FVC, low D_{LCO}	Normal or basilar atelectasis, elevated diaphragm	Good	CS	Respiratory muscle weakness from myopathies
Thromboembolic disease	—	Rare	Acute	Dyspnea, pleurisy, hemoptysis, fever, pleural rub	CXR, normal or effusion; spiral computed tomography; ventilation/ perfusion scan; D-dimer	Variable	Anticoagulation	Infection, pleurisy, PTX, AH or ALP
Pulmonary hypertension	5%–14%	20%–30%	Chronic	Dyspnea, chest discomfort, right heart failure, pericardial effusion, elevated BNP, low D_{LCO} with stable FVC	CXR, normal or per	Variable	Pulmonary vasodilators (ETRA, prostanoids, 5′PDE inhibitors), anticoagulation; CYC and CS in select cases	Infection, interstitial lung disease

Abbreviations: AH, alveolar hemorrhage; ALP, acute lupus pneumonitis; AZA, azathioprine; BNP, brain natriuretic peptide; CS, corticosteroids; CXR, chest radiograph; CYC, cyclophosphamide; D_{LCO}, diffusing capacity; ETRA, endothelin receptor antagonist; FVC, forced vital capacity; HRCT, high-resolution computed tomography; IPH, idiopathic pulmonary hemosiderosis; LIP, lymphocytic interstitial pneumonia; MCTD, mixed connective tissue disease; N/A; NSAID, nonsteroidal anti-inflammatory drug; PE, pulmonary embolus; PPh, plasmapheresis; PTX, pneumothorax; SLS, shrinking lung syndrome.

Adapted from Rabinovich CE. Paediatr Respir Rev. 2012 Mar;13(1):29-36. https://doi.org/10.1016/j.prrv.2011.05.005. Epub 2011 Jun 22. PMID: 22208791 Review; with permission.

antiphospholipid antibody syndrome with rapid multiple organ involvement has rarely been described in children.

Shrinking lung syndrome is a rare manifestation of SLE, but has been reported in cSLE.[14] Patients characteristically present with progressive dyspnea, orthopnea, and a restrictive lung pattern on PFT. Chest radiographs may reveal reduced lung volumes, elevated diaphragms, and bibasilar atelectasis. Progressive pleural fibrosis may result in restrictive lung disease.

The airways are infrequently affected in SLE, but rare cases of bronchiolitis obliterans associated with cryptogenic organizing pneumonia (formerly bronchiolitis obliterans organizing pneumonia)[6,15] have been reported. Cryptogenic organizing pneumonia is characterized histologically by nonspecific inflammatory changes within the terminal and respiratory bronchioles, alveolar ducts, and, primarily, the alveolar walls, with resultant obstructive lung disease. Patients present with dyspnea and may have associated fever, cough, and interstitial infiltrates. Open lung biopsy is often needed to confirm the diagnosis. Corticosteroids are often effective treatment.[15]

Because infection is the major cause of mortality in cSLE, children with pulmonary manifestations require thorough investigation and treatment of infectious complications. It is also important to exclude other causes of pulmonary complications in cSLE, such as drug toxicity and the impact of cardiac or renal disease.

MIXED CONNECTIVE TISSUE DISEASE

MCTD is an overlap syndrome; manifestations are a mixture of features of SLE, rheumatoid arthritis (RA), dermatomyositis, and scleroderma.[16] The defining serologic feature of MCTD is the presence of antiribonucleoprotein autoantibodies.

Prospective studies now suggest that the insidious development of ILD or PAH results in a substantial increase in morbidity and mortality in adults for a subset (20%–30%) of patients with MCTD.[16] ILD, pleuritis, and PAH are the most common and clinically important forms of pulmonary complications of MCTD (see **Table 1**). Progressive esophageal dysmotility is increased in MCTD compared with SLE, increasing the risk for aspiration pneumonia, aspiration-associated bronchoconstriction, and/or pulmonary fibrosis. Inflammatory and fibrosing ILD affects up to 66% of adult patients with MCTD, but is less common in children, with one pediatric cohort reporting a 27% prevalence of mainly mild, asymptomatic ILD without much progression over time, albeit severe disease has been reported.[17–19] The lower rate of progressive pulmonary fibrosis differentiates lung disease in MCTD from ILD found in scleroderma.

Typical presentation is progressive dyspnea on exertion with nonproductive cough. PFTs demonstrate a restrictive pattern with reduced lung volumes and diffusing capacity of lung for carbon monoxide (D_{LCO}). Characteristic high-resolution chest computed tomography (HRCT) findings include septal thickening and ground glass opacities with peripheral and basilar lung zone predominance.[1,20] Traction bronchiectasis and honeycomb changes develop later in the course of the disease, typically with a basilar, subpleural distribution. Bronchoalveolar lavage (BAL) may show a neutrophilic or eosinophilic predominance in the cell count while excluding infection. Patients who develop dyspnea and restrictive pattern on PFTs or experience a decrease in D_{LCO} should undergo HRCT of the chest. If the result is unremarkable and no other explanation is available for the pulmonary decline, BAL may be indicated to confirm the presence of inflammation and exclude infection.

The leading cause of death in adults with MCTD is PAH.[16] PAH develops in nearly one-third of patients with MCTD and occurs in children and adults.[16,20] The histologic features in MCTD are identical to those observed in PAH associated with scleroderma.

In all patients who develop PAH, routine screening for underlying secondary causes should be undertaken, including screening for chronic venous thromboembolic disease, human immunodeficiency virus, sickle cell disease, and congenital heart disease. Screening with an echocardiogram, PFTs, serum brain-natriuretic peptide, and 6-minute-walk tests are important in MCTD disease management. PAH may develop as late as 20 years following diagnosis.[21] The rate of response to immunosuppressive therapy suggests that treatment of PAH in patients with MCTD should incorporate a course of corticosteroids and CYC or mycophenolate mofetil (MMF).[10] Clinicians with expertise in managing PAH should be consulted.

SJÖGREN SYNDROME

Sjögren syndrome is a chronic autoimmune disease that primarily affects the lacrimal and salivary glands.[22] The cardinal clinical features are parotitis, keratoconjunctivitis sicca, and xerostomia, with variable systemic involvement, including ILD in adults. The hallmark autoantibody findings include a positive ANA, Ro (SS-A), La (SS-B), and rheumatoid factor (RF). In the pediatric population, Sjögren syndrome is rare with a mean age of onset of 10 years. A review of 145 pediatric cases reported parotid enlargement in 70%, eye involvement in 66%, and xerostomia in 43%.[23] In contrast to adults, pulmonary involvement is rare in children but may include ILD. Evaluation and management are similar to MCTD.

JUVENILE IDIOPATHIC ARTHRITIS

Juvenile idiopathic arthritis (JIA) is the most common rheumatic disease in childhood. JIA is characterized by arthritis, which begins less than 16 years of age, persisting for at least 6 weeks, and for which no specific cause may be found. It is twice as common in girls than in boys. Its cause is unknown, but it is associated with articular and extra-articular manifestations. The International League Against Rheumatism has categorized JIA into the following subtypes[24]:

- Polyarticular JIA, RF negative: involvement of five or more inflamed joints in the first 6 months of disease.
- Polyarticular JIA, RF positive: same as above but with two positive RF tests 3 months apart in first 6 months of disease.
- Oligoarticular: involvement of less than five inflamed joints in the first 6 months of disease
    - Persistent: does not affect greater than four joints throughout the course of disease.
    - Extended: affects greater than four joints after the first 6 months of disease.
- Systemic arthritis: fever, rash, hepatosplenomegaly.
- Psoriatic arthritis: arthritis and psoriasis or arthritis with two of the following: dactylitis, nail pits, and family history.
- Enthesitis-related arthritis: inflammation where ligaments, tendons, or joint capsules attach to the bones, typically develops in boys with lower limb arthritis (knee and heel). This may be the forerunner of ankylosing spondylitis later in life.
- Undifferentiated: does not fill criteria for any of the above or fulfills criteria for more than one category.

Lung complications of adult RA are well recognized and most commonly present as ILD with a 10% to 20% associated mortality.[25] PFTs show a restrictive defect with decreased D_{LCO}. This manifestation is rare in children. However, in a study of 32 asymptomatic children with all subsets of JIA, up to 60% of patients have abnormalities on PFTs,[26] consistent with a restrictive lung pattern: decreased forced vital capacity (FVC), forced expiratory pressure in 1 second, and DLCO, but preserved forced expiratory pressure in 1 second/FVC ratio.[26,27] An inverse relationship was reported between PFTs and RF titer, erythrocyte sedimentation rate, disease duration, and treatment with methotrexate, implying an association between disease severity, duration, and pulmonary function.[28,29] Restrictive lung function including reduced DLCO may affect up to 30% with JIA.[30,31] There also exists an association between JIA and decreased maximum inspiratory and expiratory pressures, which correlate with respiratory muscle strength.[26] This suggests that respiratory muscle weakness, potentially related to decreased levels of physical fitness and chest wall mobility in children with JIA, may also be contributing factors to PFT abnormalities.[28–31] Prevalence of lung disease remains low in children with JIA.[27,32,33]

Juvenile ankylosing spondylitis (JAS) is classified within the enthesitis-related arthritis subgroup of JIA. Sacroiliitis is the hallmark of JAS and evolves over the years, often until after adolescence, when it becomes radiographically evident to establish the diagnosis. Pleuropulmonary manifestations in ankylosing spondylitis occur in approximately 1% of patients.[34] These may include bilateral pleural thickening without effusion, fibrous, and bullous disease. PFTs reveal a restrictive pattern, which may improve with anti–tumor necrosis factor therapy.[35,36] Children with JAS rarely have symptoms of pulmonary complications. However, in one study of 18 asymptomatic JAS patients with normal chest radiographs, 30% had a restrictive pattern on PFTs with reduced DLCO.[37] In these patients, no association was found between lung function and chest expansion, disease severity, or duration.

SYSTEMIC JUVENILE IDIOPATHIC ARTHRITIS

Systemic JIA (sJIA) is the rarest subset of JIA (about 10%), defined as inflammatory arthritis plus fever for 2 weeks, daily for at least 3 days of fevers, evanescent rash, generalized lymphadenopathy, hepatosplenomegaly, or serositis.[24] Patients with sJIA often have marked elevation of inflammatory markers and are at increased risk for macrophage activation syndrome, a form of secondary hemophagocytic lymphohistiocytosis.[38] Of all subtypes, sJIA has the highest morbidity and mortality.[39,40] However, with the use of interleukin-1 and interleukin-6 inhibitors (eg, anakinra and tocilizumab), the prognosis has improved dramatically.[41]

Pulmonary involvement in JIA is uncommon. sJIA, followed by RF-positive polyarticular arthritis, is the most common subtype associated with lung complications. Pleuritis is a well-reported manifestation of sJIA, usually accompanied by pericarditis.[42] Pleural fluid findings suggest an exudate: lymphocytosis, low glucose, elevated lactate dehydrogenase and protein, and depressed complements.[23] Primary PAH has rarely been reported in sJIA.[43]

Until recently, further descriptions of pulmonary manifestations in sJIA were limited to case reports.[43,44] However, descriptions of more severe complications, such as PAH, ILD, and pulmonary alveolar proteinosis (PAP), or lipoid pneumonia have started emerging. With the increasing prevalence of these previously rare, and often fatal complications, much effort has been made to further understand their clinical presentation, pathology, and cause.

Clinically, patients with sJIA lung disease (sJIA-LD) may be asymptomatic or may present with shortness of breath, exertional dyspnea, cough, or clubbing. In one case series of 18 children, 96% of patients with sJIA-LD endorsed symptoms.[45] In another series of 45 children with sJIA-LD, acute onset of clubbing was reported in 60%, half of those associated with digital erythema; patients were found to be hypoxemic 40% of the time.[46] Other clinical findings included pruritic, nonevanescent rashes (56%); peripheral eosinophilia (37%); severe abdominal pain (16%); and a history of anaphylaxis to tocilizumab (38% of those exposed). Initial reports suggest a sJIA-LD prevalence of 6.8%.[47]

HRCT, the preferred imaging modality, shows ground glass opacities that may evolve into peripheral septal thickening, a finding common of ILD, most often affecting the lower lung zones, anterior upper lobes, or perihilar or perimediastinal zones.[46,48] Despite these common features in other forms of ILD, findings of pulmonary fibrosis are rarely seen.[46]

In lipoid pneumonia, multiple pulmonary nodules consisting of intra-alveolar and interstitial cholesterol granulomas are seen, most often in the centrilobular region.[48] Crazy-paving, pleural thickening, peribronchovascular thickening, tree-in-bud opacities, and peripheral consolidation and prominent hyperenhancing lymphadenopathy have also been reported.[46,47]

BAL may help in excluding infectious causes; however, its utility is otherwise limited. BAL results do not correlate with biopsy-proven PAP secondary to sJIA-LD,[47] consistent with adult RA-related ILD data.[49]

The most common radiographic finding in sJIA-LD, septal thickening with ground glass opacities, is most associated with NSIP (Nonspecific Interstitial Pneumonia). However, in patients with sJIA-LD who undergo open lung biopsy, histology is most consistent with PAP.[46,47] The alveolar space and airway lumens are filled with eosinophilic proteinaceous material, foamy macrophages, and cholesterol clefts.[46,47] In comparison with other forms of autoimmune PAP, these findings are most abundant in sJIA-LD.[47] In addition, a predominantly lymphocytic infiltrate, type II alveolar cell hyperplasia, chronic lung injury, collagenous fibrosis, and arterial wall thickening are commonly reported.[46,47]

A genetic mutation associated with sJIA-LD has not been identified. Risk factors for sJIA-LD include: diagnosis at less than 2 years of age; trisomy 21; a history of macrophage activation syndrome; and history of adverse reactions to cytokine blockade, most often interleukin-6 blockade with tocilizumab.[46,47]

Optimal treatment of this recently described phenomenon is poorly understood, but with a 5-year survival rate of 42%,[46] there is urgent need for further understanding of this unusual complication to better the understanding of how to prevent and treat it.

METHOTREXATE

The pulmonary toxicities of medications used to treat JIA, especially methotrexate, add a level of complexity when assessing the impact of the disease. Methotrexate is one of the most commonly used medications in JIA. It has been used for years in JIA without reports of significant lung damage. However, a recent cross-sectional study of PFTs in 49 children with JIA (70 control subjects) showed no difference in parameters except for DLCO, which was decreased in the JIA population (87% vs 99%).[27] Those with active disease, higher methotrexate doses, and longer duration of therapy had the lowest DLCO values. Analysis of covariance did show a weak independent effect of methotrexate use, but not disease activity on DLCO reduction. These findings are concerning for methotrexate-induced chronic progressive fibrosis.

An uncommon but concerning pulmonary complication of methotrexate therapy is hypersensitivity pneumonitis. Methotrexate pneumonitis is more prevalent in adult patients than in children. Estimates of pneumonitis in adults using low doses of methotrexate (<25 mg/wk) range from 0.5% to 12%, and a lack of association between RA-ILD and methotrexate pneumonitis has recently been described.[50] Manifestations of methotrexate pneumonitis include dyspnea, dry cough, tachypnea, fever,[51] and bibasilar crackles on lung auscultation.[52] Peripheral eosinophilia may be found, but is neither sensitive nor specific. Chest radiographs frequently reveal interstitial and/or alveolar infiltrates. Computed tomography scans often identify ground glass opacities, interstitial, or alveolar infiltrates.[51,52] BAL with a predominance of $CD4^+$ lymphocytes supports a diagnosis of methotrexate pneumonitis.[49,52] Lung pathology is nonspecific, but include interstitial infiltrates, fibrosis, granulomas, and diffuse alveolar damage.[51,52]

SCLERODERMA

Scleroderma, better known as systemic sclerosis (SSc), is an inflammatory and fibrotic disorder of the skin and other organs with morbidity resulting from excess collagen production.[53] It is divided into two categories: juvenile localized scleroderma (jLS) and juvenile SSc (jSSc). jLS almost exclusively involves the skin, is free of pulmonary manifestations, and may be classified into one of five categories based on disease extent and morphology.[54] It has an incidence of 0.34 to 2.7 cases per 100,00 per year and is far more common that jSSc, which has an estimated incidence of 0.27 per million per year.[53]

Although less common than jLS, it is estimated that 10% of all cases of SSc begin in childhood.[55] There is not a clear gender or racial predilection for jSSc but pulmonary manifestations are of concern in jSSc. Validated diagnostic criteria do not exist for jSSc; however, provisional criteria for classification of jSSc proposed in 2007 may aid in diagnosis.[56] Per these criteria, skin induration proximal to the metatarsophalangeal or metacarpophalangeal joints must be present, in addition to two other minor criteria.[56] Cases of jSSC may be further subdivided into limited cutaneous SSc should skin involvement be confined distal to the elbows, knees, and neck or diffuse cutaneous SSc should skin involvement also include involvement proximal to the elbows, knees, and neck or involve the chest and abdomen.[53] A third subcategory, overlap SSc, includes those with features or another rheumatic disease.

Pulmonary fulfillment of minor criteria includes evidence of pulmonary fibrosis on HRCT or chest radiograph, decreased DLCO, or evidence of PAH. In jSSc, pulmonary involvement occurs in 34% to 55% and is usually characterized by restrictive lung disease, decreased DLCO, and fibrosis rather than PAH.[57,58] PAH occurs less commonly in jSSC than SSc, but it remains an ominous sign given high association with mortality. In one study, PAH was fatal in all four children who developed this complication.[58] Less common lung manifestations in SSc have been reported including shrinking lung syndrome and pulmonary-renal syndrome with renal failure and diffuse alveolar hemorrhage.[59,60]

Overall, children with jSSC have improved survival rates compared with adults.[58] Unlike their adult counterparts, in whom pulmonary involvement, specifically pulmonary fibrosis and PAH, is the leading cause of disease-related death, patients with jSSc are more likely to experience disease-related cardiac death.[58,61–63] Children with limited cutaneous SSc have better prognosis compared with those with diffuse cutaneous SSc, with improved 20-year survival and a lower incidence of pulmonary fibrosis.[63] Factors negatively affecting survival in children include fibrosis on chest radiograph, pericarditis, and raised creatinine levels; diffuse disease with rapid progression exemplifies a typical pediatric fatal course.[64]

Autoantibodies may also aid the clinician in stratifying a patient's risk of pulmonary involvement. In adult patients, anti-Scl-70/antitopoisomerase antibody has been associated with the development of ILD.[53] The anticentromere antibody, however, may be protective against development of ILD, but may be associated with the development of PAH.[65–67]

The pathology of SSc-associated ILD (SSc-ILD) is that of an initial alveolitis with interstitial edema and patchy inflammation of alveolar walls. This leads to thinning and rupture of alveolar walls, with resultant cyst formation, interstitial, and peribronchial fibrosis.[68] An increase in memory T cells likely contributes to the evolution of pulmonary injury and remodeling.[69] As a result, lung volumes and DLCO progressively decrease. Lung inflammation has been shown to be associated with the evolution of progressive restrictive lung disease.[70]

Diagnosis of ILD remains a clinical challenge because children may underreport symptoms. The most common clinical manifestation in children is chronic nonproductive cough.[71] In a group of children with proven ILD, only 2 of 11 reported dyspnea on exertion.[70] Chest radiographs are often normal until later in the disease course, but use of HRCT as an imaging tool has improved detection.[70] Common findings include ground glass opacities, honeycombing, bronchiectasis, subpleural nodules, subpleural cysts, and interlobular septal thickening giving a reticular pattern.[72] Ground glass appearance is indicative of cellular infiltration, whereas a reticular pattern correlates with fibrosis (**Fig. 1**).[73]

In addition to HRCT, PFTs may detect pulmonary involvement and follow treatment response.[74] PFTs show decreased FVC and DLCO. A decreased FVC correlates with the presence of honeycombing and ground glass appearance on HRCT.[70,72] A decreased DLCO best reflects the extent of fibrosing alveolitis, but may also be reflective of PAH.[75] Findings on BAL suggestive of active alveolitis include polymorphonuclear leukocytes (≥4%) and/or eosinophils (≥2%).[76] BAL abnormalities may be suggestive of more severe ILD and early mortality, but otherwise does not correlate with disease progression or treatment response.[76–78] Thus, BAL fluid analysis may be abnormal early in disease course and may help to exclude infection, but it has little prognostic value with no indication to perform serial studies.

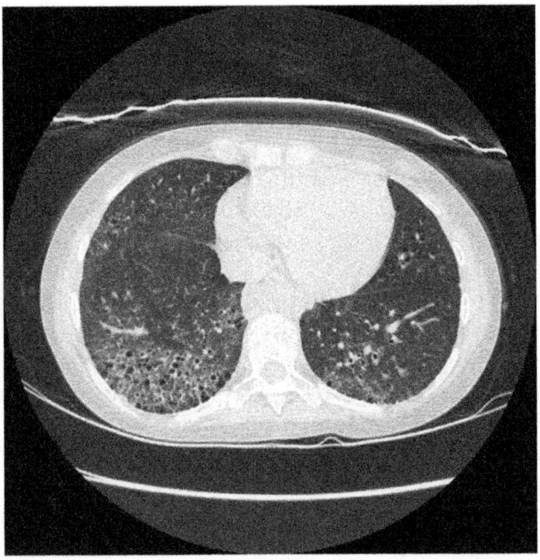

Fig. 1. HRCT in an adolescent with juvenile systemic sclerosis. Note honeycombing and ground glass opacities.

Treatment of SSc-ILD should be initiated early in disease course. Oral, daily CYC was the first therapy to be studied prospectively and showed significant improvements in lung function, dyspnea, skin scores, and health-related quality of life.[79,80] However, side effects were common. Azathioprine maintenance therapy following 6 months of intravenous CYC showed a nonsignificant trend toward improvement in FVC.[81] Most recently, MMF was compared with oral CYC in a prospective, randomized controlled trial. Although there was no difference in lung function, dyspnea, imaging, or skin findings between the two arms, there were fewer side effects in the MMF arm, supporting the use of MMF in treatment of SSc-ILD as an equivalent therapy to CYC with fewer side effects.[82] Improvements with rituximab have been reported in case series and it may represent a promising treatment option; however, data from randomized controlled trials are still pending.[83] Tocilizumab has also been studied and shown to prevent decline in FVC,[84] as has the antifibrotic agent, pirfenidone.[83,85] Stem cell transplant may be beneficial for those with rapidly progressive disease; however, its significant treatment-associated side effects must be carefully considered.[86]

Aggressive and early treatment of SSc-associated PAH (SSc-PAH) has dramatically increased life expectancy.[87] However, data guiding treatment of SSc-PAH are largely extrapolated from studies conducted on heterogeneous populations of PAH. European League Against Rheumatism current treatment recommendations for SSc-PAH include intravenous epoprostenol for severe cases. For less severe cases, the endothelin receptor antagonists ambrisentan, bosentan, and macitentan, phosphosdiesterase-5 inhibitors sildenafil, tadalafil, and riociguat, all approved for treatment of PAH associated with connective tissue disease, or prostacyclin analogues are recommended.[86] Bosentan has been reported to be efficacious in treating PAH in the pediatric age group.[88] In addition to these targeted therapies, supportive measures include correction of hypoxemia with oxygen therapy, regulation of intravascular volume statues with fluid/sodium restriction or diuretics, digitalis, anticoagulation, and prevention of pulmonary infections with vaccinations for influenza and pneumococcal pneumonia.[87]

JUVENILE DERMATOMYOSITIS

Juvenile dermatomyositis (JDMS) is a chronic autoimmune inflammatory disorder of skin and muscle characterized by a typical rash, proximal muscle weakness, and elevation of muscle enzymes.[89] In rare cases, when the rash is absent, the term polymyositis is applied. Pulmonary involvement with JDMS in children is rare. The characteristic histopathology of JDMS is a small vessel vasculitis. With severe muscle involvement, respiratory failure from thoracic muscle fatigue may result.

Classical signs of respiratory distress, such as retractions or tachypnea, may not herald the onset of respiratory failure.[89] Therefore, children with severe weakness should be monitored in the hospital for respiratory muscle weakness (negative inspiratory force in younger children), vital capacity in older children, and/or carbon dioxide retention (end tidal capnography or arterial blood gas measurements).

There have been specific autoantibodies associated with ILD in JDMS including the anti-tRNA synthetase antibodies (anti-Jo-1, anti-PL-12) and anti-Ro52 and anti-MDA-5.[90–93] The pulmonary pathology is largely extrapolated from adults with dermatomyositis, because although 30% to 50% of adults have ILD, the pulmonary expression of JDMS is rarer in children, affecting up to 14%.[92,94] The lung histopathology is devoid of vasculitic contribution. The characteristic lung fibrosis may present either as interstitial/alveolar (usual interstitial pneumonitis) or small airways obstruction (bronchiolitis obliterans with organizing pneumonia).

Acute respiratory distress syndrome may be an alternative presentation with the pathophysiologic process associated with vascular leak, such as alveolar edema, and the formation of hyaline membranes. However, there is recent evidence that the lung disease in JDMS is subclinical and is characterized by decreased total lung capacity and DLCO with 37% having HRCT abnormalities including ILD (14%), chest wall calcinosis (14%), and airway disease (15%).[95] HRCT abnormality in these children correlated with cumulative organ damage and health-related quality of life.

Although much progress has been made in the therapy for JDMS with current mortality less than 10%, treatment strategies are not grounded in prospective, controlled data. Corticosteroid therapy remains the mainstay, although methotrexate is increasingly used as a first-line therapy.[96] More severe disease, such as weakness of the thoracic musculature, is often treated with pulse methylprednisolone. Hydroxychloroquine is used to control skin manifestations and may permit steroid sparing. Alternative immunomodulatory therapies for JDMS have included intravenous immunoglobulin, rituximab, azathioprine, CYC, and cyclosporine.[89]

SARCOIDOSIS

Sarcoidosis is a chronic multisystem inflammatory disorder of unknown cause characterized by the development of noncaseating granulomas in a wide range of tissues.[97,98] Because of this, sarcoidosis, like tuberculosis, may mimic a variety of clinical disorders varying from asymptomatic to life threatening. Commonly affected organs include thoracic lymph nodes, lungs, liver, spleen, eyes, bones, joints, salivary and lacrimal glands, central nervous system, and skin. Sarcoidosis affects boys and girls equally, with an incidence in the United States estimated at 5 per 100,000 in Whites and 40 per 100,000 in African Americans.[99,100]

Sarcoidosis in the preschool age group presents with a triad of a granulomatous skin rash, uveitis, and arthritis, and is known as Blau syndrome.[101] Mutations are seen in the caspase recruitment domain-15 (CARD-15)/nucleotide-binding oligomerization domain-2 (NOD2) proteins, members of the NOD family of proteins.[102] These mutations are associated with the activation of nuclear factor-κB, associated with the upregulation of several inflammatory cytokines. The response to therapy for Blau syndrome is often disappointing and challenging.[101]

The more common presentation of sarcoidosis occurs in the third and fourth decades of life and includes combinations of lung disease, lymphadenopathy, fever, weight loss, and hypercalcemia.[98] Variations of this phenotype occur throughout childhood and occur most commonly in adolescents. School-aged children are more likely to have pulmonary parenchymal involvement in addition to hilar or paratracheal adenopathy.[98,100] Multiorgan disease expression in children is typical.[100]

The classical lesion of sarcoidosis on tissue biopsy is a noncaseating granuloma.[100] A typical lesion consists of an organized ring of epithelioid cells that are radially arranged, and are populated with Langerhans-type giant cells surrounded by lymphocytes.[98] Noncaseating granulomas may also be seen in certain toxic exposures (beryllium), viral and fungal infections, tuberculosis, and in lymph nodes draining sites of cancer, so that careful analysis of the differential is critical.[97] There are recent reports of sarcoid granulomas in multiple organs after E-cigarette or marijuana vaping in adolescents.[103]

The immune inflammatory response responsible for the evolution of the granulomas is thought to originate with the presentation of antigens by macrophages to T lymphocytes, which then causes proliferation and activation of T cells, resulting in cytokine and chemokine elaboration with additional recruitment of monocytes and macrophages causing an exaggerated and amplified immune response.[98,100] Granulomas may resolve, or heal with fibrosis, causing end-tissue damage. The granulomas are known to be capable of secreting and activating vitamin D, explaining the observed complications of hypercalcemia and hypercalciuria and their frequently positive response to treatment with corticosteroid therapy.[104]

Respiratory symptoms are often subtle and include cough, dyspnea, chest pain, and/or sputum production. Signs often are absent, but include coarse or muffled breath sounds, wheezing, or crackles.[100] In contrast, chest radiographs are often abnormal. In a published series of 19 children with sarcoidosis, nearly all cases demonstrated parabronchial adenopathy with most demonstrating paratracheal adenopathy with parenchymal involvement.[105] Typical HRCT features include reticulonodular and interstitial patterns; less typical features include alveolar filling processes, distinct nodules, fibrotic phenotypes, or more dramatic changes, such as pneumothorax, pleural thickening, or atelectasis.[106]

The adult radiographic staging of chest radiographs has been adopted for use in evaluating children: stage 0 is a normal chest radiograph, stage 1 has parabronchial adenopathy, stage 2 includes parabronchial adenopathy along with parenchymal infiltrates, stage 3 has parenchymal infiltrates without parabronchial adenopathy, and stage 4 is characterized by fibrotic lesions and bullous emphysema.[97,107] Disease progression follows the sequence of the radiographic staging with worsening prognosis in the more advanced stages.

The most consistently seen PFT abnormality is a restrictive pattern in which total lung capacity and functional residual capacity are reduced.[106,108] Decreases in D_{LCO} are also seen.[107] Syndromes of airway hyperresponsiveness and airway obstruction are common in sarcoidosis, thus bronchodilators and inhaled corticosteroids may be helpful.[109] In rare cases, granulomas may involve any of the structures of the larynx and upper airway, producing hoarseness, stridor, dyspnea, obstructive sleep apnea, cough, or dysphagia.[97]

The diagnosis of sarcoidosis in children is the same as that in adults and is based on criteria published in a joint consensus statement of the American Thoracic Society and European Respiratory Society in 1999.[107] The diagnosis requires (1) a compatible clinical profile, (2) histologic evidence of noncaseating granulomas, and (3) exclusion of other disease processes that potentially mimic sarcoidosis. The critical parts are the requirement of tissue confirmation and the elimination of confounding candidates. Bronchoscopy with cultures is sometimes necessary to exclude infection. In addition, BAL fluid with ratio of $CD4^+$ to $CD8^+$ lymphocytes of greater than 3.5, although insensitive (53% detection), has been determined to be highly specific (94%) for the diagnosis of sarcoidosis.[103] Tissue biopsy source may be a suspicious lesion anywhere on the body; superficial targets, such a skin or conjunctival lesions, are preferred.[98] The feasibility of fine-needle aspiration of lung or mediastinal lymph nodes has been demonstrated in adolescent patients.

Supportive diagnostic studies are not specific. The erythrocyte sedimentation rate is usually elevated in active disease. Levels of serum angiotensin-converting enzyme are elevated in up to 80% of children with sarcoidosis and may be helpful in following disease activity. However, several diseases, including diabetes, liver disease, and neoplasms, are also associated with elevated angiotensin-converting enzyme levels. Angiotensin-converting enzyme levels in children may be up to 50% greater than in adults, so that pediatric-specific normal values should be applied.[110]

The cornerstone of therapy for sarcoidosis is daily oral or parenteral corticosteroids with demonstrated short-term improvement; however, data are still lacking for evidence for long-term success.[98] Many with mild disease recover without intervention. Sarcoidosis that is refractory to usual therapy may respond to methotrexate or to pharmacologic blockade of tumor necrosis factor-α; pentoxifylline may have a corticosteroid-sparing role.[98] The outcome for most school-aged children seems to be favorable, albeit there is evidence that those less than 10 years of age (without Blau syndrome) do better than those older than 10 years.[103,111] The prognoses for school-aged children with more advanced pulmonary disease and younger children with Blau syndrome are more guarded. For patients with pulmonary disease there is a need for multicenter controlled trials of therapy with corticosteroids and alternative candidate therapies.

SUMMARY

Pulmonary involvement in the pediatric rheumatic diseases is rare, often initially asymptomatic, but can cause significant morbidity and mortality. Those at risk should undergo periodic screening with PFTs; BAL and HRCT are adjunctive diagnostic modalities. There has been recent recognition of a highly fatal lung disease in systemic onset JIA; risk factors include onset of JIA less than 2 years of age, history of macrophage activation syndrome, presence of trisomy 21, and history of anaphylactic reaction to biologic therapy. Treatment of lung disease in children with rheumatic diseases should be targeted with ultimate prognosis in mind.

CLINICAL CARE POINTS

- Children with pulmonary involvement of their rheumatic disease are often clinically asymptomatic.
- As such, a high index of suspicion must be maintained and clinicians must not be overly reassured by minimal symptoms.
- PFTs and chest Xray are useful modalities to begin the evaluation for pulmonary involvement for those at risk, and High-resolution chest CT may be indicated for further evaluation.

DISCLOSURE

The authors have nothing to disclose.

REFERENCES

1. Rabinovich CEFE, Shanahan J, Majure JM, et al. Pulmonary manifestations of rheumatoid diseases. In: Turcios NLFR, editor. Pulmonary manifestations of pediatric diseases. Philadelphia (PA): Saunders; 2009. p. 202–4.
2. Bundhun PK, Kumari A, Huang F. Differences in clinical features observed between childhood-onset versus adult-onset systemic lupus erythematosus: a systematic review and meta-analysis. Medicine (Baltimore) 2017;96(37):e8086.
3. Veiga CS, Coutinho DS, Nakaie CMA, et al. Subclinical pulmonary abnormalities in childhood-onset systemic lupus erythematosus patients. Lupus 2016;25(6): 645–51.
4. Tavangar-Rad F, Ziaee V, Moradinejad M-H, et al. Morbidity and mortality in Iranian children with juvenile systemic lupus erythematosus. Iran J Pediatr 2014; 24(4):365–70.

5. Delgado EA, Malleson PN, Pirie GE, et al. The pulmonary manifestations of childhood onset systemic lupus erythematosus. Semin Arthritis Rheum 1990; 19(5):285–93.
6. Murin S, Wiedemann HP, Matthay RA. Pulmonary manifestations of systemic lupus erythematosus. Clin Chest Med 1998;19(4):641–65.
7. Haupt HM, Moore GW, Hutchins GM. The lung in systemic lupus erythematosus. Am J Med 1981;71(5):791–8.
8. Pan TL-T, Thumboo J, Boey ML. Primary and secondary pulmonary hypertension in systemic lupus erythematosus. Lupus 2000;9(5):338–42.
9. Anuardo P, Verdier M, Gormezano NWS, et al. Subclinical pulmonary hypertension in childhood systemic lupus erythematosus associated with minor disease manifestations. Pediatr Cardiol 2017;38(2):234–9.
10. Jais X, Launay D, Yaici A, et al. Immunosuppressive therapy in lupus- and mixed connective tissue disease–associated pulmonary arterial hypertension: a retrospective analysis of twenty-three cases. Arthritis Rheum 2008;58(2):521–31.
11. Zamora MR, Warner ML, Tuder R, et al. Diffuse alveolar hemorrhage and systemic lupus erythematosus: clinical presentation, histology, survival, and outcome. Medicine (Baltimore) 1997;76(3):192–202.
12. Todd DJ, Costenbader KH. Dyspnoea in a young woman with active systemic lupus erythematosus. Lupus 2009;18(9):777–84.
13. Campos LM, Kiss MH, D'Amico ÉA, et al. Antiphospholipid antibodies and antiphospholipid syndrome in 57 children and adolescents with systemic lupus erythematosus. Lupus 2003;12(11):820–6.
14. Ferguson PJ, Weinberger M. Shrinking lung syndrome in a 14-year-old boy with systemic lupus erythematosus. Pediatr Pulmonol 2006;41(2):194–7.
15. Min JK, Hong YS, Park SH, et al. Bronchiolitis obliterans organizing pneumonia as an initial manifestation in patients with systemic lupus erythematosus. J Rheumatol 1997;24(11):2254–7.
16. Burdt MA, Hoffman RW, Deutscher SL, et al. Long-term outcome in mixed connective tissue disease: longitudinal clinical and serologic findings. Arthritis Rheum 1999;42(5):899–909.
17. Mier RJ, Shishov M, Higgins GC, et al. Pediatric-onset mixed connective tissue disease. Rheum Dis Clin North Am 2005;31(3):483–96.
18. Castelino FV, Varga J. Interstitial lung disease in connective tissue diseases: evolving concepts of pathogenesis and management. Arthritis Res Ther 2010; 12(4):213.
19. Hetlevik SO, Flatø B, Rygg M, et al. Long-term outcome in juvenile-onset mixed connective tissue disease: a nationwide Norwegian study. Ann Rheum Dis 2017; 76(1):159–65.
20. Michels H. Course of mixed connective tissue disease in children. Annu Mediaev 1997;29(5):359–64.
21. Vegh J, Szodoray P, Kappelmayer J, et al. Clinical and immunoserological characteristics of mixed connective tissue disease associated with pulmonary arterial hypertension. Scand J Immunol 2006;64(1):69–76.
22. Talal N. Sjögren's syndrome: historical overview and clinical spectrum of disease. Rheum Dis Clin North Am 1992;18(3):507–15.
23. Shiel BWC, Prete PE. Pleuropulmonary manifestations of rheumatoid arthritis. Semin Arthritis Rheum 1984;13(3):235–43.
24. Petty RE, Southwood TR, Manners P, et al. International league of associations for rheumatology classification of juvenile idiopathic arthritis: second revision, Edmonton, 2001. J Rheumatol 2004;31(2):390–2.

25. O'Dwyer DN, Armstrong ME, Cooke G, et al. Rheumatoid arthritis (RA) associated interstitial lung disease (ILD). Eur J Intern Med 2013;24(7):597–603.
26. Alkady EAM, Helmy HAR, Mohamed-Hussein AAR. Assessment of cardiac and pulmonary function in children with juvenile idiopathic arthritis. Rheumatol Int 2012;32(1):39–46.
27. Attanasi M, Lucantoni M, Rapino D, et al. Lung function in children with juvenile idiopathic arthritis: a cross-sectional analysis. Pediatr Pulmonol 2019;54(8): 1242–9.
28. Metin G, Oztürk L, Kasapçopur O, et al. Cardiopulmonary exercise testing in juvenile idiopathic arthritis. J Rheumatol 2004;31(9):1834–9.
29. Kwon H-J, Kim YL, Lee HS, et al. A study on the physical fitness of children with juvenile rheumatoid arthritis. J Phys Ther Sci 2017;29(3):378–83.
30. Knook LMe, de Kleer Im, van der Ent CK, et al. Lung function abnormalities and respiratory muscle weakness in children with juvenile chronic arthritis. Eur Respir J 1999;14(3):529.
31. Noyes BE, Albers GM, deMello DE, et al. Early onset of pulmonary parenchymal disease associated with juvenile rheumatoid arthritis. Pediatr Pulmonol 1997; 24(6):444–6.
32. Athreya BH, Doughty RA, Bookspan M, et al. Pulmonary manifestations of juvenile rheumatoid arthritis. A report of eight cases and review. Clin Chest Med 1980;1(3):361–74.
33. Raimundo K, Solomon JJ, Olson AL, et al. Rheumatoid arthritis–interstitial lung disease in the United States: prevalence, incidence, and healthcare costs and mortality. J Rheumatol 2019;46(4):360–9.
34. Rosenow E, Strimlan CV, Muhm JR, et al. Pleuropulmonary manifestations of ankylosing spondylitis. Mayo Clin Proc 1977;52(10):641–9.
35. Sampaio-Barros PD, Cerqueira EMFP, Rezende SM, et al. Pulmonary involvement in ankylosing spondylitis. Clin Rheumatol 2007;26(2):225–30.
36. Dougados M, Braun J, Szanto S, et al. Efficacy of etanercept on rheumatic signs and pulmonary function tests in advanced ankylosing spondylitis: results of a randomised double-blind placebo-controlled study (SPINE). Ann Rheum Dis 2011;70(5):799–804.
37. Camiciottoli G, Trapani S, Ermini M, et al. Pulmonary function in children affected by juvenile spondyloarthropathy. J Rheumatol 1999;26(6):1382–6.
38. Ravelli A, Grom AA, Behrens EM, et al. Macrophage activation syndrome as part of systemic juvenile idiopathic arthritis: diagnosis, genetics, pathophysiology and treatment. Genes Immun 2012;13(4):289–98.
39. Hashkes PJ, Wright BM, Lauer MS, et al. Mortality outcomes in pediatric rheumatology in the US. Arthritis Rheum 2010;62(2):599–608.
40. Nigrovic PA. Storm warning: lung disease in systemic juvenile idiopathic arthritis. Arthritis Rheum 2019;71(11):1773–5.
41. Nigrovic PA, Mannion M, Prince FH, et al. Anakinra as first-line disease-modifying therapy in systemic juvenile idiopathic arthritis: report of forty-six patients from an international multicenter series. Arthritis Rheum 2011;63(2):545–55.
42. de Benedetti F, Schneider R. Systemic juvenile idiopathic arthritis. In: Petty RE, Laxer RM, Lindsley C, et al, editors. Textbook of pediatric rheumatology. 7th edition. Philadelphia: Elsevier, Inc; 2016. p. 205–16.
43. Padeh S, Laxer RM, Silver MM, et al. Primary pulmonary hypertension in a patient with systemic-onset juvenile arthritis. Arthritis Rheum 2010;34(12):1575–9.
44. Schultz R, Mattila J, Gappa M, et al. Development of progressive pulmonary interstitial and intra-alveolar cholesterol granulomas (PICG) associated with

therapy-resistant chronic systemic juvenile arthritis (CJA). Pediatr Pulmonol 2001;32(5):397–402.
45. Kimura Y, Weiss JE, Haroldson KL, et al. Pulmonary hypertension and other potentially fatal pulmonary complications in systemic juvenile idiopathic arthritis. Arthritis Care Res (Hoboken) 2013;65(5):745–52.
46. Saper VE, Chen G, Deutsch GH, et al. Emergent high fatality lung disease in systemic juvenile arthritis. Ann Rheum Dis 2019;78(12):1722–31.
47. Schulert GS, Yasin S, Carey B, et al. Systemic juvenile idiopathic arthritis-associated lung disease: characterization and risk factors. Arthritis Rheum 2019;71(11):1943–54.
48. García-Peña P, Boixadera H, Barber I, et al. Thoracic findings of systemic diseases at high-resolution CT in children. Radiographics 2011;31(2):465–82.
49. Biederer J, Schnabel A, Muhle C, et al. Correlation between HRCT findings, pulmonary function tests and bronchoalveolar lavage cytology in interstitial lung disease associated with rheumatoid arthritis. Eur Radiol 2004;14(2):272–80.
50. Fragoulis GE, Conway R, Nikiphorou E. Methotrexate and interstitial lung disease: controversies and questions. A narrative review of the literature. Rheumatology (Oxford) 2019;58(11):1900–6.
51. Zisman DA, McCune WJ, Tino G, et al. Drug-induced pneumonitis: the role of methotrexate. Sarcoidosis Vasc Diffuse Lung Dis 2001;18(3):243–52.
52. Kremer JM, Alarcon GS, Weinblatt ME, et al. Clinical, laboratory, radiographic, and histopathologic features of methotrexate-associated lung injury in patients with rheumatoid arthritis: a multicenter study with literature review. Arthritis Rheum 1997;40(10):1829–37.
53. Li SC. Scleroderma in children and adolescents: localized scleroderma and systemic sclerosis. Pediatr Clin North Am 2018;65(4):757–81.
54. Laxer RM, Zulian F. Localized scleroderma. Curr Opin Rheumatol 2006;18(6):606–13.
55. Uziel Y, Miller ML, Laxer RM. Scleroderma in children. Pediatr Clin North Am 1995;42(5):1171–203.
56. Zulian F, Woo P, Athreya BH, et al. The pediatric rheumatology European Society/American College of Rheumatology/European League Against Rheumatism provisional classification criteria for juvenile systemic sclerosis. Arthritis Rheum 2007;57(2):203–12.
57. Stevens BE, Torok KS, Li SC, et al. Clinical characteristics and factors associated with disability and impaired quality of life in children with juvenile systemic sclerosis: results from the Childhood Arthritis and Rheumatology Research Alliance Legacy Registry. Arthritis Care Res (Hoboken) 2018;70(12):1806–13.
58. Scalapino K, Arkachaisri T, Lucas M, et al. Childhood onset systemic sclerosis: classification, clinical and serologic features, and survival in comparison with adult onset disease. J Rheumatol 2006;33(5):1004–13.
59. Scirè CA, Caporali R, Zanierato M, et al. Shrinking lung syndrome in systemic sclerosis: letters. Arthritis Rheum 2003;48(10):2999–3000.
60. Naniwa T, Banno S, Sugiura Y, et al. Pulmonary-renal syndrome in systemic sclerosis: a report of three cases and review of the literature. Mod Rheumatol 2007;17(1):37–44.
61. Varga J, Abraham D. Systemic sclerosis: a prototypic multisystem fibrotic disorder. J Clin Invest 2007;117(3):557–67.
62. Tyndall AJ, Bannert B, Vonk M, et al. Causes and risk factors for death in systemic sclerosis: a study from the EULAR scleroderma trials and research (EUSTAR) database. Ann Rheum Dis 2010;69(10):1809–15.

63. Foeldvari I, Nihtyanova SI, Wierk A, et al. Characteristics of patients with juvenile onset systemic sclerosis in an adult single-center cohort. J Rheumatol 2010; 37(11):2422–6.
64. Martini G, Vittadello F, Kasapçopur O, et al. Factors affecting survival in juvenile systemic sclerosis. Rheumatology (Oxford) 2009;48(2):119–22.
65. Cottin V, Brown KK. Interstitial lung disease associated with systemic sclerosis (SSc-ILD). Respir Res 2019;20(1):13.
66. Nunes JPL, Cunha AC, Meirinhos T, et al. Prevalence of auto-antibodies associated to pulmonary arterial hypertension in scleroderma: a review. Autoimmun Rev 2018;17(12):1186–201.
67. Bonhomme O, André B, Gester F, et al. Biomarkers in systemic sclerosis-associated interstitial lung disease: review of the literature. Rheumatology (Oxford) 2019;58(9):1534–46.
68. Harrison NK, Myers AR, Corrin B, et al. Structural features of interstitial lung disease in systemic sclerosis. Am Rev Respir Dis 1991;144(3_pt_1):706–13.
69. Wells AU, Lorimer S, Majumdar S, et al. Fibrosing alveolitis in systemic sclerosis: increase in memory T-cells in lung interstitium. Eur Respir J 1995;8(2):266–71.
70. Seely JM, Jones LT, Wallace C, et al. Systemic sclerosis: using high-resolution CT to detect lung disease in children. Am J Roentgenol 1998;170(3):691–7.
71. Garty BZ, Athreya BH, Wilmott R, et al. Pulmonary functions in children with progressive systemic sclerosis. Pediatrics 1991;88(6):1161–7.
72. Valeur NS, Stevens AM, Ferguson MR, et al. Multimodality thoracic imaging of juvenile systemic sclerosis: emphasis on clinical correlation and high-resolution CT of pulmonary fibrosis. AJR Am J Roentgenol 2015;204(2):408–22.
73. Wells AU, Hansell DM, Corrin B, et al. High resolution computed tomography as a predictor of lung histology in systemic sclerosis. Thorax 1992;47(9):738–42.
74. Remy-Jardin M, Remy J, Wallaert B, et al. Pulmonary involvement in progressive systemic sclerosis: sequential evaluation with CT, pulmonary function tests, and bronchoalveolar lavage. Radiology 1993;188(2):499–506.
75. White B. Interstitial lung disease in scleroderma. Rheum Dis Clin North Am 2003; 29(2):371–90.
76. Witt C, Borges AC, John M, et al. Pulmonary involvement in diffuse cutaneous systemic sclerosis: bronchoalveolar fluid granulocytosis predicts progression of fibrosing alveolitis. Ann Rheum Dis 1999;58(10):635–40.
77. Goh NSL, Veeraraghavan S, Desai SR, et al. Bronchoalveolar lavage cellular profiles in patients with systemic sclerosis–associated interstitial lung disease are not predictive of disease progression. Arthritis Rheum 2007;56(6):2005–12.
78. Strange C, Bolster MB, Roth MD, et al. Bronchoalveolar lavage and response to cyclophosphamide in scleroderma interstitial lung disease. Am J Respir Crit Care Med 2008;177(1):91–8.
79. Tashkin DP, Elashoff R, Clements PJ, et al. Cyclophosphamide versus placebo in scleroderma lung disease. N Engl J Med 2006;354(25):2655–66.
80. Khanna D, Yan X, Tashkin DP, et al. Impact of oral cyclophosphamide on health-related quality of life in patients with active scleroderma lung disease: results from the scleroderma lung study. Arthritis Rheum 2007;56(5):1676–84.
81. Hoyles RK, Ellis RW, Wellsbury J, et al. A multicenter, prospective, randomized, double-blind, placebo-controlled trial of corticosteroids and intravenous cyclophosphamide followed by oral azathioprine for the treatment of pulmonary fibrosis in scleroderma. Arthritis Rheum 2006;54(12):3962–70.
82. Tashkin DP, Roth MD, Clements PJ, et al. Mycophenolate mofetil versus oral cyclophosphamide in scleroderma-related interstitial lung disease (SLS II): a

randomised controlled, double-blind, parallel group trial. Lancet Respir Med 2016;4(9):708–19.
83. Mackintosh JA, Stainer A, Barnett JL, et al. Systemic sclerosis associated interstitial lung disease: a comprehensive overview. Semin Respir Crit Care Med 2019;40(2):208–26.
84. Khanna D, Denton CP, Lin CJF, et al. Safety and efficacy of subcutaneous tocilizumab in systemic sclerosis: results from the open-label period of a phase II randomised controlled trial (faSScinate). Ann Rheum Dis 2018;77(2):212–20.
85. Khanna D, Albera C, Fischer A, et al. An open-label, phase II study of the safety and tolerability of pirfenidone in patients with scleroderma-associated interstitial lung disease: the LOTUSS trial. J Rheumatol 2016;43(9):1672–9.
86. Kowal-Bielecka O, Fransen J, Avouac J, et al. Update of EULAR recommendations for the treatment of systemic sclerosis. Ann Rheum Dis 2017;76(8): 1327–39.
87. Galiè N, Torbicki A, Barst R, et al. Guidelines on diagnosis and treatment of pulmonary arterial hypertension. The task force on diagnosis and treatment of pulmonary arterial hypertension of the European Society of Cardiology. Eur Heart J 2004;25(24):2243–78.
88. Beghetti M. Current treatment options in children with pulmonary arterial hypertension and experiences with oral bosentan. Eur J Clin Invest 2006;36(Suppl 3): 16–24.
89. Batthish M, Feldman BM. Juvenile dermatomyositis. Curr Rheumatol Rep 2011; 13(3):216–24.
90. Sakurai N, Nagai K, Tsutsumi H, et al. Anti-CADM-140 antibody-positive juvenile dermatomyositis with rapidly progressive interstitial lung disease and cardiac involvement. J Rheumatol 2011;38(5):963–4.
91. Sabbagh S, Pinal-Fernandez I, Kishi T, et al. Anti-Ro52 autoantibodies are associated with interstitial lung disease and more severe disease in patients with juvenile myositis. Ann Rheum Dis 2019;78(7):988–95.
92. Kobayashi N, Takezaki S, Kobayashi I, et al. Clinical and laboratory features of fatal rapidly progressive interstitial lung disease associated with juvenile dermatomyositis. Rheumatology (Oxford) 2015;54(5):784–91.
93. Rider LG, Shah M, Mamyrova G, et al. The myositis autoantibody phenotypes of the juvenile idiopathic inflammatory myopathies. Medicine (Baltimore) 2013; 92(4):223–43.
94. Fathi M. Interstitial lung disease, a common manifestation of newly diagnosed polymyositis and dermatomyositis. Ann Rheum Dis 2004;63(3):297–301.
95. Sanner H, Aaløkken TM, Gran JT, et al. Pulmonary outcome in juvenile dermatomyositis: a case-control study. Ann Rheum Dis 2011;70(1):86–91.
96. Stringer E, Bohnsack J, Bowyer SL, et al. Treatment approaches to juvenile dermatomyositis (JDM) across North America: the Childhood Arthritis and Rheumatology Research Alliance (CARRA) JDM treatment survey. J Rheumatol 2010; 37(9):1953–61.
97. Dell SD, Schneider R, Yeung RSM. Sarcoidosis. Kendig's disorders of the respiratory tract in children. 9th edition. Philadelphia: Elsevier; 2019. p. 850–75.
98. Iannuzzi MC, Fontana JR. Sarcoidosis: clinical presentation, immunopathogenesis, and therapeutics. JAMA 2011;305(4):391–9.
99. Torrington KG, Shorr AF, Parker JW. Endobronchial disease and racial differences in pulmonary sarcoidosis. Chest 1997;111(3):619–22.
100. Shetty AK, Gedalia A. Childhood sarcoidosis: a rare but fascinating disorder. Pediatr Rheumatol Online J 2008;6:16.

101. Rosé CD, Wouters CH, Meiorin S, et al. Pediatric granulomatous arthritis: an international registry. Arthritis Rheum 2006;54(10):3337–44.
102. Kanazawa N. Early-onset sarcoidosis and CARD15 mutations with constitutive nuclear factor-B activation: common genetic etiology with Blau syndrome. Blood 2004;105(3):1195–7.
103. Chiu B, Chan J, Das S, et al. Pediatric sarcoidosis: a review with emphasis on early onset and high-risk sarcoidosis and diagnostic challenges. Diagnostics (Basel) 2019;9(4):160.
104. Reichel H, Koeffler HP, Barbers R, et al. Regulation of 1,25-dihydroxyvitamin D3 production by cultured alveolar macrophages from normal human donors and from patients with pulmonary sarcoidosis. J Clin Endocrinol Metab 1987;65(6): 1201–9.
105. Marcille R, McCarthy M, Barton JW, et al. Long-term outcome of pediatric sarcoidosis with emphasis on pulmonary status. Chest 1992;102(5):1444–9.
106. Abehsera M, Valeyre D, Grenier P, et al. Sarcoidosis with pulmonary fibrosis: CT patterns and correlation with pulmonary function. AJR Am J Roentgenol 2000; 174(6):1751–7.
107. American Thoracic Society. Statement on sarcoidosis. Joint statement of the American Thoracic Society (ATS), the European Respiratory Society (ERS) and the World Association of Sarcoidosis and other Granulomatous Disorders (WASOG) adopted by the ATS board of directors and by the ERS executive committee, 1999. Am J Respir Crit Care Med 1999;160(2):736–55.
108. Winterbauer RH, Hutchinson JF. Use of pulmonary function tests in the management of sarcoidosis. Chest 1980;78(4):640–7.
109. Bechtel JJ, Starr T 3rd, Dantzker DR, et al. Airway hyperreactivity in patients with sarcoidosis. Am Rev Respir Dis 1981;124(6):759–61.
110. Bénéteau-Burnat B, Baudin B, Morgant G, et al. Serum angiotensin-converting enzyme in healthy and sarcoidotic children: comparison with the reference interval for adults. Clin Chem 1990;36(2):344–6.
111. Nathan N, Marcelo P, Houdouin V, et al. Lung sarcoidosis in children: update on disease expression and management. Thorax 2015;70(6):537–42.

Pulmonary Manifestations of Systemic Vasculitis in Children

Muserref Kasap Cuceoglu, MD, Seza Ozen, MD*

KEYWORDS

• Child • Vasculitis • Pulmonary features • Lung

KEY POINTS

- Vasculitides are defined and classified according to the vessel size they involve. Lung vessels may be involved as well.
- Pulmonary involvement is common in granulomatous polyangiitis (GPA, Wegener granulomatosis) and may present with cavities, nodules, or infiltrates. Eosinophilic granulomatosis with polyangiitis (Churg-Strauss syndrome) is rare in childhood but also presents with pulmonary involvement.
- Involvement of lung vessels is very rare in the common childhood vasculitides: IgA vasculitis (Henoch Schonlein purpura) and Kawasaki disease, although case reports describe occasional involvement.

INTRODUCTION

Systemic vasculitides are a heterogenous group of uncommon diseases in children. A diagnosis is often made on the basis of clinical presentation, serologic studies, and diagnostic imaging, but pathologic evaluation biopsy may be necessary in some cases to ascertain the precise diagnosis.

Chapel Hill Classification 2012 introduced a new nomenclature of vasculitides based on the vessels mainly involved and partly on pathogenesis.[1] However, the most widely accepted classification for childhood vasculitides is the Ankara 2008 Consensus Criteria endorsed by the European League Against Rheumatism (EULAR) and the Pediatric Rheumatology European Society (PRES).[2]

Despite intensive investigation, the pathogenesis of vascular inflammation remains unknown in most cases. The cause of vasculitides is probably multifactorial. It may include genetic predisposition, environmental factors (infection and inhalation of particulate matter), and other yet unknown factors.

Department of Pediatric Rheumatology, Hacettepe University, Sihhiye Campus, Ankara 06100, Turkey

* Corresponding author.

E-mail address: sezaozen@gmail.com

Pediatr Clin N Am 68 (2021) 167–176
https://doi.org/10.1016/j.pcl.2020.09.014

TAKAYASU ARTERITIS

Takayasu arteritis (TA) is a rare form of vasculitis of unknown cause that involves the aorta and its major branches.[3] It is characterized by granulomatous inflammation that affects all parts of the vessel wall. TA may result in stenotic, blocked arteries, aneurysms, or vascular remodeling.[4] It is more common in girls and women of 10 to 30 years of age (80%–90%). Although clinical manifestations are nonspecific at onset, as the TA vascular insufficiency progresses, pediatric patients often present with hypertension, headaches, fever, and weight loss.

There is no specific laboratory marker for TA. Common inflammatory markers, such as erythrocyte sedimentation rate and C-reactive protein, are often elevated. Conventional angiography is the major diagnostic modality of TA. The thoracic aorta and abdominal aorta are the vessels most often involved in childhood TA. Other vascular imaging methods include magnetic resonance angiography and computed tomography (CT) angiography.[2]

Corticosteroids are still the mainstay of treatment. They are effective for most patients with active TA. Surgical procedures may be performed in these patients once the inflammation has been suppressed.

A lightly modified classification suggested by the Ankara 2008 criteria includes characteristic angiographic abnormalities in the aorta or its main branches and pulmonary arteries (stenosis, occlusion, dilatation/aneurysm, or arterial wall thickening not owing to fibromuscular dysplasia) and at least one of the 5 features given below:

- Pulse deficit (lost/decreased/unequal peripheral artery pulse or pulses) and/or claudication induced by activity
- Systolic blood pressure difference greater than 10 mm Hg between any limbs
- Bruits or thrills over the aorta and/or its major branches
- Hypertension
- Elevated acute-phase reactants

Pulmonary involvement is rare. Cough, dyspnea, hemoptysis, chest pain, and manifestations of pulmonary hypertension are the symptoms most commonly seen in patients with TA and pulmonary involvement.[5] Pulmonary artery involvement has been reported in nearly 7% of adults patients with TA.[6] In children, pulmonary artery involvement is very rare. In a series of patients 16 to 50 years of age, Sharma and colleagues[7] reported angiographic evidence of pulmonary involvement in only 14.3% of the patients with TA. Segmental and subsegmental branches in the upper lobes were the mainly involved vessels.

KAWASAKI DISEASE

Kawasaki disease (KD) is a childhood vasculitis with predominantly medium-sized artery involvement. The coronary arteries are the most frequently involved. KD is a disease of early childhood. The cause of KD has not been fully clarified yet.[8,9] There are no specific laboratory tests to confirm the diagnosis of KD; therefore, it is considered based on clinical criteria. Diagnosis is based on the presence of fever longer than 5 days along with 4 of the 5 following features at the same time or during the course of the disease[10,11]:

- Bilateral nonpurulent conjunctivitis
- Oropharyngeal changes
- Unilateral cervical lymphadenopathy
- Polymorphic rash
- Changes in extremities

However, if coronary artery involvement is present, 4 criteria are not required.[12] Some patients may have atypical findings and involvement of other medium-sized arteries.[13]

Pulmonary involvement in KD is quite rare, and it might be due to inflammation of vessels leading to increased vascular permeability. Singh and colleagues[14] reported 11 cases with KD: there was radiographic evidence of parenchymal consolidation in all patients, pleural effusion in 6 patients, empyema in 3 patients, and pneumothorax in 2 patients. Lee and colleagues[15] observed chest radiographic abnormalities in 51.2% of patients with KD. Pleural effusion, empyema, and pneumothorax findings were reported in 54.5%, 27.3%, and 18.2%, respectively.

POLYARTERITIS NODOSA

Polyarteritis nodosa (PAN) is a systemic necrotizing vasculitis with aneurysm formation affecting small- and medium-sized arteries. The Ankara 2008 classification criteria require pathologic evidence of necrotizing vasculitis in the biopsy specimen of small- and medium-sized arteries or the presence of aneurysms and stenoses in angiography without fibromuscular dysplasia as a mandatory criterion. In order to classify the child as PAN, at least one of the 5 systemic features listed in **Box 1**)[2,10,16] should be observed.

Although most of the medium-sized arteries of any organ system may be affected, pulmonary involvement is very rare in PAN, although it has been reported in an adult series.[17]

GRANULOMATOSIS WITH POLYANGIITIS (WEGENER)

Granulomatosis with polyangitis (GPA) is a multisystemic necrotizing granulomatous vasculitis of unknown cause. The disease mostly involves the upper- (sinuses, larynx, and ear) and lower- (trachea) respiratory tract, lungs, and kidneys. In contrast to the other vasculitis, the most common and probably the most aggressive involvement is the pulmonary vasculitis.[18]

Ankara (2008) proposed consensus criteria (final European League Against Rheumatism/Pediatric Rheumatology European Society/Paediatric Rheumatology INternational Trials Organisation [EULAR/PRINTO/PRES] Wegener granulomatosis [WG]

Box 1
European League Against Rheumatism/Pediatric Rheumatology European Society/Paediatric Rheumatology INternational Trials Organisation–endorsed Ankara 2008

Classification criteria for childhood PAN

- Skin involvement (livedo reticularis, tender subcutaneous nodules, superficial or deep skin infarctions)
- Myalgia or muscle tenderness
- Hypertension
- Peripheral neuropathy
- Renal (medium-sized artery) involvement

Data from Ozen S, Pistorio A, Iusan SM, et al. EULAR / PRINTO / PRES criteria for Henoch – Schönlein purpura , childhood polyarteritis nodosa , childhood Wegener granulomatosis and childhood Takayasu arteritis: Ankara 2008. Part II: Final classifi cation criteria. 2010;(1):798-806.

criteria) to classify a child as GPA (WG) having at least 3 of the 6 conditions presented below:

- Upper-airway involvement (chronic purulent or bloody nasal discharge or recurrent epistaxis/crusts/granulomata, nasal septum perforation or saddle nose deformity, chronic or recurrent sinus inflammation)
- Renal involvement (proteinuria >0.3 g/24 hours or >30 mmol/mg of urine albumin/creatinine ratio on a spot morning sample, hematuria, or red blood cell casts >5 red blood cells/high power field or red blood cells casts in the urinary sediment or $\geq$2+ on dipstick necrotizing pauci-immune glomerulonephritis)
- Pulmonary involvement (chest radiography or CT showing the presence of nodules, cavities, or fixed infiltrates)
- Laryngotracheobronchial involvement (subglottic, tracheal, or bronchial stenosis)
- Antineutrophil cytoplasmic autoantibody (ANCA) positivity by immunofluorescence or by enzyme-linked immunosorbent assay (MPO/p or proteinase 3 [PR3]/c ANCA)
- Granulomatous inflammation within the wall of an artery or in the perivascular or extravascular area

Lung involvement is one of the main features of the disease. Other organ involvement includes kidneys, skin, peripheral and central nervous system, eyes, heart, and gastrointestinal tract.

Patients with GPA (WG) may present with involvement of airways or pulmonary parenchyma causing hoarseness, cough, dyspnea, stridor, wheezing, hemoptysis, or pleuritic pain.[19–21] These symptoms may be accompanied by pulmonary consolidation and/or pleural effusion. These patients may also develop pulmonary fibrosis and pulmonary arterial hypertension.[21] Laryngotracheobronchial involvement may include tracheal or subglottic stenosis presenting with stridor.

The chest radiographic findings are variable. Common manifestations include nodules, patchy or diffuse opacities, fleeting infiltrates, and hilar adenopathy.[22] Pulmonary nodules are often multiple, bilateral, and cavitated. Cavities typically occur in nodules larger than 2 cm in diameter. GPA (WG) should be considered in cases when thick-walled cavitary infiltrates are detected.

c-ANCA positivity, especially against PR3 target antigen, has a specificity of 80% to 100%, and sensitivity of 28% to 92% in GPA (WG). PR3-ANCA levels are considered to be associated with activity, and high titers are usually associated with the risk of exacerbation. Although parenchymal lung nodules are a well-recognized radiographic manifestation, ANCA-associated vasculitis may occasionally present as tumorlike masses.[23]

GPA (WG) is fatal in untreated cases. The conventional induction treatment was cyclophosphamide + corticosteroids. However, recent studies have shown that Rituximab (anti-CD20 antibody) is an effective alternative treatment.[24,25] Plasmapheresis and intravenous immunoglobulin are used as required. Once remission is achieved, maintenance treatment should be started with azathioprine or other suggested immunosuppressives and steroid tapering. The SHARE group have suggested some treatment recommendations for pediatric patients with GPA.[26] Prophylactic cotrimoxazole is also recommended to prevent *Pneumocystis jirovecii* (previously P. carinii) pneumonia and upper-respiratory tract relapses in GPA.[27]

IgA VASCULITIS (HENOCH SCHONLEIN PURPURA)

IgA vasculitis (Henoch Schonlein purpura) (IgAV [HSP]) is one of the most common vasculitis of childhood.[28,29] Its incidence is 22 per 100,000. Boys are affected twice as often as girls. The disease is characterized by palpable purpura, arthritis and arthralgia, abdominal pain, gastrointestinal bleeding, and glomerulonephritis.[2] The cause of IgAV (HSP) is not yet known, but it usually follows an upper-respiratory infection. Group A streptococcus has been shown as a trigger for IgAV (HSP) because antistreptolysin O antibodies may be increased in patients with IgAV (HSP).[30] Circulating immune complexes (CICs) containing IgA are the hallmark of the pathogenesis, and accumulation of IgA immune complex in the vascular walls and renal mesangium is typical for the disease. Pulmonary manifestations are rare; however, diffuse alveolar hemorrhage and interstitial pneumonitis have been reported.[31] Other reported cases include pleural effusion and chylothorax.

The Ankara 2008 (final EULAR/PRINTO/PRES IGAV [HSP] criteria) suggested the mandatory criterion is purpura (usually palpable and in clusters) or petechiae, with lower-limb predominance and without thrombocytopenia or coagulopathy, and also one or more of the conditions given below must be seen in a patient:

- Abdominal pain (diffuse abdominal colicky pain with acute onset assessed by history and physical examination, may include intussusception and gastrointestinal bleeding)
- Histopathology (leukocytoclastic vasculitis with predominant IgA deposit or proliferative glomerulonephritis with predominant IgA deposit)
- Arthritis or arthralgias (arthritis of acute onset defined as joint swelling or joint pain with limitation on motion, arthralgia of acute onset defined as joint pain without joint swelling or limitation on motion)
- Renal involvement (proteinuria >0.3 g/24 hours or >30 mmol/mg of urine albumin/creatinine ratio on a spot morning sample, hematuria or red blood cell casts: >5 red blood cells/high power field or red blood cells casts in the urinary sediment or ≥2+ on dipstick).

Pulmonary involvement is also rare in IgAV (HSP). In a cohort of French adult patients hospitalized for IgAV (HSP), impaired carbon monoxide diffusion capacity (DLCO) and mild interstitial changes on chest radiographs were found in most patients (97% and 69%, respectively) despite the absence of significant respiratory symptoms.[32] In this study, 70% of patients had radiographic evidence for mild interstitial lung changes. Similarly, Cazzato and colleagues[33] found impaired DLCO in IgAV (HSP) patients who did not have clinical or radiologic evidence of lung involvement compared with age-matched control patients.

Pulmonary hemorrhage is very rare in patients with IgAV (HSP) and is primarily reported in adults and adolescents.[31,34] Diffuse alveolar bleeding is indeed a serious complication associated with IgAV (HSP), albeit very rare. Pulmonary bleeding is secondary to disruption of the small alveolar arteries-capillaries by CICs. A study reported that 8 out of 28 patients under 20 years of age with IgAV (HSP) had widespread alveolar hemorrhage with pleural effusion.[35] The youngest patient with IgAV (HSP)-related lung disease was a 5-month-old infant with widespread alveolar hemorrhage and interstitial fibrosis.[35] The first choice of treatment for pulmonary involvement is prednisone. Severe cases are managed as a systemic vasculitis, and cyclophosphamide would be added.[32,36]

MICROSCOPIC POLYANGITIS

Microscopic polyangiitis (MPA), involving arterioles, venules, and capillaries, is a small vessel vasculitis characterized by rapidly progressing glomerulonephritis and pulmonary capillaritis. The incidence is approximately 1:100,000 in adults and is very rare in children.

The main target organ is the kidney with focal segmental and sometimes necrotizing glomerulonephritis. Crescent formation may be observed. Unlike classical PAN, microaneurysms do not occur in the renal vessels in MPA, and there is no granulomatous inflammation.

Lung involvement is less frequent, manifested by dyspnea, cough, and hemoptysis. Pulmonary hemorrhage is a very serious condition and is associated with poor prognosis. Lung involvement is reported to occur in about one-third of adult patients with MPA. Chest CT findings in 51 adult patients with MPO-ANCA–positive showed ground-glass attenuation in greater than 90% with areas of consolidation and bronchovascular thickening. Pathologic correlation showed that these findings were due to pulmonary hemorrhage, interstitial inflammation, and fibrosis.

ANCA is a diagnostic test for MPA. ANCA is positive in 90% to 95% of patients, and approximately 70% is MPO-ANCA. Treatment of microscopic polyangitis is the same as for GPA (WG).

EOSINOPHILIC GRANULOMATOSIS WITH POLYANGIITIS

Churg-Strauss Syndrome

Eosinophilic granulomatosis with polyangiitis (EGPA) (Churg-Strauss syndrome) is a rare disease characterized by asthma, necrotizing vasculitis affecting mainly small-sized arteries and veins, involvement of 2 or more extrapulmonary organs with systemic vasculitis, and peripheral blood eosinophilia.[37] It is suspected that children with EGPA are less likely than adult patients to have positive ANCA titers, but more likely to have pulmonary involvement and experience higher mortalities.[38] Gendelman and colleagues[38] in a retrospective study of pediatric patients with EGPA reported 9 patients all had eosinophilia, upper-airway disease (allergic rhinitis, chronic sinusitis, and nasal polyps), and pulmonary involvement defined as asthma, nonfixed pulmonary infiltrates, pleural effusions, alveolar hemorrhage, laryngeal or tracheobronchial stenosis, or lung nodules. Pulmonary function testing revealed predicted values compatible with restrictive lung disease, obstructive lung disease, and/or decreased DLCO.[38] Abnormal chest radiographic or chest CT findings included nonfixed infiltrates, nodules, effusions, or cavitary lesions. Systemic corticosteroids are the mainstay of treatment.

Behçet Disease

Behçet disease (BD) is a vasculitis with autoinflammatory features that may affect arteries and veins of all sizes. Recurrent oral and genital ulcers and eye involvement are among the main features of the disease.[39] Skin features, arthritis/arthralgia, neurologic, vascular, and gastrointestinal system involvements may occur as well. Behçet described this disease with the trilogy of oral and genital ulcers and uveitis.[40] BD is very common in Eastern Mediterranean and Asia countries, located around the ancient trade route called the “Silk Road.” Turkey has an incidence of as high as 1/250 in young adults.[41] The disease is most often observed between the ages of 20 and 40.[42] It is rare in young children and individuals over 50 years of age; however, it is estimated that 5% of overall cases are adolescents.[43]

Vascular involvement in BD is the main cause of morbidity and mortality. Vascular involvement in BD was found to be 14.3% and 12.8% in Turkey and China, respectively.[44,45] Among the vascular involvements, pulmonary artery aneurysm has the highest morbidity and mortality; hence, early diagnosis is critical.[46] Indeed, pulmonary aneurysms involving the large proximal branches are the most common pulmonary vascular lesion in BD, rarely seen in other diseases.[46] The typical finding is thrombotic aneurysms of the pulmonary arteries.

Hemoptysis is the most common manifestation of pulmonary involvement. Other symptoms include cough, shortness of breath, fever, and pleuritic pain.[47] In adults with BD, other pulmonary findings, such as pleural effusion, bronchial stenosis, chronic bronchitis, pulmonary infarction, bleeding, and both organized and eosinophilic pneumonias, have been reported.[48]

Demir and colleagues[49] successfully treated 2 pediatric patients' BD and pulmonary aneurysms with early and aggressive combined immunosuppressive therapy of intravenous cyclophosphamide, systemic steroids, and interferon infusions.

CLINICS CARE POINTS

- Patients with granulomatosis with polyangiitis (Wegener granulomatosis) may present with involvement of airways or pulmonary parenchyma, causing hoarseness, cough, dyspnea, stridor, wheezing, hemoptysis, or pleuritic pain.
- As in adults, both C-ANCA and P-ANCA should be studied in patients suspected to have granulomatosis with polyangiitis (Wegener granulomatosis). C-ANCA positivity, especially against proteinase 3 target antigen, has a specificity of 80% to 100%, and sensitivity of 28% to 92% in granulomatosis with polyangiitis (Wegener granulomatosis).
- Pulmonary involvement is rare in the other childhood vasculitides.
- Pulmonary artery involvement is associated with high morbidity p-ANCA and mortality in Behçet disease, thus requires early diagnosis and treatment.

DISCLOSURE

The authors have nothing to disclose related to this work. However, Dr S. Ozen has received consultation and speaker fees from Novartis and SOBI.

REFERENCES

1. Jennette JC, Falk RJ, Bacon PA, et al. 2012 revised International Chapel Hill Consensus Conference Nomenclature of Vasculitides. Arthritis Rheum 2013; 65(1):1–11.
2. Ozen S, Pistorio A, Iusan SM, et al. EULAR/PRINTO/PRES criteria for Henoch-Schönlein purpura, childhood polyarteritis nodosa, childhood Wegener granulomatosis and childhood Takayasu arteritis: Ankara 2008. Part II: final classification criteria. Ann Rheum Dis 2010;69:798–806.
3. Johnston SL, Lock RJ, Gompels MM. Takayasu arteritis: a review. J Clin Pathol 2002;55(7):481–6.
4. Kalyoncu S. Takayasu arteritis: differential diagnosis. Turkiye Klin J Cardiovasc Sci 2009;21(3):499–501.
5. Nakajima N. Takayasu arteritis: consideration of pulmonary involvement. Ann Vasc Dis 2008;1(1):7–10.

6. Bicakcigil M, Aksu K, Kamali S, et al. Takayasu's arteritis in Turkey – clinical and angiographic features of 248 patients. Clin Exp Rheumatol 2008;27(1 Suppl 52): S59–64.
7. Sharma S, Kamalakar T, Rajani M, et al. The incidence and patterns of pulmonary artery involvement in Takayasu's arteritis. Clin Radiol 1990;42:177–81.
8. Rowley AH, Wolinsky SM, Relman DA, et al. Search for highly conserved viral and bacterial nucleic acid sequences corresponding to an etiologic agent of Kawasaki disease. Pediatr Res 1994;36(5):567–71.
9. Rowley AH. The etiology of Kawasaki disease: superantigen or conventional antigen? Pediatr Infect Dis J 1999;18(1):69–70.
10. Ozen S, Ruperto N, Dillon MJ, et al. EULAR/PReS endorsed consensus criteria for the classification of childhood vasculitides. Ann Rheum Dis 2006;936–41. https://doi.org/10.1136/ard.2005.046300.
11. Bolger AF. Diagnosis, treatment, and long-term management of Kawasaki disease: a scientific statement for health professionals from the American Heart Association. Circulation 2017. https://doi.org/10.1161/CIR.0000000000000484.
12. Council on Cardiovascular Disease in the Young, Committee on Rheumatic Fever, Endocarditis, and Kawasaki Disease, American Heart Association. Diagnostic guidelines for Kawasaki disease. Circulation 2001;103(2):335–6.
13. Sonobe T, Kawasaki T. Atypical Kawasaki disease. Prog Clin Biol Res 1987;250: 367–78. Available at: https://www.ncbi.nlm.nih.gov/pubmed/3423050.
14. Singh S, Gupta A, Kumar A, et al. Pulmonary presentation of Kawasaki disease — a diagnostic challenge. Pediatr Pulmonol 2017. https://doi.org/10.1002/ppul.23885.
15. Vaidya PC, Narayanan K, Suri D, et al. Pulmonary presentation of Kawasaki disease: an unusual occurrence. Int J Rheum Dis 2017;20(12):2227-9.
16. Weiss P. Pediatric vasculitis. Pediatr Clin North Am 2012;59(2):407–23.
17. Pagnoux C, Seror R, Henegar C, et al. Clinical features and outcomes in 348 patients with polyarteritis nodosa: a systematic retrospective study of patients diagnosed between 1963 and 2005 and entered into the French Vasculitis Study Group Database. Arthritis Rheum 2010;62(2):616–26.
18. Gómez-Gómez A, Martínez-Martínez MU, Cuevas-orta E, et al. Manifestaciones pulmonares de la poliangeítis granulomatosa. Reumatol Clin 2014. https://doi.org/10.1016/j.reuma.2013.12.010.
19. Canela M, Lorente J, Pallisa E. Clinical features and therapeutic management of subglottic stenosis in patients with Wegener's granulomatosis. Lupus 2008. https://doi.org/10.1177/0961203308089693. Available at: http://lup.sagepub.com/.
20. Ben Ameur S, Niaudet P, Baudouin V, et al. Lung manifestations in MPO-ANCA associated vasculitides in children. Pediatr Pulmonol 2014;49(3):285–90.
21. Gómez-Puerta JA, Hernández-Rodríguez J, López-Soto A, et al. Antineutrophil cytoplasmic antibody-associated vasculitides and respiratory disease. Chest 2009;136(4):1101-11.
22. Cordier JF, Valeyre D, Guillevin L, et al. Pulmonary Wegener's granulomatosis. A clinical and imaging study of 77 cases. Chest 1990;97(4):906–12.
23. Kariv R, Sidi Y, Gur H. Systemic vasculitis presenting as a tumorlike lesion. Four case reports and an analysis of 79 reported cases. Medicine (Baltimore) 2000; 79(6):349–59.
24. Jones RB, Tervaert JWC, Hauser T, et al. Rituximab versus cyclophosphamide in ANCA-associated renal vasculitis. N Engl J Med 2010;363(3):211–20.

25. Stone JH, Merkel PA, Spiera R, et al. Rituximab versus cyclophosphamide for ANCA-associated vasculitis. N Engl J Med 2010;363:221–32.
26. de Graeff N, Groot N, Brogan P, et al. Original article European consensus-based recommendations for the diagnosis and treatment of rare paediatric vasculitides – the SHARE initiative. Rheumatology (Oxford) 2019. https://doi.org/10.1093/rheumatology/key322.
27. Stegeman CA, Tervaert JW, de Jong PE, et al. Trimethoprim-sulfamethoxazole (co-trimoxazole) for the prevention of relapses of Wegener's granulomatosis. Dutch Co-Trimoxazole Wegener Study Group. N Engl J Med 1996;335(1):16–20.
28. Ballinger S. Henoch-Schonlein purpura. Curr Opin Rheumatol 2003;15(5):591–4.
29. Tizard EJ. Henoch-Schönlein purpura. Arch Dis Child 1999;80(4):380–3.
30. Masuda M, Nakanishi K, Yoshizawa N, et al. Group A streptococcal antigen in the glomeruli of children with Henoch-Schönlein nephritis 2003;41(2):366–70.
31. Di Pietro GM, Castellazzi ML, Mastrangelo A, et al. Henoch-Schönlein purpura in children: not only kidney but also lung. Pediatr Rheumatol Online J 2019;17(1):75.
32. Kalifa G. Impairment of lung diffusion capacity in Schonlein-Henoch purpura. J Pediatr 1992;12112–6.
33. Cazzato S, Bernardi F, Cinti C, et al. Pulmonary function abnormalities in children with Henoch-Schönlein purpura. Eur Respir J 1999;13:597–601.
34. Besbas N, Duzova A, Topaloglu R, et al. Pulmonary haemorrhage in a 6-year-old boy with Henoch-Schönlein purpura. Clin Rheumatol 2001;20(4):293–6.
35. Article O. Pulmonary involvement in Henoch-Schönlein purpura. Mayo Clin Proc 2004;1151–7. https://doi.org/10.4065/79.9.1151.
36. Al-harbi NN. Henoch-Schönlein nephritis complicated with pulmonary hemorrhage but treated successfully. Pediatr Nephrol 2002;762–4. https://doi.org/10.1007/s00467-002-0926-y.
37. Gross WL. Systemic necrotizing vasculitis. Baillieres Clin Rheumatol 1997;11(2):259–84.
38. Gendelman S, Zeft A, Spalding SJ, et al. Childhood-onset eosinophilic granulomatosis with polyangiitis (formerly Churg-Strauss syndrome): a contemporary single-center cohort. J Rheumatol 2013;40(6). https://doi.org/10.3899/jrheum.120808.
39. Yazici H, Fresko I, Yurdakul S. Behçet's syndrome: disease manifestations, management, and advances in treatment. Nat Clin Pract Rheumatol 2007;3(3):148–55.
40. Tan SY, Poole PS. Hulusi Behçet (1889–1948): passion for dermatology. Singapore Med J 2016;57(7):408–9.
41. Hatemi G, Yazici Y, Yazici H. Behçet's syndrome. Rheum Dis Clin North Am 2013;39(2):245–61.
42. Karincaoglu Y, Borlu M, Toker SC, et al. Demographic and clinical properties of juvenile-onset Behçet's disease: a controlled multicenter study. J Am Acad Dermatol 2008;58(4):579–84.
43. Koné-paut I, Shahram F, Darce-bello M, et al. Consensus classification criteria for paediatric Behçet's disease from a prospective observational cohort: PEDBD. Ann Rheum Dis 2015;1–7. https://doi.org/10.1136/annrheumdis-2015-208491.
44. Sarica-kucukoglu R, Akdag-kose A, Kayabalı M, et al. Vascular involvement in Behçet's disease: a retrospective analysis of 2319 cases. Int J Dermatol 2006;45:919–21.
45. Fei Y, Li X, Lin S, et al. Major vascular involvement in Behçet's disease: a retrospective study of 796 patients. Clin Rheumatol 2013;845–52. https://doi.org/10.1007/s10067-013-2205-7.

46. Article R. Pulmonary artery aneurysms in Behçet disease: search strategies 2014;13(3):217–28.
47. Uzun O, Akpolat T, Erkan L. Pulmonary vasculitis in Behcet disease: a cumulative analysis. Chest 2005;127(6):2243–53.
48. Uzun O, Erkan L, Akpolat I, et al. Pulmonary involvement in Behçet's disease. Respiration 2008;75(3):310–21.
49. Demir S, Sag E, Akca UK, et al. The challenge of treating pulmonary vasculitis in Behçet disease: two pediatric cases. Pediatrics 2019;144(2). https://doi.org/10.1542/peds.2019-0162.

Respiratory Complications of Pediatric Neuromuscular Diseases

John R. Bach, MD[a,*], Nelson L. Turcios, MD[b], Liping Wang, MD[c]

KEYWORDS

- pediatric neuromuscular disease • noninvasive ventilation
- noninvasive ventilatory support • mechanical insufflation exsufflation
- muscular dystrophy • spinal muscular atrophy • respiratory management

KEY POINTS

- Respiratory muscle weakness is a major cause of morbidity and mortality in patients with neuromuscular diseases.
- Noninvasive ventilatory support (NVS) settings are necessary to provide optimal respiratory muscle rest and ventilatory support.
- NVS via portable ventilators or bi-level machines can prolong survival without invasive airway tubes.

INTRODUCTION

Lung failure results in hypoxemia from ventilation/perfusion mismatching, with or without hypercarbia. Pump failure leads to hypoventilation primarily manifested by hypercarbia, which is the hallmark of ventilatory failure. Pump failure may be caused by depression of the central respiratory controller, mechanical defect in the respiratory pump, and respiratory muscle weakness.[1]

VENTILATORY PUMP—NORMAL FUNCTION AND FAILURE

The ventilatory pump consists of chest wall and diaphragm, intercostal, accessory, and abdominal muscles. During quiet breathing at rest, the diaphragm, the principal muscle of inspiration, decreases intrathoracic pressure, thus drawing air into the lungs and the external intercostal muscles mainly stabilize the ribcage. Under conditions that require increased inspiratory workload (stiffness of the chest wall, obstruction

[a] Department of Physical Medicine and Rehabilitation, Rutgers University, New Jersey Medical School, Newark, NJ, USA; [b] Hackensack Meridian School of Medicine, Nutley, NJ 07110, USA; [c] Department of Neurology, Peking University Third Hospital, 49 North Garden Road, Haidian District, Beijing 100191, China
* Corresponding author. 536-28th Street, Union City, NJ 07102.
E-mail address: bachjr@njms.rutgers.edu

Pediatr Clin N Am 68 (2021) 177–191
https://doi.org/10.1016/j.pcl.2020.09.006

of the airways, or weakness of the diaphragm), additional diaphragmatic motor units and accessory inspiratory muscles are recruited.

During quiet breathing at rest, expiration is a passive process, thus expiratory muscles are inactive. During increased demands for air pumping, the major expiratory muscles (internal intercostal and abdominal muscles) are activated during expiration. Any decrease in the force of the expiratory muscles leads to air trapping—increased residual volume and decreased vital capacity (VC).

Pump failure develops when the energy supply to the respiratory muscles is reduced in the presence of increased work demands or when respiratory load requirements exceed the work capacity of normal respiratory muscles. Disorders that alter functional properties of the respiratory muscles (inspiratory, bulbar-innervated, or expiratory) include progressive neuropathic and myopathic disorders, which may be acquired or congenital.

Ventilatory pump failure leads to shallow breathing and ineffective cough.[2] Failure to clear airway secretions effectively predisposes patients with neuromuscular diseases (NMDs) to recurrent or chronic atelectasis and pneumonia, which in turn reduces lung compliance (distensibility), increases airway resistance, and increases ventilatory demands, increasing the respiratory load requirements while decreasing the work capacity of the respiratory pump.[2]

CHRONIC RESPIRATORY FAILURE

Respiratory symptoms may not correlate well with the degree of respiratory muscle fatigue. Infants with severe NMDs often present with paradoxic breathing (ie, asynchronous motion between the thorax and abdomen: the upper ribcage is drawn inwardly during inspiration instead of being elevated), accompanied by tachypnea, sleep flushing, perspiration, and frequent arousals even when apnea-hypopnea indexes are normal. These infants may develop otherwise benign respiratory tract infections that result in airway mucus plugging because of their ineffective cough that, if not promptly reversed by effective assisted coughing, results in pneumonia and respiratory failure with persistent oxyhemoglobin desaturation as measured by pulse oximetry (SpO_2 <95%).

In older children, manifestations of chronic ventilatory pump insufficiency include general fatigue and shortness of breath with activity, sleep dysfunction with frequent awakenings, nocturnal parasomnias, enuresis, profuse sweating, and daytime symptoms, such as morning headaches, hypersomnolence, impaired concentration, irritability, anxiety, poor control of upper airway secretions, and exacerbation of swallowing difficulties.[3] Often, however, because many of these patients are wheelchair confined and inactive, only fatigue, anxiety, and sleeplessness are noted. Symptoms of right heart failure due to unsuspected pulmonary hypertension may also indicate chronic sleep-related hypoxemia and hypoventilation. Nocturnal hypoventilation with an increase in CO_2 often is the first sign of chronic respiratory failure in progressive NMD.[4] Serial evaluation of ventilatory pump function is necessary to predict or recognize the first signs of chronic respiratory muscle fatigue in these patients.[4]

CLINICAL EVALUATION

For the infant and small child, inspection usually is the only evaluation that is necessary. Most floppy infants with NMD have paradoxic breathing. The chest wall configuration, rate and amplitude of breathing, pattern of spontaneous breathing, diaphragmatic excursion during inspiration, and cough strength all are evaluated.[3]

As the relative load to breathing increases, the patient adopts an increased respiratory rate with shallow breaths to avoid fatigue. Breathing that becomes increasingly more rapid and shallow and is interrupted by a deep breath with a pause may be a sign of fatigue. Although pauses are normal in healthy children, they may signal respiratory distress, as does nasal flaring, nocturnal flushing, and perspiration. Cyanosis with brief cough or pause, drooling in the absence of airway obstruction (cannot pause to swallow), and confusion also may be signs of impending respiratory arrest (**Box 1**).

Respiratory function must be assessed annually in children with NMDs. Routine measurements of lung function usually include spirometry, static lung volumes, maximal inspiratory pressure and maximal expiratory pressure and cough peak flow (CPF), and gas exchange. The VC measured with the patient recumbent is more important than when sitting because hypoventilation begins during sleep. When below 80% in the sitting position, VC also should be measured in the supine position, to investigate for diaphragm weakness (defined by a decrease in VC >20% from the sitting position). CPF values under 270 L/min to 300 L/min in adolescents and adults may indicate that cough is ineffective and could place patients at risk of recurrent respiratory infections and respiratory failure.[5] As the supine VC decreases below 40% of predicted normal or when any symptoms of hypoventilation or sleep-disordered breathing are suspected, when symptoms are obvious, a trial of nocturnal noninvasive ventilation clearly is warranted.

When floppy infants have paradoxic breathing, they require sleep NVS at pressure support levels of 16 cm H_2O to 20 cm H_2O.[6] For children with more subtle symptoms and signs, overnight polysomnography or combined pulse oximetry and transcutaneous/end-tidal CO_2 should be obtained in children when the VC is less than normal. The importance of obtaining polysomnography stems from the recognition that sleep-disordered breathing is frequent, even before the loss of ambulation, and includes not only diaphragm weakness-related alveolar hypoventilation but also obstructive apneas.

THE NEUROMUSCULAR DISORDERS

Spinal Muscular Atrophy

Spinal muscular atrophy (SMA) is an autosomal recessive degenerative motor neuron disorder causing progressive weakness of the skeletal and respiratory muscles.[7] It has an approximate incidence of 1 in 11,000. SMAs are neuropathies caused by a deficient survival motor neuron (SMN) protein, encoded by 2 genes, *SMN1* and *SMN2*. *SMN1* is the only gene that produces the full-length SMN. SMAs are due to a mutation of the

Box 1
Laboratory evaluation of ventilatory pump function.

Oximetry and end-tidal CO_2

Polysomnogram with transcutaneous CO_2

Pulmonary function tests: lung volumes and spirometry (forced VC sitting and supine), air stacking capacity (lung volume recruitment)

Assisted and unassisted CPF

Maximal inspiratory pressure at mouth, sniff inspiratory pressure, maximal expiratory pressure at mouth (transdiaphragmatic pressure)

Chest radiographs (full expiration and inspiration)

Data from 4- Praud J-Paul and Redding GJ. Chest Wall and Respiratory Muscle Disorders. Kendig's Disorders of the Respiratory Tract in Children. Edited by Wilmott RW, Bush A. 2019, Philadelphia: Elsevier, 1044-1061.

SMN1 gene, which results in the degeneration of the anterior horn cells of the spinal cord and often of the bulbar motor nuclei, leading, in turn, to skeletal muscle weakness and atrophy.

The SMAs are classified clinically by age of onset and highest motor milestone achieved. SMA type 1 is the most severe and most common type. Infants with this disease typically present with marked trunk and proximal limb weakness in the first 6 months of life and the inability to roll over or sit independently. Chest radiographs show a reduced intrathoracic volume and a bell-shaped thorax. Affected infants suffer from hypoventilation, swallowing disorders, and aspiration pneumonia and are at risk of recurrent respiratory failure with viral respiratory infections.

The prognosis is poor, with 95% of infants dying from respiratory failure by the age of 18 months without intensive respiratory support, an important part in the management of symptomatic patients with SMA type 1.

In SMA type 2, muscle weakness usually begins after the age of 6 months. The child may sit but cannot walk. Swallowing disorders, gastroesophageal reflux, recurrent atelectasis, and respiratory infections carry the risk of respiratory failure. In a majority of older children, scoliosis further aggravates respiratory function. Recurrent pulmonary infections precede nocturnal hypoxemia, nocturnal hypoventilation, and then daytime hypoventilation. Half of these patients have paradoxic breathing and require sleep NVS. Those who do not have paradoxic breathing usually do not need NVS but do need mechanical insufflation-exsufflation (MIE) to clear airway secretions during intercurrent upper respiratory infections (URIs). With adequate respiratory management tailored to respiratory involvement and the prevention of respiratory infections, a good quality of life and life span into adulthood is expected for most patients.

Patients with SMA type 3 usually present with proximal limb weakness and the ability to walk sometime in childhood. They often go into respiratory failure during URIs as early as age 2 years, but usually much later, and may require continuous NVS and aggressive MIE to avoid hospitalization and intubation during URIs.

Disorders of Muscles

Duchenne muscular dystrophy

Duchenne muscular dystrophy (DMD) presents in boys, with proximal muscle weakness at 2 years to 4 years of age. It is the most common and severe of the muscular dystrophies that afflict humans, with an estimated incidence of 1:3500 male births.[7] The gene responsible is localized in the X chromosome (Xp21), and a protein product, termed *dystrophin*, is lacking in DMD. Weakness progresses linearly and the patient becomes confined to a wheelchair at 10 years to 12 years of age. Impairment of respiratory function is accelerated after the loss of ambulation. A restrictive syndrome due to muscle weakness characterizes the pulmonary compromise in these patients. The first sign of chronic respiratory failure is nocturnal hypoventilation, which may be aggravated by obstructive sleep-disordered breathing, a frequent occurrence in patients with DMD, even in the first decade of life. With proper noninvasive management average life expectancy approaches 40 years with some patients living well in their 50s.[7]

Myotonic muscular dystrophy

Myotonic muscular dystrophy (MyD) is the second most common muscular dystrophy. MyD is an autosomal dominant, inherited disease, with an estimated frequency of 1:30,000.[7] Myotonia, a very slow relaxation of muscle after contraction, and muscle weakness are the prominent features. Many other organ systems also may be affected. Involvement of the respiratory system is the major contributor to morbidity and mortality.

Congenital myotonic dystrophy

This form of myotonic dystrophy develops in a small group of infants born to mothers, and rarely to fathers, with myotonic dystrophy.[7] Prominent manifestations include hypotonia along with feeding and respiratory difficulties. Myotonia is absent. Examining the parents and finding the repeat segment of DNA on the myotonic dystrophy gene may confirm the diagnosis. Polyhydramnios, prematurity, severe weakness, pleural effusions, and pulmonary hypoplasia presumably due to the absence of fetal movements account for the intrauterine onset of the disease. Diagnosis of this disease is suspected when the newborn is recognized to be difficult to wean from the ventilator for unknown reasons. The condition usually improves in early childhood. If ventilatory support is needed beyond 4 weeks of life in the neonatal period, the prognosis is poor, with the risk of sudden death in survivors, even without apparent respiratory exacerbation.

Management Objectives

Important concerns in the management of NMD are enhancement of airway clearance and the role of NVS in improving morbidity, mortality, and quality of life.

WHAT ARE PHYSICAL MEDICINE RESPIRATORY MUSCLE AIDS?

Inspiratory and expiratory muscle aids are devices and techniques that involve the application of forces to the body or pressure changes to the airway to assist inspiratory or expiratory muscle function. Body ventilators act on the body to assist inspiration just as an abdominal thrust may assist coughing. For example, the intermittent abdominal pressure ventilator (**Fig. 1**) is a corset with an air bladder inside. A ventilator on the back of a wheelchair delivers air to the air bladder under the user's clothing, it then presses on the abdomen, moves the diaphragm up, and its descent by gravity ventilates the lungs. Negative pressure applied to the airway during expiration also assists the expiratory muscles for coughing, just as positive pressure applied to the airway during inhalation, or noninvasive intermittent positive pressure ventilation, assists the inspiratory muscles. Continuous positive airway pressure assists neither inspiratory muscles nor expiratory muscles thus rarely, if ever, should be used for these patients.

ENHANCE AIRWAY CLEARANCE

The Normal Cough

Adequate expiratory muscle function is critical for creating the CPF necessary to clear airway secretions and bronchial mucus plugs. A normal cough begins with a deep inspiration or insufflation to approximately 85% of total lung capacity. This maneuver not only increases the airway diameter but also places the expiratory muscles in a favorable position of their length-tension curve. The glottis then closes for approximately 200 ms while the expiratory muscles contract, resulting in a rapid increase in thoracoabdominal pressures sufficient to generate an explosive decompression of the chest at glottic opening and CPF exceeding 5 L/s.[8]

Impairment of any phase of cough may have deleterious effects on clearance of secretions from central airways: inspiratory muscle weakness limits precough inspiration and volume-dependent flow velocity; bulbar dysfunction (whether from neurologic disease or the presence of a tracheostomy) impairs the compressive phase of cough; and expiratory muscle weakness diminishes the velocity of expiratory air flow.

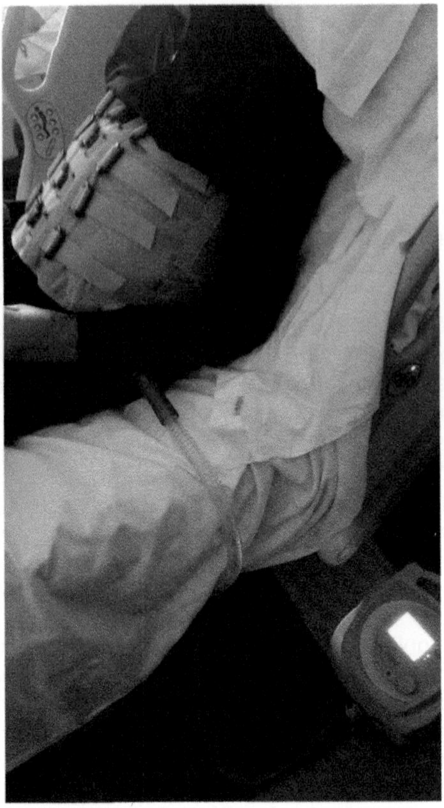

Fig. 1. Intermittent abdominal pressure ventilator for diurnal ventilatory support for adolescents and adults, worn under the clothing except for demonstration purposes in this image.

Assisted Coughing

Chest percussion and vibration are not alternatives to coughing. Bulbar-innervated, inspiratory, and expiratory, muscles are needed for coughing. The oximetry feedback respiratory aid protocol uses an oximeter to monitor Spo_2 to keep it greater than 94% by maintaining effective alveolar ventilation and airway secretion elimination by using inspiratory and/or expiratory aids, that is, up to continuous NVS and assisted coughing. This is most important during respiratory tract infections and when extubating patients with little or no breathing tolerance.

Bach and Saporito[9] assessed factors that would predict successful removal of endotracheal or tracheostomy tubes in adult subjects with primarily neuromuscular ventilatory insufficiency. Of all factors considered, only the ability of subjects to generate a CPF greater than 160 L/min with assisted or unassisted cough predicted successful extubation or decannulation. Bach and colleagues[5,10,11] suggested that patients with less than 5 L/s (300 L/min) of unassisted CPF may benefit from assisted coughing and MIE.

Manually assisted cough

A manually assisted cough involves the application of abdominal thrust, which may be combined with an anterior chest wall compression timed to glottic opening to augment expiratory muscle activity.[9] For small children, 1 hand or only a few fingers may be used. For adolescents or adults with less than 1.5 L of VC, a maximal insufflation or air stacking precedes the manually assisted maneuver. Breath stacking may be accomplished with glossopharyngeal breathing (GPB) or a manual resuscitation bag with or without a 1-way valve. Manually assisted cough is less effective in the presence of chest wall distortion and scoliosis and should not be used for 1 hour after meals or for patients after abdominal trauma or surgery.

Mechanical insufflation-exsufflation

If lung function, chest wall distortion, or unstable chest wall precludes the use of manually assisted cough, MIE may be used to produce effective expiratory flows to expel secretions. MIE involves passive lung expansion with the use of a positive-pressure insufflation followed rapidly by exsufflation with negative pressure to generate an expiratory flow velocity high enough to shear secretions from the airway wall and move them upward where they can be expectorated or suctioned. Insufflation and exsufflation pressures usually are set at +55 cm H_2O to -55 cm H_2O. Similar pressures have been used without untoward effects in young children.[12] At present, the best indicators for whether a young child with NMD requires assistance with cough are a history of recurrent pneumonia and the qualitative assessment of a weak cough. The use of MIE has been shown to have a dramatic effect on CPF and hence is considered an effective means of assisting cough in individuals with NMD.

One treatment consists of approximately 5 cycles of MIE followed by a period of normal breathing or ventilator use for 20 seconds to 30 seconds to avoid hyperventilation. Five or more treatments are given in 1 sitting and the treatments are repeated until no further secretions are expelled and mucus plug triggered Spo_2 desaturations are reversed. MIE sessions may be repeated every 5 minutes to 10 minutes as needed. It is used via noninvasive (facial interface or mouthpiece) or invasive interfaces (endotracheal and tracheostomy tubes). It is less uncomfortable than invasive tracheal suctioning.[13] The use of MIE allows extubation of patients with little or no ventilator-free breathing ability (VFBA) to NVS. It also may avert intubation for patients with URIs. Barotrauma with the use of MIE is rare.

APPROACHES TO MOBILIZE SECRETIONS

Incentive spirometry or deep breathing is ineffective because they expand the lungs to no more than the VC. A variety of techniques have been used to mobilize secretions from the peripheral to the more central airways, where they may then be coughed out or suctioned. These include intrapulmonary percussive ventilation, high-frequency chest wall oscillator (HFCWO), and the use of mucoactive agents to alter the properties of secretions.

Intrapulmonary Percussive Ventilation

Intrapulmonary percussive ventilation provides low-amplitude bursts of air at frequencies in the range of 50 cycles/min to 550 cycles/min, with pressures of 5 cm H_2O to 35 cm H_2O applied over the patient's own breathing frequency. The percussions of gas are delivered directly and continuously to the airways via mouthpiece, face mask, or artificial airway (endotracheal or tracheostomy tube) through a Venturi device (Phasitron [Percussionaire Corp., Sandpoint, ID, USA]), powered with compressed gas at pressures of 20 pounds per square inch (psi) to 40 psi. The positive pressure oscillations cause airway walls to vibrate and the lungs to expand allowing gas to fill distal lung areas beyond the obstructing secretions. It provides a mechanical means for loosening and mobilizing secretions. It also may be used to simultaneously deliver medications to the lower airways.[14]

High-Frequency Chest Wall Oscillator

HFCWO uses extrathoracic oscillations generated by forces external to the respiratory system. These oscillations are applied using an inflatable vest attached by hoses to an air pressure generator. The generator rapidly injects and withdraws small volumes of air into and out of the vest, inflating and deflating it to produce chest compressions at frequencies and pressures selected by the operator. The frequencies typically used range between 5 Hz and 25 Hz. The Monarch Airway Clearance System (Hill-Rom, Inc., St. Paul, MN) uses oscillating discs, which provide targeted kinetic energy to the lungs to generate air flow and mobilize mucus from the airways; the Vibralung Acoustical Percussor (Westmed, Inc., Tucson, AZ) transfers acoustic energy-generated vibrations to the airways during inspiration and expiration to mobilize secretions.[15] HFCWOs are considered a mucus-mobilization technique. The effectiveness of HFCWOs has been demonstrated in patients with cystic fibrosis[16,17] but the experience in patients with NMD is limited.

Mucoactive Agents

The characteristics of mucus and airway-lining fluid affect how effectively either mucociliary clearance or cough clears the respiratory tract of secretions. The more elastic the mucus, the better mucociliary clearance, whereas cough clearance is optimized when mucus has high viscosity.

Medications that alter the properties of mucus have been grouped into expectorants, mucolytics, mucokinetics, and mucoregulators. Although several agents may alter the physical properties of mucus or the airway-lining fluid, all pharmacologic therapies directed at enhancing airway clearance, including the use of hyperosmolar agents like hypertonic saline; mucolytics like dornase alfa; mucokinetics like β_2-agonists; and mucoregulators like anticholinergics, are considered off-label for children with NMD.[18]

SLEEP-DISORDERED BREATHING IN PATIENTS WITH NEUROMUSCULAR DISEASES

Under normal circumstances, sleep is responsible for significant changes in lung mechanics and respiratory muscle control. The supine position leads to a decrease in FRC, mainly due to the cephalad displacement of the abdominal contents. Sleep decreases the ventilatory response to both hypoxemia and hypercapnia compared with wakefulness.[19–21] Sleep also leads to a decrease in tonic activity of upper airway and intercostal muscles, especially during rapid-eye-movement sleep, eliminating their contribution to inspiration and accentuating the dependence of gas exchange on diaphragm contraction. Neuromuscular weakness amplifies these alterations in breathing and thus leads to significant sleep-related hypercapnia and hypoxemia, often before daytime ventilatory impairment is recognized.[4]

The myriad problems that may occur during sleep in patients with NMD and sleep-disordered breathing include hypoventilation, hypoxemia, central and obstructive hypopneas and apneas, frequent arousals, sleep fragmentation, decreased sleep efficiency, and even seizures.[22–24] As patients develop respiratory muscle weakness significant enough to affect gas exchange, they compensate for hypoventilation with an arousal response. The arousal limits the extent of hypoxemia and hypercapnia by changing the sleep state, recruiting respiratory and upper-airway muscular activity, and depth of ventilation.[22] With persistent hypoventilation and its accompanying arousals, sleep fragmentation and deprivation increase; eventually, the ventilatory chemoreceptor responses become blunted, resulting in fewer arousals, longer periods of rapid-eye-movement sleep, and longer periods of hypoventilation with hypoxemia. This sequence of events leading to progressive hypoventilation is common among patients with NMD. Current guidelines for evaluation of patients with NMDs recommend both diurnal oximetry and capnography and sleep oximetry and either end-tidal or transcutaneous CO_2 monitoring.[25]

NONINVASIVE VENTILATORY SUPPORT IN NEUROMUSCULAR DISEASES

In general, the objectives of NVS in patients with NMD are to normalize gas exchange, relieve dyspnea, correct sleep-disordered breathing and abnormal sleep architecture, prevent or reverse cor pulmonale, improve daytime function, promote and sustain growth and development, improve quality of life, and prolong survival. The addition of NVS in this patient population has changed the natural history of their diseases.[26–32]

NVS is applied with a variety of interfaces and ventilators, at full ventilator support settings to optimally rest respiratory muscles, which low-span bilevel positive airway pressure and continuous positive airway pressure do not achieve. The interface has a major impact on patient comfort during NVS. The most commonly used interfaces are nasal, oronasal, and mouthpieces (**Fig. 2**). A variety of sizes and designs are available, as both disposable and reusable designs (**Table 1**).

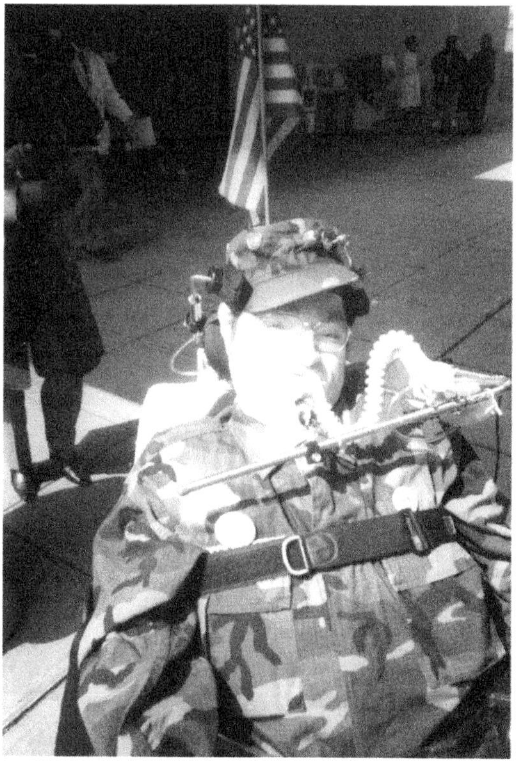

Fig. 2. A 41-year-old with DMD who required CNVS since age 14 and began NVS at age 12. Here he is seen using NVS via a 15-mm angled mouthpiece during daytime hours.

Table 1
Commonly used noninvasive ventilatory support interfaces

	Advantages	Disadvantages
Nasal	Less risk of aspiration Easier secretion clearance Less claustrophobia Easier speech Patient may be able to eat Easy to fit and secure Less dead space	Mouth leak Higher resistance through nasal passages Less effective with nasal obstruction Nasal irritation and rhinorrhea Mouth dryness
Oronasal	Better oral leak control More effective in mouth breathers	Increased dead space Claustrophobia Increased aspiration risk Increased difficulty speaking and eating Asphyxiation with ventilator malfunction
Mouthpiece	Less interference with speech Very little dead space May not require headgear	Less effective if patient cannot maintain mouth seal Usually requires nasal or oronasal interface at night Nasal leak

The Ventilator for Noninvasive Ventilatory Support

Any ventilator may be attached to a face mask or other NVS interface, rather than an artificial airway. Critical-care ventilators may be used to provide NVS in the hospital setting, with the advantages of precise control of fraction of inspired oxygen (F_{IO_2}), various modes and inspiratory flow patterns, and separation of inspiratory and expiratory gases to limit rebreathing. Critical-care ventilators have numerous monitors and alarms, which may be desirable during invasive ventilation but may be distracting and annoying for patients and clinicians during NVS.

Conventional home-care ventilators have been used to provide NVS. Newer home-care ventilators, however, are much improved and offer a variety of modes and features. Some are battery-powered, small, and light-weight and thus portable.

Pressure support ventilation also is available on portable ventilators and bilevel machines. The latter may be used at NVS settings but rarely is so these patients ultimately develop respiratory failure. Their major advantage is the ability to function correctly with leaks. When volume limited, they are blowers that vary inspiratory and expiratory pressure in response to patient demand. They also gush air into the patient throat and disrupt sleep. They do not allow air stacking for deep breaths to speak louder and to increase cough flows the way volume preset ventilators does.

NVS may be achieved by high-span bilevel settings with inspiratory positive airway pressure (IPAP) is at least 15 cm H_2O greater than expiratory positive airway pressure (EPAP). The IPAP minus the EPAP is the level of pressure support for optimal muscle rest. Pressure-assist control on portable ventilators may be used with or without positive end-expiratory pressure (PEEP).[33]

When portable pressure ventilators use single hoses that do not have exhalation valves, there is a potential for CO_2 rebreathing.[34] This is not a problem at NVS settings. Patients also exhale into the atmosphere instead of into the tubing.

Supplemental oxygen usually is unnecessary in patients NMD who require NVS. If needed, newer ventilators allow a precisely set F_{IO_2}.

Mode

There are advantages and disadvantages to volume-controlled ventilation (VCV), pressure-support ventilation (PSV), and pressure-controlled (PCV) for NVS (**Box 2**).

Settings for Noninvasive Ventilatory Support

Selection of settings for NVS often is done empirically and is symptom-based. For infants, initially, the NVS settings are selected based on short-term symptoms and reversing paradoxic breathing. Patients with ventilatory pump failure usually do not require PEEP. Moreover, higher PEEP results in higher inspiratory pressure, which may decrease patient tolerance. Although for most patients with NMD and otherwise normal lung function, pressure support of approximately 15 to 20 cm H_2O usually is adequate, because of the potential for ineffective triggers and central apnea, a backup rate should be set at approximately 12 breaths/min.

Newer ventilator triggers are very sensitive to patient effort, so auto-triggering may occur because of leaks, which is less of a problem with a bilevel ventilator. Pressurization rate (rise time) refers to the amount of time required to reach the pressure target at the onset of inhalation with PSV and PCV. In patients with NMD, a slower rise time often is tolerated better. Rise time should be set to maximize patient comfort. The term, *cycle*, refers to the changeover from the inspiratory phase to the expiratory phase. During PSV, the inspiratory phase terminates when flow falls to a predetermined fraction of peak inspiratory flow. In some modern ventilators, the flow cycle may be adjusted to minimize issues with leaks.[35]

Dryness and nasal stuffiness commonly occur during noninvasive ventilation, particularly with the use a nasal mask. These symptoms may be addressed by use of an oronasal mask or heated humidification. If symptoms persist despite adequate humidification, saline spray or topical nasal decongestants may be applied.

Glossopharyngeal Breathing

GPB (frog breathing) involves the use of the tongue and pharyngeal muscles to produce a tidal volume by projecting boluses of air past the glottis into the lungs. The glottis closes with each gulp of air. Each breath usually consists of 6 gulps to 9 gulps of 60 mL to 100 mL each. GPB may provide an individual who has little or no

Box. 2
Comparison of volume ventilator and pressure ventilator for noninvasive ventilatory support for patients with neuromuscular diseases

Volume ventilation
- More complicated to use
- Wide range of alarms
- Constant high-delivered volumes (allow patient's ventilatory drive to vary tidal volume)
- Breath stacking possible
- No leak compensation
- May be used without PEEP
- Rebreathing minimized

Pressure ventilation
- Limited alarms depending on ventilator
- Variable tidal volume
- Breath stacking not possible
- Leak compensation

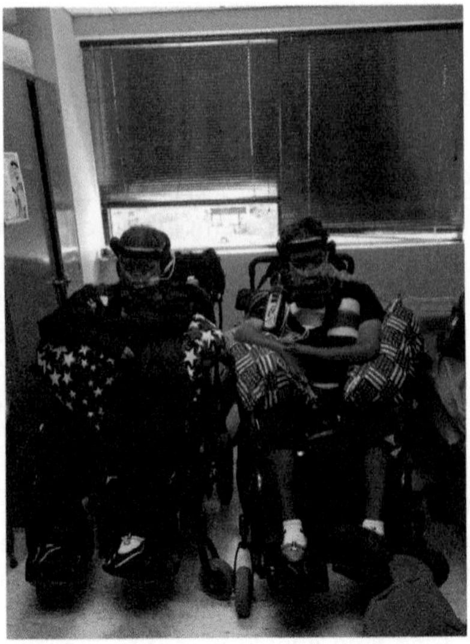

Fig. 3. A 25 year old and 23 year old with Werdnig-Hoffmann's disease, dependent on nasal continuous NVS since 8 months and 4 months of age with no VFBA.

measurable VC with normal lung ventilation throughout daytime hours and perfect safety in the event of ventilator failure day or night.[35]

LUNG VOLUME RECRUITMENT

The patient uses a mouthpiece to air stack consecutively delivered volumes from a volume-cycling ventilator or a manual resuscitator multiple times, 3 times daily. If the lips or cheeks are too weak to allow air stacking via a mouthpiece, it then is done via a nasal interface or lip cover phalange. If the bulbar-innervated muscles are too weak for deep air stacking, single deep insufflations may be provided via a CoughAssist (Philips-Respironics Inc., Murrysville, PA) at 60 cm H_2O to 70 cm H_2O 3 times a day. Most individuals need instruction and encouragement to learn this technique.

EXTUBATION AND DECANNULATION

Infants and patients of all ages who are intubated for ARF almost always can be extubated to continuous NVS (CNVS) and MIE without resort to tracheotomies.[36,37] This is true even for infants and children with SMA type 1 who have no ventilator free breathing ability (**Fig. 3**). Children who undergo tracheotomies also may be evaluated for decannulation to up to CNVS once they are old enough to understand and cooperate with the protocols.[38] This is true even for patients with no VFBA. Whereas 94% of conventionally managed SMA type 1 children fail extubation, the success rate of extubating them to CNVS and MIE is more than 90%.[36,37] Manually assisted coughing and MIE are used aggressively after extubation.

SUMMARY

Virtually all pediatric patients with NMD, including those with SMA type 1, may be managed without tracheostomies. The exceptions are those who's bulbar-innervated muscular is severely impaired in association with upper motor neuron dysfunction, which is rare in pediatric NMD. Patients may become continuously dependent on noninvasive intermittent positive pressure ventilation without ever needing hospitalization, intubation, tracheostomy, or bronchoscopy. Noninvasive methods enhance quality of life, allow the use of GPB for safety in the event of ventilator failure and reduce morbidity and mortality. Prognoses for these patients are improving due to newly available medications. Thus far, oligonucleotides like nusinersen essentially correct the RNA; gene therapy with Zolgensma (Genentech Inc., South San Francisco, CA) places the correct DNA into the cell nuclei; and Evrysdi (PTC Therapeutics, South Plainfield, NJ) modified the splicing pattern of the SMN2 gene for it to produce more full length SMN. All have been shown to improve motor function significantly for some patients with SMA. Exon skipping agents, including eteplirsen, for DMD likewise have demonstrated some benefits. Similar potential therapies are in the pipeline for many other NMDs, including myotonic dystrophy, the limb-girdle and other muscular dystrophies, and congenital myopathies. These may make noninvasive respiratory management only easier.

CLINICS CARE POINTS

- Patients with myopathic or lower motor neuron diseases of all ages can be managed by up to continuous noninvasive ventilatory support and use mechanical insufflation exsufflation to clear airways indefinitely and without resort to tracheostomy tubes.
- Institution of sleep nasal noninvasive ventilatory support (NVS) for children with ventilatory pump failure normalizes diurnal blood gases until further muscle deterioration causes patients to extend sleep NVS into daytime hours.
- Patients using sleep nasal noninvasive ventilatory support (NVS) usually become and remain asymptomatic until diurnal hypoventilation causes the oxyhemoglobin saturation to decrease below 95% and may then begin to use daytime NVS.
- Using up to continuous noninvasive ventilatory support (CNVS) patients with Duchenne muscular dystrophy are now surviving over 45 years, infants with severe spinal muscular atrophy type 1 over 25 years, and children with milder neuromuscular conditions, likewise, and without resort to tracheotomies.

DISCLOSURE

The authors have nothing to disclose.

REFERENCES

1. Roussos C, Macklem PT. The respiratory muscles. N Engl J Med 1982;307(13): 786–97.
2. Perrin C, Unterborn JN, Ambrosio CD, et al. Pulmonary complications of chronic neuromuscular diseases and their management. Muscle Nerve 2004;29(1):5–27.
3. J-Paul P, Redding GJ. Chest wall and respiratory muscle disorders. In: Wilmott RW, Bush A, editors. Kendig's disorders of the respiratory tract in children. Philadelphia (PA): Elsevier; 2019. p. 1044–61.
4. Bendit JO. Pathophysiology of neuromuscular respiratory diseases. Clin Chest Med 2018;39(2):297–308.
5. Bach JR, Martinez D. Duchenne muscular dystrophy: continuous noninvasive ventilatory support prolongs survival. Respir Care 2011;56(6):744–50.

6. Bach JR, Bianchi C. Prevention of pectus excavatum for children with spinal muscular atrophy type 1. Am J Phys Med Rehabil 2003;82(10):815–9.
7. Bach JR. Physical medicine and rehabilitation interventions for skeletal and cardiopulmonary muscle dysfunction: In: Bach JR, Chiou M, editors. Volume 1 – physical and medical concerns, 2020 Ventilamed.com, ISBN 978-1-7336008-1-1
8. Leith DE. The development of cough. Am Rev Respir Dis 1985;131(5):S39–42.
9. Bach JR, Saporito LR. Criteria for extubation and tracheostomy tube removal for patients with ventilatory failure: a different approach to weaning. Chest 1996; 110(6):1566–71.
10. Bach JR, Ishikawa Y, Kim H. Prevention of pulmonary morbidity for patients with Duchenne muscular dystrophy. Chest 1997;112(4):1024–8.
11. Bach JR. Mechanical insufflation-exsufflation: comparison of peak expiratory flows with manually assisted and unassisted coughing techniques. Chest 1993; 104:1553–62.
12. Homnick DN. Mechanical insufflation-exsufflation for airway mucus clearance. Respir Care 2007;52(10):1296–305.
13. Miske LJ, Hickey EM, Kolb SM, et al. Use of the mechanical in-exsufflator in pediatric patients with neuromuscular disease and impaired cough. Chest 2004; 125(4):1406–12.
14. Toussaint M, De Win H, Steens M, et al. Effect of intrapulmonary percussive ventilation on mucus clearance in Duchenne muscular dystrophy patients: a preliminary report. Respir Care 2003;48(10):940–7.
15. Fitzgerald K, Dugre J, Pagala S, et al. High-frequency chest wall compression therapy in neurologically impaired children. Respir Care 2014;59(1):107–12.
16. Arens R, Gozal D, Omlin KJ, et al. Comparison of high frequency chest compression and conventional chest physiotherapy in hospitalized patients with cystic fibrosis. Am J Respir Crit Care Med 1994;150(4):1154–7.
17. Warwick WJ, Hansen LG. The long-term effect of high-frequency chest compression therapy on pulmonary complications of cystic fibrosis. Pediatr Pulmonol 1991;11(3):265–71.
18. Rogers DF. Mucoactive agents for airway mucus hypersecretory diseases. Respir Care 2007;52(9):1176–93.
19. Alves RS, Resende MB, Skomro RP, et al. Sleep and neuromuscular disorders in children. Sleep Med Rev 2009;13(2):133–48.
20. Arens R, Muzumdar H. Sleep, sleep disordered breathing, and noc- turnal hypoventilation in children with neuromuscular diseases. Paediatr Respir Rev 2010; 11(1):24–30.
21. Piper A. Sleep abnormalities associated with neuromuscular disease: pathophysiology and evaluation. Semin Respir Crit Care Med 2002;23(3):211–9.
22. Dhand UK, Dhand R. Sleep disorders in neuromuscular diseases. Curr Opin Pulm Med 2006;12(6):402–8.
23. Labanowski M, Schmidt-Nowara W, Guilleminault C. Sleep and neuromuscular disease: frequency of sleep-disordered breathing in a neuromuscular disease clinic population. Neurology 1996;47(5):1173–80.
24. Katz SL. Assessment of sleep-disordered breathing in pediatric neuromuscular diseases. Pediatrics 2009;123(Suppl 4):S222–5.
25. Bach JR, Gonçalves MR, Hon AJ, et al. Changing trends in the management of end-stage respiratory muscle failure in neuromuscular disease: current recommendations of an international consensus. Am J Phys Med Rehabil 2013;92(3): 267–77.

26. Bach JR, Alba AS. Management of chronic alveolar hypoventilation by nasal ventilation. Chest 1990;97:52–7.
27. Bach JR, Alba AS, Bohatiuk G, et al. Mouth intermittent positive pressure ventilation in the management of post-polio respiratory insufficiency. Chest 1987;91: 859–64.
28. McKim DA, Griller N, LeBlanc C, et al. Twenty-four hour noninvasive ventilation in Duchenne muscular dystrophy: a safe alternative to tracheostomy. Can Respir J 2013;20(1):e5–9.
29. Tzeng AC, Bach JR. Prevention of pulmonary morbidity for patients with neuromuscular disease. Chest 2000;118:1390–6.
30. Gomez-Merino E, Bach JR. Duchenne muscular dystrophy: prolongation of life by noninvasive respiratory muscle aids. Am J Phys Med Rehabil 2002;81:411–5.
31. Bach JR. Point: is non-invasive ventilation always the most appropriate manner of long-term ventilation for infants with spinal muscular atrophy type 1? Yes, almost always? Chest 2016;151(5):962–5.
32. Goncalves MR, Bach JR, Ishikawa Y, et al. Continuous noninvasive ventilatory support outcomes for neuromuscular disease: a multicenter collaboration and literature review. Rev Port Pneumol 2019. [Epub ahead of print]. https://doi.org/10.1016/j.pulmoe.2019.05.006.
33. Highcock MP, Morrish E, Jamieson S, et al. An overnight comparison of two ventilators used in the treatment of chronic respiratory failure. Eur Respir J 2002; 20(4):942–5.
34. Hill NS, Carlisle C, Kramer NR. Effect of a nonrebreathing exhalation valve on long-term nasal ventilation using a bilevel device. Chest 2002;122(1):84–91.
35. Bach JR. Update and perspectives on noninvasive respiratory muscle aids: part 1: the inspiratory aids. Chest 1994;105(4):1230–40.
36. Bach JR, Gonçalves MR, Hamdani I, et al. Extubation of unweanable patients with neuromuscular weakness: a new management paradigm. Chest 2010;137(5): 1033–9.
37. Bach JR, Sinquee D, Saporito LR, et al. Efficacy of mechanical insufflation-exsufflation in extubating unweanable subjects with restrictive pulmonary disorders. Respir Care 2015;60(4):477–83.
38. Bach JR, Saporito LR, Shah HR, et al. Decanulation of patients with severe respiratory muscle insufficiency: efficacy of mechanical insufflation-exsufflation. J Rehabil Med 2014;46:1037–41.

Pulmonary Manifestations of Parasitic Diseases in Children

Teena Huan Xu, MD[a], Nair Lovaton, MD[b], Jose Serpa, MD, MS[a], Theresa J. Ochoa, MD, PhD[c,*]

KEYWORDS

- Parasite • Loeffler syndrome • Protozoa • Cestodes • Trematodes • Nematodes
- Tropical pulmonary eosinophilia

KEY POINTS

- Parasites cause respiratory symptoms through 3 main mechanisms: hypersensitivity stimulus, direct invasion of the lung parenchyma or pleural space, and migration from other infected organs.
- Parasitic lung disease can be focal (hydatidosis, amebiasis, paragonimiasis) or diffuse (ascariasis, toxocariasis, ancylostomiasis, strongyloidiasis, schistosomiasis, toxoplasmosis, malaria, tropical pulmonary eosinophilia).
- Pulmonary symptoms associated with peripheral eosinophilia or gastrointestinal, hepatobiliary, or cutaneous symptoms should raise suspicion for a parasitic process.
- Diagnosis is typically made through microscopic examination of stool or respiratory tract samples or serologic testing.
- With early identification, most parasitic lung diseases are curable with medical treatment (antiparasitic drugs).

INTRODUCTION

Parasitic diseases are a major cause of morbidity and mortality in the tropical and subtropical areas of the world. Infection or infestation can occur in children of all ages. Children develop parasitic diseases by ingestion of contaminated food or water, contact with animal and pets, ingestion of soil contaminated with infected animal or human feces, and direct contact with larvae in soil. Two main classes of parasites

[a] Section of Infectious Diseases, Department of Medicine, Baylor College of Medicine, One Baylor Plaza. BCM 285, Houston, TX 77030, USA; [b] Department of Pediatrics, Faculty of Medicine, Universidad Peruana Cayetano Heredia, Av. Honorio Delgado 430, San Martin de Porres, Lima 15102, Peru; [c] Department of Pediatrics, Faculty of Medicine, Instituto de Medicina Tropical Alexander von Humboldt, Universidad Peruana Cayetano Heredia, Av. Honorio Delgado 430, San Martin de Porres, Lima 15102, Peru
* Corresponding author.
E-mail address: Theresa.J.Ochoa@uth.tmc.edu

Pediatr Clin N Am 68 (2021) 193–207
https://doi.org/10.1016/j.pcl.2020.09.007

cause pulmonary disease: protozoa (microscopic, unicellular organisms) and helminths (large, multicellular organisms). The latter includes cestodes (tapeworms), trematodes (flukes), and nematodes (roundworms). Soil-transmitted helminths are of major importance in developing countries, affecting the poorest and most disadvantaged communities. Intestinal parasites can cause diarrhea, abdominal pain, intestinal obstruction, and anemia. They are associated with growth impairment and developmental delay. Pulmonary involvement can be a major feature of some parasitic infections. Lung pathology is often a complication of transpulmonary larval migration during the acute migratory phase of parasite life cycles. With increasing travel and human migration, it is important to consider parasitic infections as mimickers of more common lung diseases such as tuberculosis and malignancy, as they may share similar clinical and radiological features. When pulmonary symptoms are associated with peripheral eosinophilia or gastrointestinal (abdominal pain, diarrhea), hepatobiliary (jaundice, nausea, vomiting), or cutaneous (rash, skin nodules, migratory skin lesions) symptoms, an underlying parasitic process should be suspected.

CLINICAL APPROACH

Parasites can cause fever and nonspecific respiratory symptoms such as cough, dyspnea, wheezing, chest pain, and hemoptysis. The degree of lung involvement will depend on the characteristics and location of the parasite, as well as the host's immune response. Many clinical features are due to the host immune response to parasite antigens, which may be protective or deleterious.[1]

Parasites can produce respiratory symptoms through 3 main mechanisms: (1) hypersensitivity stimulus during their life cycle, (2) direct invasion of the lung parenchyma or pleural space during a hematogenous phase, and (3) migration from other infected organs.

Radiologic findings in parasitic lung disease can be divided into 2 groups based on degree of involvement: focal and diffuse.[2]

Focal Lung Involvement

Common focal findings include cystic lesions, coinlike nodular lesions, consolidation, and pleural effusions.[2] Parasitic syndromes presenting with focal lung lesions include hydatidosis, amebiasis, paragonimiasis, and dirofilariasis. Hydatidosis causes single or multiple cystic lesions (**Fig. 1**). Most children with an intact hydatid lung cyst are asymptomatic.[3] Pulmonary amebiasis, the most frequent complication of an amebic liver abscess, can produce pleural effusions with or without empyema, pneumonitis, consolidation, or lung abscess.[4] Although rare in children, pulmonary paragonimiasis is frequently confused with tuberculosis. It typically presents as a pleural effusion without parenchymal involvement.[5] Pulmonary dirofilariasis presents as a single, subpleural, coinlike lesion that can mimic malignancy.[2] It is rarely described in children.

Diffuse Lung Involvement

Diffuse findings may be transient in nature, appearing as alveolar or interstitial infiltrates. Transpulmonary larval migration can precipitate an acute eosinophilic pneumonitis (Loeffler syndrome), most commonly seen in ascariasis, toxocariasis, ancylostomiasis, and strongyloidiasis. Patients present with fever, dry cough, wheezing, dyspnea, and rarely hemoptysis. Diffuse migratory infiltrates and occasional localized nodular lesions are evident on chest imaging. The onset and exacerbation of childhood asthma are associated with toxocariasis and strongyloidiasis.[6,7] In severe cases, *Strongyloides* hyperinfection can result in acute respiratory distress

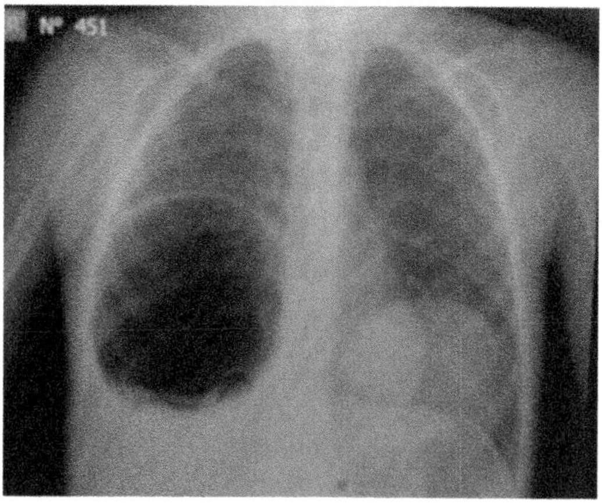

Fig. 1. Chest radiograph of a 5-year-old girl from a rural community in the Andes of Peru. Bilateral cystic lesions: right lung, air-filled water-lily sign consistent with ruptured hydatid cyst. Left lung, fluid density consistent with unruptured cyst. (*Courtesy of* A. Clinton White, MD, FACP FIDSA FASTMH, Galveston, Texas.)

syndrome (ARDS), alveolar hemorrhage, and gram-negative bacterial pneumonia. During its pulmonary migration, *Strongyloides* larvae enter alveoli, creating interstitial and alveolar lesions on chest radiograph.[8,9] This radiologic pattern is also seen with pulmonary schistosomiasis, particularly during the acute phase of infection (Katayama fever).[10] In chronic schistosomiasis, pulmonary fibrosis, vasculature obliteration, and pulmonary hypertension can lead to cor pulmonale.[11] Radiologically, there are diffuse reticular and reticulonodular infiltrates and chronic cardiomegaly.[12]

MOST RELEVANT PARASITES

Clinical manifestations and management of the most relevant parasites associated with pulmonary manifestation are discussed in this section. Epidemiology, transmission, and incubation period of each parasite are presented in **Table 1**. Pulmonary symptoms, chest imaging, and diagnostics tools are summarized in **Table 2**.

Protozoa

Malaria

Malaria is globally endemic to the tropics with an estimated 228 million cases; children younger than 5 years account for 67% of malaria deaths.[13] Human malaria, transmitted through female Anopheline mosquitoes, is caused by 5 *Plasmodium* species: *Plasmodium falciparum, Plasmodium vivax, Plasmodium ovale, Plasmodium malariae,* and *Plasmodium knowlesi*.

Clinical manifestations Malaria presents as an acute febrile illness with intermittent paroxysms coinciding with the release of merozoites into the bloodstream.[14] Cough is present in 20% to 50% of uncomplicated malaria cases.[15] Pulmonary symptoms are generally associated with *P falciparum* but also reported with *P vivax* and *P knowlesi*. A unique feature of *P falciparum* is its ability to infect erythrocytes of all stages, leading to high parasitemia and severe disease through sequestration of infected erythrocytes within the microvasculature of major organs. Sequestration within pulmonary microvasculature causes impaired gas exchange and decreased diffusion

Table 1
General characteristics of the main parasites associated with pulmonary manifestations

Parasite	Epidemiology	Transmission	Incubation Period
Malaria: *Plasmodium falciparum, Plasmodium vivax, Plasmodium ovale, Plasmodium malariae, Plasmodium knowlesi*	Tropical and subtropical areas of Africa, South America, Asia, and Oceania	*Anopheles* mosquito bite	7–30 d (*P falciparum*), 14 d to months (*P vivax, P ovale*), 18 d (*P malariae*)
Amebiasis: *Entamoeba histolytica*	Worldwide; tropical areas with poor sanitation, institutionalized individuals, men who have sex with men	Fecal-oral through contaminated food or water, sexual transmission	2–4 wk
Toxoplasmosis: *Toxoplasma gondii*	Worldwide	Ingestion of contaminated food or water, mother-to-fetus, organ transplantation	5–23 d
Echinococcus: *Echinococcus granulosus*	Mediterranean, East and Central Asia, sub-Saharan Africa, Russia, China, South America	Ingestion of contaminated food or water	Months to years
Ascariasis: *Ascaris lumbricoides*	Worldwide; tropics and subtropics	Fecal-oral (soil)	4–8 wk
Hookworm: *Necator americanus, Ancylostoma duodenale*	Worldwide; highest prevalence in sub-Saharan Africa, Asia, Latin America, Caribbean	Direct skin contact (soil), fecal-oral (*A duodenale*)	1–2 wk
Strongyloidiasis: *Strongyloides stercoralis*	Worldwide; subtropics and tropics	Direct skin contact (soil)	Days to years
Toxocariasis: *Toxocara canis, Toxocara cati*	Worldwide; tropics	Ingestion of contaminated food or water	Several weeks
Tropical pulmonary eosinophilia: *Brugia malayi, Wuchereria bancrofti, Brugia timori*	Asia, sub-Saharan Africa, Latin America, Caribbean	Mosquito bites	Years
Paragonimiasis: *Paragonimus westermani*	East Asia, Southeast Asia, Latin America, Africa	Ingestion of raw or undercooked crab or crayfish	1–27 mo
Schistosomiasis: *Schistosoma mansoni, Schistosoma haematobium, Schistosoma japonicum, Schistosoma mekongi*	Africa, South America, East Asia, Southeast Asia	Direct skin contact (water)	14–84 d

Table 2
Pulmonary symptoms and chest imaging of the main parasites associated with pulmonary manifestations

Disease	Pulmonary Symptoms	Chest Imaging	Diagnostic Tools
Protozoa			
Malaria	Fever, chills, cough, dyspnea, chest tightness, tachypnea, respiratory failure	Noncardiogenic pulmonary edema, pleural effusion, diffuse interstitial edema, lobar consolidation	• Antigen detection • Microscopy: thick and thin blood smears
Amebiasis	Productive cough (anchovy paste sputum), chest pain, dyspnea, hemoptysis	Right-sided pleural effusion, consolidation (right lower and middle lobes), lung abscess, empyema, hepatobronchial fistula	• Eosinophilia (–) • Serology (positive after 1 wk) • Microscopy (trophozoites): sputum, pleura, tissue
Toxoplasmosis	Fever, dyspnea, cough	Acute interstitial pneumonia, pneumonitis, micronodular infiltrates, cavitary lesions, lobar pneumonia	• Serology (detectable within 1–2 wk) • Microscopy (tachyzoites): tissue or body fluid
Cestodes			
Cystic echinococcus (hydatidosis)	Chest pain, cough, dyspnea hypersensitivity reaction with cyst rupture (fever, wheezing, hemoptysis)	Single or multiple cysts, endocyst floating in partially fluid-filled cyst (water-lily sign), pleural effusion, hydropneumothorax	• Eosinophilia (–), unless unstable cyst • Serology • Microscopy (protoscolices, hooklets): fluid aspirate
Nematodes			
Ascariasis	Fever, cough, wheezing, dyspnea, chest pain, hemoptysis, rash (Loeffler syndrome)	Migratory bilateral nodular infiltrates	• Microscopy (eggs): sputum, gastric samples
Hookworm	Fever, cough, wheezing, dyspnea, chest pain (Loeffler syndrome)	Migratory bilateral nodular infiltrates	• Eosinophilia (+) • Microscopy (eggs): stool
Strongyloidiasis	Acute: fever, cough, sore throat, rash, wheezing, chest pain, hemoptysis (Loeffler syndrome) Hyperinfection syndrome: respiratory failure, shock, alveolar hemorrhage	Acute: migratory bilateral nodular opacities Hyperinfection: lobar or segmental infiltrates, diffuse alveolar infiltrates, miliary nodules, lung abscess, pleural effusion	• Eosinophilia (+) • Serology • Microscopy (larvae): stool, sputum, bronchoalveolar lavage, duodenal aspirate

(*continued on next page*)

Table 2
(*continued*)

Disease	Pulmonary Symptoms	Chest Imaging	Diagnostic Tools
Toxocariasis	Fever, cough, wheezing, dyspnea, respiratory failure (visceral larva migrans)	Diffuse ground-glass opacities, bilateral nodular infiltrates, consolidations, linear opacities	• Eosinophilia (+) • Serology • Microscopy (larvae): tissue
Tropical pulmonary eosinophilia	Fever, cough, dyspnea, wheezing, weight loss	Migratory nodular opacities, mediastinal lymphadenopathy	• Eosinophilia (+) • Serology
Trematodes			
Schistosomiasis	Fever, cough, dyspnea, rash, arthralgias (Katayama fever); Loeffler syndrome, chronic dyspnea	Migratory bilateral infiltrates, pulmonary hypertension, pulmonary arteriovenous fistulae	• Eosinophilia (+) • Serology • Antigen test (serum, urine) • Microscopy (eggs): stool, urine, sputum, feces
Paragonimiasis	Fever, cough, pleuritic chest pain, Loeffler syndrome, hemoptysis, chronic bronchitis	Migratory unilateral infiltrates, ring shadow with crescent-shaped opacity, calcified cystic lesions, nodules, cysts, pleural effusion, pneumothorax	• Serology • Microscopy (eggs): stool, sputum

capacity, causing dyspnea, tachypnea, and hypoxia. Severe malaria can trigger an inflammatory cascade, resulting in a rapidly progressive capillary leak syndrome with ARDS. In young children, compensatory tachypnea for severe metabolic acidosis and anemia can be profound.[16] Other complications include superimposed pneumonia, acute lung injury from concomitant bacterial sepsis, aspiration pneumonia, and iatrogenic pulmonary edema.

Management Treatment should be initiated at the time of diagnosis.[17] Identifying the geographic area of acquisition is important for determining risk of drug resistance. Uncomplicated disease is treated with oral antimalarials determined by *Plasmodium* species, risk of chloroquine resistance, and drug availability. Severe malaria should be managed in the hospital.

Amebiasis

Amebiasis is endemic worldwide and caused by *Entamoeba histolytica*, a protozoan that lives within the colonic lumen of humans.

Clinical manifestations Fecal-oral transmission of *E. histolytica* cysts or trophozoites can result in asymptomatic carrier states or invasive disease. Trophozoite invasion of colonic epithelial cells results in amebic colitis. Subsequent hematogenous spread leads to extraintestinal disease, a rare complication in children. Liver abscess, the most common form of extraintestinal disease, is associated with pleuropulmonary disease in 10% to 15% of cases.[4,18] Pulmonary manifestations include right-sided atelectasis, pleural effusion, pneumonia, lung abscess, and empyema.[19,20] "Anchovy paste" sputum is seen in individuals with hepatobronchial fistula. A combination of serologic testing with stool antigen detection or polymerase chain reaction analysis is likely to provide the greatest diagnostic yield.

Management Treatment of pulmonary amebiasis includes metronidazole or tinidazole followed by a luminal agent for cyst eradication (paromomycin). Consider surgical management in individuals not responding to therapy or at high risk of abscess rupture.

Toxoplasmosis

Infection with *Toxoplasma gondii* occurs through contact with infected cat feces, ingestion of undercooked meat infected with tissue cysts, blood transfusion, and organ transplantation.

Clinical manifestations Primary toxoplasmosis is typically subclinical, but 10% to 20% may develop a self-limited, flulike syndrome.[21] Pulmonary disease is rare in immunocompetent individuals and may be associated with more virulent *T gondii* strains in South America.[22,23] Manifestations include acute interstitial pneumonia, micronodular infiltrates, cavitary lesions, and lobar pneumonia.[24] Pneumonitis has been observed with untreated acute congenital toxoplasmosis.[21] Individuals with impaired cell-mediated immunity can reactivate latent toxoplasmosis to develop severe disease such as pneumonia.[25] Lung histopathology generally shows a necrotizing pneumonitis.

Management Primary toxoplasmosis in immunocompetent individuals will generally self-resolve. Treatment is indicated in severe disease, end-organ damage (eg, pneumonitis), immunosuppression, pregnancy, and congenital disease. Combination of pyrimethamine with leucovorin and sulfadiazine is effective, although optimal duration of treatment is not well established.

Cestodes

Cystic echinococcus

Hydatid disease and cystic echinococcus is primarily caused by the canine tapeworm, *Echinococcus granulosus*. Infection occurs through ingestion or inhalation of eggs in canine feces. Intermediate hosts include sheep, goats, camels, cervids, horses, cattle, and swine, although humans can become accidently infected. After entering the gastrointestinal tract, eggs hatch into larvae and translocate through mucosa into the circulatory system. They travel to the liver and lungs and develop into hydatid cysts that enlarge over time, producing protoscolices and daughter cysts.

Clinical manifestations Cystic echinococcosis is often asymptomatic and incidentally discovered when a cystic liver or lung lesion is found on imaging (see **Fig. 1**). Isolated pulmonary cysts are more common in children.[26] Pulmonary disease develops through direct inhalation, lymphohematogenous spread, or transdiaphragmatic seeding from a ruptured liver cyst. Over time, enlargement of cysts can compress adjacent structures, causing abdominal pain, cough, or chest pain. Cysts can destabilize and rupture, releasing antigenic material and protoscolices that seed body cavities and trigger hypersensitivity reactions with fever, wheezing, and rarely anaphylaxis.[27] Peripheral eosinophilia is present in 25% of cases and may herald cyst leakage.[28] Rupture of cysts into the tracheobronchial tree can cause hemoptysis and expectoration of cyst contents. Other complications include pneumothorax, pleural effusion, and secondary infection leading to empyema and lung abscess.

Diagnosis relies on radiologic and serologic tests in the context of epidemiologic risk factors. Chest imaging of unruptured pulmonary cysts reveal well-demarcated, homogenous oval or round masses, with shape variability on inspiratory and expiratory films. Pulmonary cysts are typically solitary and more frequently found in the base of the right lung.[28] Unlike hepatic cysts, pulmonary cysts rarely calcify. Bronchial erosion and cyst rupture may produce a crescent or meniscus sign due to the introduction of air.[20] Other radiologic features of pulmonary echinococcosis such as water-lily sign, characterized as an endocyst floating in a partially fluid-filled cyst, are infrequently seen. Percutaneous aspiration for evaluation of protoscolices, hooklets, or hydatid membranes is generally avoided with pulmonary cysts due to risk for rupture.

Management Surgical excision remains the treatment of choice for pulmonary echinococcosis, although smaller cysts have been successfully managed with antiparasitic therapy alone. Adjunctive albendazole or mebendazole with or without praziquantel decreases the risk of intraoperative dissemination and recurrence.[27] Nonoperable cases should be treated with prolonged courses of albendazole (preferred) or mebendazole.

Nematodes

Ascariasis

Ascariasis, caused by the human roundworm *Ascaris lumbricoides*, is the most common helminth infection worldwide. It is a significant cause of childhood morbidity through deleterious impact on nutrition and is associated with development of primary lung diseases such as asthma.[29] Infection occurs through ingestion of eggs in contaminated soil, water, and food. Ingested eggs hatch into larvae in the small intestines and translocate into the portal vasculature or lymphatics. After dissemination to the lungs, larvae migrate into alveoli, ascend the tracheobronchial tree, and are ingested. Adult worms develop within the small intestine (**Fig. 2**).

Clinical manifestations Pulmonary ascariasis is more prominent in children.[30] It occurs within 4 to 16 days of infection during the acute migratory phase and self-resolves over weeks. Transpulmonary migration of larvae causes a Loeffler syndrome, manifesting with fever, wheezing, cough, dyspnea, chest pain, hemoptysis, rash, and peripheral hypereosinophilia.[31,32] Chest imaging shows migratory bilateral nodular infiltrates. Although pulmonary disease is not typically seen in chronic ascariasis, young children with high worm burden can develop severe intestinal disease from mechanical obstruction.[33]

Management Individuals diagnosed with ascariasis can be treated with oral benzimidazoles (metronidazole, albendazole), although efficacy during acute migration is unknown. Ivermectin can also be used, but data in children weighing less than 15 kg are limited.

Hookworm

Human hookworm infection is caused by 2 species, *Necator americanus* and *Ancylostoma duodenale*. Chronic hookworm infection is a major cause of pediatric anemia worldwide.[34] Transmission occurs when infective larvae enter the body through skin penetration or ingestion (*A duodenale* only). Larvae migrate into the circulatory system and travel to the lungs, where they cross into alveoli and ascend the respiratory tract until coughed up and swallowed. Adult worms develop within the small intestines, where they attach to the mucosa and cause chronic blood loss.

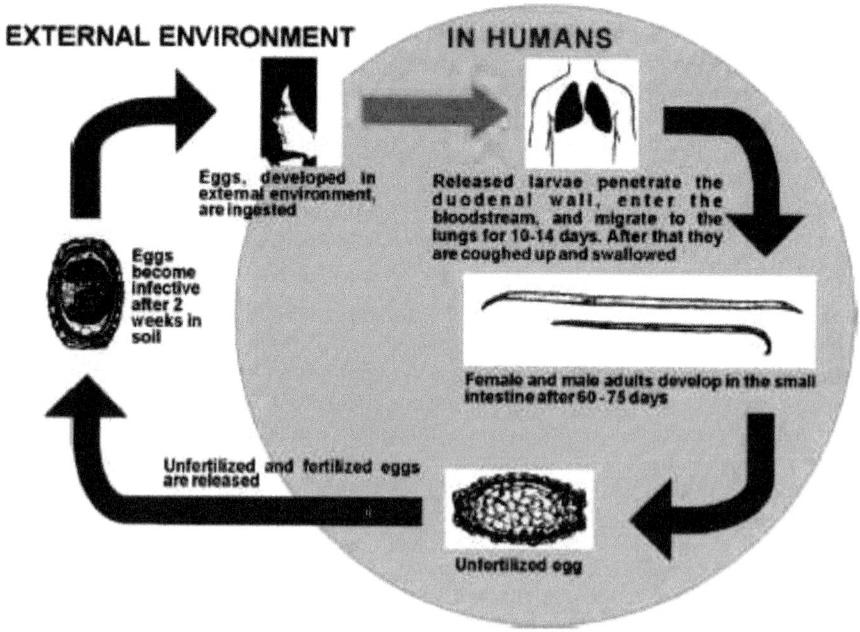

Fig. 2. Life cycle of *Ascaris lumbricoides*. (*From* Martinez S. et al. Thoracic manifestations of tropical parasitic diseases: A pictorial review. Radiographics 2005;25:135-55; with permission.)

Clinical manifestations Individuals with low burden of infection are frequently asymptomatic. During the initial stages of infection, a pruritic, serpiginous rash, or "ground itch" can develop at sites of entry.[18] Transpulmonary migration of larvae causes a Loeffler syndrome, typically less severe than ascariasis.[2] Transient diffuse lung infiltrates are seen on chest imaging.[2]

Management A single dose of albendazole is generally effective, but treatment failure is observed when disease burden is high.[31]

Strongyloidiasis

Strongyloides stercoralis is a soil-transmitted nematode that can persist in humans for years after exposure by means of autoinfection. Primary infection occurs when infective larvae (filariform) enter circulation through direct contact with skin or ingestion of contaminated food or water. Filariform larvae migrate through tissue to reach the venous system. They travel to pulmonary vasculature and cross into alveoli, eventually ascending the respiratory tract to be coughed up and swallowed. Adult worms develop within the small intestine. They release eggs that hatch into noninfective larvae (rhabditiform) that are excreted in stool. Alternatively, molting into infective larvae can occur within the intestinal tract, resulting in autoinfection. Impaired cell-mediated immune function (eg, corticosteroid use) allows for increased cycles of autoinfection, resulting in massive extraintestinal dissemination of filariform larvae.[35] This hyperinfection syndrome is a significant cause of morbidity and mortality in individuals with immunosuppression, malnutrition, and coinfection with human T-cell lymphotropic virus type I.

Clinical manifestations Clinical manifestations of strongyloidiasis depends on stage of infection, disease burden, and underlying host immune status. Although chronic strongyloidiasis is typically subclinical, in children, it can cause a malabsorption syndrome and is associated with poorly controlled asthma. During primary infection, some patients develop a mild Loeffler syndrome that self-resolves over weeks.[36] Cough, sore throat, dyspnea, wheezing, chest pain, and hemoptysis may occur as larvae travel through the respiratory tract. Transpulmonary migration during hyperinfection syndrome causes alveolar hemorrhage, ARDS, pleural effusion, and secondary bacterial infections such as pneumonia, empyema, and lung abscess. During hyperinfection, translocation of enteric flora can cause gram-negative or polymicrobial sepsis. Detection of larvae in extraintestinal sites supports a diagnosis of hyperinfection. Chest imaging can show migratory pulmonary infiltrates, miliary nodules, pleural effusions, and consolidation.[37]

Management Strongyloidiasis should be treated due to the risk of hyperinfection syndrome. Before immunosuppression, people who have traveled to endemic regions should be screened for subclinical disease. Weight-based ivermectin is the drug of choice. A single dose eradicates uncomplicated disease in 86% of cases.[38] Multiple doses may be considered in individuals with higher disease burden or risk for hyperinfection. In hyperinfection syndrome, some experts advocate for prolonged ivermectin therapy with or without albendazole for several weeks. Decrease in antibody titers at 6 months suggests cure.[39]

Toxocariasis

Toxocariasis occurs through accidental infection of humans with *Toxocara canis* (dog roundworm) or *Toxocara cati* (cat roundworm). Young children are commonly exposed to infectious eggs when playing in sandboxes and playgrounds contaminated by animal feces.

Toxocara eggs can remain infective in the environment for months to years. Humans become infected after ingesting infectious eggs. Within the small intestine, eggs hatch into larvae that migrate through villi to reach circulation. Visceral dissemination occurs over several months. Pathogenesis is driven by the host immune response to migration and death of larvae.

Clinical manifestations Human toxocariasis is typically subclinical but can manifest as 3 clinical syndromes: ocular larva migrans, covert toxocariasis, and visceral larva migrans (VLM).[40] Covert toxocariasis without visceral or ocular involvement has been linked to childhood asthma, chronic lung disease, and developmental delay. VLM, the most severe form of human toxocariasis, presents in preschool children and is caused by the multisystemic migration of larvae.[41] Classically, patients have fever, hepatomegaly, and hypereosinophilia (up to 80%). Pulmonary manifestations, such as pneumonitis, occur in 20% to 80% of children.[32] Symptoms include dry cough, wheezing, dyspnea, crackles, and rhonchi.[42] Although fulminant disease is uncommon, recovery from VLM is protracted and can take 1 to 2 years.[43] Chest imaging can show ground-glass opacities (most common), solid nodules, consolidations, and linear opacities.[44]

Management VLM is typically self-resolving. Supportive care with antiinflammatory agents can temper the host immune response and hypereosinophilia. The role of antihelminth therapy (eg, albendazole, mebendazole) is unclear, and paradoxic worsening with treatment is possible.[42]

TROPICAL PULMONARY EOSINOPHILIA

Tropical pulmonary eosinophilia (TPE) is a clinical syndrome associated with lymphatic filariasis (*Brugia malayi, Wuchereria bancrofti, Brugia timori*). It is caused by a robust host immune response to microfilariae trapped in the lungs.[45] TPE is rare in children.

Clinical manifestations include fever, cough, nocturnal asthma, weight loss, lymphadenopathy, and diffuse migratory pulmonary nodules. Diagnosis is supported by elevated antifilarial antibodies in the setting of hypereosinophilia (>3000/mL). Diethylcarbamazine, which is active against adult worms and microfilariae, is the treatment of choice. Untreated TPE can progress to interstitial pulmonary fibrosis and irreversible restrictive lung disease.[2]

Trematodes

Paragonimiasis

There are more than 20 million cases of paragonimiasis (lung fluke disease) worldwide. *Paragonimus westermani* is responsible for most cases. Other important species include *Paragonimus mexicanus, Paragonimus africanus, Paragonimus heterotremus, Paragonimus skrjabini,* and *Paragonimus kellicotti. P westermani* life cycle is complex and involves 2 intermediate hosts. Humans are infected through ingestion of raw or undercooked crab or crayfish. Parasites excyst in the duodenal lumen, cross into the peritoneal cavity, and traverse the diaphragm to reach the lungs. Seeding of extrapulmonary sites during migration can occur. Within the lungs, parasites burrow into small airways and mature into adult worms. Several weeks later, eggs are released into the airway and expectorated. Some are swallowed and passed in stool.

Clinical manifestations Paragonimiasis classically manifests as pleuropulmonary disease.

During the early migratory phase, patients are typically asymptomatic. Migration across the pleura and lungs can cause a mild Loeffler syndrome with pleural effusion. Symptoms include fever, pleuritic chest pain, cough, dyspnea, malaise, and night sweats.[46] Bronchitis or bronchiectasis are features of chronic disease. Cough can be dry or productive of mucoid, rust-colored, or blood tinged sputum. Episodic hemoptysis may occur. Destructive inflammation and secondary bacterial infections may lead to bronchopneumonia, lung abscess, empyema, pneumothorax, pleural adhesions, pulmonary fibrosis, and alveolar hemorrhage.[47,48] Chest imaging may be normal in early infection.[20] Pleural effusion and pneumothorax can be seen during pleural migration. Parenchymal invasion causes patchy airspace consolidation that may cavitate over time. After resolution of consolidation, a “ring shadow” may appear as a crescent-shaped opacity along the inner cyst border.[32] This is representative of the adult worm.

Management Praziquantel is the treatment of choice.

Schistosomiasis

Schistosomiasis is mainly caused by 3 trematode species: *Schistosoma mansoni, Schistosoma japonicum,* and *Schistosoma haematobium.* Freshwater snails harbor and release cercariae that infect humans through contact with skin and hematogenously circulate until reaching their target venous plexus.

Clinical manifestations Acute schistosomiasis (Katayama fever) is a self-limited disease that begins 2 to 12 weeks after exposure.[2] Patients may develop high fever, cough, dyspnea, abdominal pain, diarrhea, rash, arthralgias, hepatosplenomegaly, lymphadenopathy, pneumonitis, and eosinophilia. Transpulmonary parasite migration can cause severe larval pneumonitis in children. Chest imaging reveals diffuse pulmonary nodules with miliary features. Chronic schistosomiasis involving the mesenteric plexus (*S. mansoni* or *S japonicum*) can lead to advanced hepatosplenic disease and portal hypertension. This results in diversion of eggs into the pulmonary circulation. Patients can develop localized granulomas, obliterative arteritis, pulmonary hypertension, pulmonary arteriovenous fistulae, and cor pulmonale.[20] Clinical features include dyspnea, exercise intolerance, hypoxemia, and clubbing. Peripheral eosinophilia is common during acute infection.

Management Treatment of choice is praziquantel, with adjunctive corticosteroids in severe pneumonitis or Katayama fever.[24]

SUMMARY AND FUTURE DIRECTIONS

Parasitic infections account for significant childhood morbidity and disproportionately affect children in low- and middle-income countries. Pulmonary manifestations occur on a spectrum of disease, ranging from transient and self-limited syndromes to chronic and serious lung pathology. Early diagnosis and treatment can prevent long-term pulmonary sequelae. Although major advancements have been made in human parasitology in recent years, several high-priority areas for research and intervention remain: (1) development of rapid (point-of-care), accurate, and low-cost diagnostic tests and validated clinical algorithms; (2) elimination of soil-transmitted helminths (ascariasis, trichuriasis, hookworm) and other neglected tropical diseases through expansion and implementation of mass drug administration programs among preschool and school-age children in endemic areas; (3) development of effective and safe treatment options for strongyloidiasis in young children; (4) prevention of transmission and reinfection through investment in public health educational campaigns and infrastructure (provision of adequate sanitation and hygiene); (5) development of vaccines against the most prevalent parasitic infections.

CLINICAL CARE POINTS

- Parasitic infections may mimic common lung diseases such as tuberculosis (eg, Paragonimus), asthma (eg, Ascaris) and malignancy (e.g. Dirofilaria), as they share similar clinical and radiological features.
- Loeffler syndrome, which is associated with several helminths (Ascaris, hookworms, strongyloides, etc), manifests with fever, wheezing, cough, dyspnea, chest pain, hemoptysis, rash, and peripheral hypereosinophilia.
- Corticosteroid use and human T-cell lymphotropic virus type (HTLV-I) infection may result in increased cycles of Strongyloides autoinfection, resulting in massive extraintestinal dissemination of larvae (hyperinfection syndrome).
- Before immunosuppression, people who have lived or traveled to endemic regions should be screened for Strongyloidiasis due to the risk of hyperinfection syndrome. Ivermectin is the drug of choice for treatment.
- Surgical excision remains the treatment of choice for pulmonary echinococcosis.
- Tropical pulmonary eosinophilia is a clinical syndrome associated with lymphatic filariasis characterized by fever, cough, wheezing, weight loss, lymphadenopathy, and diffuse migratory pulmonary nodules.

DISCLOSURE

The authors have nothing to disclose.

REFERENCES

1. Zumla AI, James DG. Immunologic aspects of tropical lung disease. Clin Chest Med 2002;23(2):283-287.

2. Kunst H, Mack D, Kon OM, et al. Parasitic infections of the lung: a guide for the respiratory physician. Thorax 2011;66(6):528–36.
3. Petropoulos AS, Chatzoulis GA. Echinococcus granulosus in childhood: a retrospective study of 187 cases and newer data. Clin Pediatr (Phila) 2019;58(8): 864–88.
4. Shamsuzzaman SM, Hashiguchi Y. Thoracic amebiasis. Clin Chest Med 2002;23: 479–92.
5. Gong Z, Miao R, Shu M, et al. Paragonimiasis in Children in Southwest China: A retrospective case reports review from 2005 to 2016. Medicine (Baltimore) 2017; 96(25):e7265.
6. Li L, Gao W, Yang X, et al. Asthma and toxocariasis. Ann Allergy Asthma Immunol 2014;113(2):187–92.
7. Momen T, Esmaeil N, Reisi M. Seroprevalence of toxocara canis in asthmatic children and its relation to the severity of diseases - a case-control study. Med Arch 2018;72(3):174–7.
8. Pereira A dos S, Marques AG, Doi AM, et al. Challenge in the diagnosis of pulmonary strongyloidiasis. Einstein 2019;17(1):eAI4441.
9. Nabeya D, Haranaga S, Parrott GL, et al. Pulmonary strongyloidiasis: assessment between manifestation and radiological findings in 16 severe strongyloidiasis cases. BMC Infect Dis 2017;17(1):320.
10. Ross AG, Bartley PB, Sleigh AC, et al. Schistosomiasis. N Engl J Med 2002; 346(16):1212–20.
11. Verjee MA. Schistosomiasis: still a cause of significant morbidity and mortality. Res Rep Trop Med 2019;10:153–63.
12. Schwartz E, Rozenman J, Perelman M. Pulmonary manifestations of early schistosome infection among nonimmune travelers. Am J Med 2000;109(9):718–22.
13. World Health Organization. World malaria report. 2019. Available at: https://www.who.int/publications-detail/world-malaria-report-2019. Accessed March 18, 2020.
14. Taylor WR, White NJ. Malaria and the lung. Clin Chest Med 2002;23(2):457–68.
15. Taylor WRJ, Hanson J, Turner GDH, et al. Respiratory manifestations of malaria. Chest 2012;142(2):492–505.
16. Cohee LM, Laufer MK. Malaria in Children. Pediatr Clin North Am 2017;64(4): 851–66.
17. Centers for Disease Control and Prevention. Treatment of malaria: guidelines for clinicians (United States) 2019. Available at: https://www.cdc.gov/malaria/diagnosis_treatment/clinicians1.html.
18. Alter SJ, Turcios NL. Pulmonary manifestations of parasitic diseases. In: Turcios NL, Fink RJ, editors. Pulmonary manifestations of pediatric diseases. 1st edition. Philadelphia: Saunders Elsevier; 2009. p. 274–93.
19. Stanley SL. Amoebiasis. Lancet 2003;361:1025–34.
20. Martínez S, Restrepo CS, Carrillo JA, et al. Thoracic manifestations of tropical parasitic infections: a pictorial review. Radiographics 2005;25(1):135–55.
21. McAuley JB. Congenital Toxoplasmosis. J Pediatr Infect Dis Soc 2014;3(Suppl 1): S30–5.
22. Leal FE, Cavazzana CL, de Andrade HF Jr, et al. Toxoplasma gondii pneumonia in immunocompetent subjects: case report and review. Clin Infect Dis 2007;44(6): e62–6.
23. Demar M, Hommel D, Djossou F, et al. Acute toxoplasmoses in immunocompetent patients hospitalized in an intensive care unit in French Guiana. Clin Microbiol Infect 2012;18(7):E221–31.

24. Cheepsattayakorn A, Cheepsattayakorn R. Parasitic pneumonia and lung involvement. Biomed Res Int 2014;2014:874021.
25. Pomeroy C, Filice GA. Pulmonary toxoplasmosis: a review. Clin Infect Dis 1992; 14(4):863–70.
26. Serpa JA, Cabada MM, White C Jr. Cestodes. In: Cherry JD, Harrison GJ, Kaplan SL, et al, editors. Feigin and Cherry's textbook of pediatric infectious diseases. 8th edition. Philadelphia: Saunders Elsevier; 2018. p. 2242–54.
27. Morar R, Feldman C. Pulmonary echinococcosis. Eur Respir J 2003;21(6): 1069–77.
28. Sarkar M, Pathania R, Jhobta A, et al. Cystic pulmonary hydatidosis. Lung India 2016;33(2):179–91.
29. Hawlader MD, Ma E, Noguchi E, et al. Ascaris lumbricoids Infection as a Risk Factor for Asthma and Atopy in Rural Bangladeshi Children. Trop Med Health 2014;42(2):77–85.
30. Khuroo MS. Ascariasis. Gastroenterol Clin North Am 1996;25(3):553–77.
31. Mejia R, Weatherhead J, Hotez PJ. Intestinal nematodes (roundworms). In: Bennett JE, Dolin R, Blaser MJ, editors. Mandell, Douglas, and Bennett's principles and practices of infectious diseases. 9th edition. Philadelphia: Elsevier Churchill Livingstone; 2019. p. 774–83.
32. Chitkara RK, Krishna G. Parasitic pulmonary eosinophilia. Semin Respir Crit Care Med 2006;27(2):171–84.
33. Jourdan PM, Lamberton PHL, Fenwick A, et al. Soil-transmitted helminth infections. Lancet 2018;391(10117):252–65.
34. Hotez PJ, Brooker S, Bethony JM, et al. Hookworm infection. N Engl J Med 2004; 351(8):799–807.
35. Keiser PB, Nutman TB. Strongyloides stercoralis in the Immunocompromised Population. Clin Microbiol Rev 2004;17(1):208–17.
36. Mokhlesi B, Shulzhenko O, Garimella PS, et al. Pulmonary strongyloidiasis: the varied clinical presentations. Clin Pulm Med 2004;11(1):6–13.
37. Kuzucu A. Parasitic diseases of the respiratory tract. Curr Opin Pulm Med 2006; 12(3):212–21.
38. Buonfrate D, Salas-Coronas J, Muñoz J, et al. Multiple-dose versus single-dose ivermectin for Strongyloides stercoralis infection (Strong Treat 1 to 4): a multicentre, open-label, phase 3, randomised controlled superiority trial. Lancet Infect Dis 2019;19(11):1181–90.
39. Salvador F, Sulleiro E, Sánchez-Montalvá A, et al. Usefulness of Strongyloides stercoralis serology in the management of patients with eosinophilia. Am J Trop Med Hyg 2014;90(5):830–4.
40. Lee RM, Moore LB, Bottazzi ME, et al. Toxocariasis in North America: a systematic review. PLoS Negl Trop Dis 2014;8(8):e3116.
41. Despommier D. Toxocariasis: clinical aspects, epidemiology, medical ecology, and molecular aspects. Clin Microbiol Rev 2003;16(2):265–72.
42. Ranasuriya G, Mian A, Boujaoude Z, et al. Pulmonary toxocariasis: a case report and literature review. Infection 2014;42(3):575–8.
43. Hotez PJ. Parasitic Nematode Infections. In: Cherry JD, Harrison GJ, Kaplan SL, et al, editors. Feigin and Cherry's textbook of pediatric infectious diseases. 8th edition. Philadelphia: Saunders Elsevier; 2018. p. 2229–40.
44. Lee KH, Kim TJ, Lee KW. Pulmonary toxocariasis: initial and follow-up CT findings in 63 patients. AJR Am J Roentgenol 2015;204(6):1203–11.
45. Vijayan VK. Tropical pulmonary eosinophilia: pathogenesis, diagnosis and management. Curr Opin Pulm Med 2007;13(5):428–33.

46. Keiser J, Utzinger J. Food-borne trematodiases. Clin Microbiol Rev 2009;22(3): 466–83.
47. Zarrin-Khameh N, Citron DR, Stager CE, et al. Pulmonary paragonimiasis diagnosed by fine-needle aspiration biopsy. J Clin Microbiol 2008;46(6):2137–40.
48. Yoshida A, Doanh PN, Maruyama H. Paragonimus and paragonimiasis in Asia: an update. Acta Trop 2019;199:105074.

Pulmonary Manifestations of Renal Disorders in Children

Laura Malaga-Dieguez, MD, PhD[a,*], Howard Trachtman, MD[a],
Robert Giusti, MD[b]

KEYWORDS

- Congenital abnormalities of the kidney and urinary tract • Oligohydramnios
- Pulmonary hypoplasia • Urinothorax • Acute kidney injury • Nephrotic syndrome
- Acute glomerulonephritis • Renal replacement therapies

KEY POINTS

- Kidney disease in children resulting from congenital abnormalities of the kidney and urinary tract (CAKUT) may have a significant impact on lung development and are associated with pulmonary hypoplasia.
- The most common pulmonary manifestations of kidney disease in children are related to fluid overload.
- Fluid leaks and accumulation in the pleural space are important complications of renal replacement in children.
- Sleep disorders are frequent complications in children with chronic kidney disease.
- Collaboration among pediatric nephrologists, pulmonologists, and intensivists is key to manage complications related to kidney disease treatment including dialysis and transplantation.

OVERVIEW AND CLINICAL ASSESSMENT

The causes of kidney disease in pediatric patients are evenly divided between congenital abnormalities of the kidney and urinary tract (CAKUT) and acquired disorders. It is estimated that nearly 10% to 15% of adults in the United States have chronic kidney disease (CKD). There are no comparable data about the prevalence of CKD in children. Regardless of the age of the patient, CKD is a systemic problem that affects every organ system in the body including the lung. In the following sections, we review

[a] Division of Pediatric Nephrology, Department of Pediatrics, NYU School of Medicine, Hassenfeld Children's Hospital at NYU Langone, 550 First Avenue, New York, NY 10016, USA; [b] Division of Pediatric Pulmonology, Department of Pediatrics, NYU School of Medicine, Hassenfeld Children's Hospital at NYU Langone, 550 First Avenue, New York, NY 10016, USA
* Corresponding author. 403 E 34th Street, Suite 104, New York, NY 10016.
E-mail address: laura.malaga-dieguez@nyulangone.org

Pediatr Clin N Am 68 (2021) 209–222
https://doi.org/10.1016/j.pcl.2020.09.008 pediatric.theclinics.com

the diagnostic tests used to evaluate kidney disease and the main clinical syndromes that are likely to be encountered to aid the pulmonology consultant who is asked to assess these patients.

DIAGNOSTIC TESTS

Urinalysis

This is an accessible and low cost screening test that may be used to identify patients with renal disease or to monitor severity in children with known kidney disease.[1] The most common elements of dipstick testing include specific gravity, pH, blood, protein, leukocytes, and nitrites. There is *no* normal specific gravity and urinary concentration should be evaluated in clinical context based on the expected response to the state of hydration. Urinary pH varies depending on dietary protein intake. In patients with lung disease and chronic respiratory acidosis or respiratory alkalosis, urine pH will reflect primary change in P_{CO_2} and adaptive renal responses. Children should have a *negative* dipstick result and at most 3 to 5 red blood cells or white blood cells per high power field in the urine. Hematuria may be glomerular or nonglomerular in origin and this distinction can only be made by microscopic examination of a spun urine sample. Red blood cell casts and dysmorphic erythrocytes indicate the presence of glomerular bleeding. Proteinuria is best assessed in a first morning urine specimen to exclude an orthostatic component. The normal value is <0.2 (mg:mg). Proteinuria may reflect glomerular or tubular injury. The amount of protein is usually greater and dominated by albuminuria in children with glomerular disease. Leukocyturia is indicative of inflammation and may be seen in patients with glomerular disease, interstitial nephritis, or urinary tract infection. The latter requires a urine culture for confirmation and a positive nitrite is supportive but not diagnostic.

Blood Pressure

High blood pressure (BP) is an important feature in pediatric patients with kidney disease, particularly in those with glomerular disease.[2] Although blood pressure is usually measured using auscultatory methods, oscillometric devices are being more widely incorporated into clinical practice. They facilitate the measurement of BP in very young children. Normal values for BP vary with age, gender, and height. Normative levels were updated in 2017 and this resource should be referenced when determining if BP is abnormal.[3] More sophisticated method to assess BP including ambulatory BP monitors are available for use in the outpatient setting and provide insight in patients with pulmonary disease or sleep disorders.

Glomerular Filtration Rate

In clinical practice, the serum concentration of creatinine is used as an index of kidney function. There are formulas that enable estimation of glomerular filtration rate (GFR) based on the patient's height and serum creatinine. The bedside version, estimated GFR (eGFR) (mL/min/1.73 m^2) = 0.413 $\times$ height (cm)/serum creatinine (mg/dL), is the most widely used version in the United States.[4] Because serum creatinine is influenced by diet and muscle mass, alternative markers of GFR are available including cystatin C. The use of cystatin C may be relevant in patients with cystic fibrosis.[5] Precise measurements of GFR using radionuclide agents are reserved for patients in whom treatment such as administration of potentially nephrotoxic drugs or agents that are cleared by the kidney is dependent on a precise measurement of GFR.

Imaging Studies

Radiographic testing is a valuable component in the assessment of children with CAKUT. This includes ultrasound, computed tomography (CT), and MRI. Voiding cystourethrograms with contrast or radionuclide agents may be performed in children with hydronephrosis and/or urinary tract infections. The use of contrast agents, both iodinated compounds for CT scans and gadolinium for MRIs, should be carefully considered in children with intrinsic kidney disease.

CLINICAL SYNDROMES

Hypertension

Hypertension may be a primary disorder or may be secondary to systemic disorders including sleep apnea syndrome. The diagnosis is established by standardized measurement of BP. In acute clinical circumstances, a single determination is sufficient, whereas in other situations repeat measurements are generally required.

Acute Kidney Injury

Acute kidney injury (AKI) reflects a sudden decrease in GFR. It arises secondary to injury to the glomeruli (acute glomerulonephritis [AGN], see later in this article), injury to the tubulointerstitium, or obstruction to urine outflow.[6] Tubular injury occurs secondary to ischemia or direct damage to the tubular epithelium. Ischemia may arise due to volume contraction, cardiac failure, sepsis, anaphylaxis, or third spacing. Toxic nephropathy may be secondary to drugs, biologicals, or diagnostic agents. Tubular interstitial inflammation may occur in response to medication or infection. There are novel biomarkers such as neutrophil gelatinase-associated lipocalin that are more sensitive to detect tubular injury and may be elevated in the absence of a decline in GFR and rise in serum creatinine concentration. Obstructive uropathy may reflect a congenital anomaly or complication of a medical or surgical procedure. Children with AKI are generally very ill and require hospitalization in an intensive care unit. They may have oliguria, hypertension, and electrolyte abnormalities. There are no corrective therapies and management is supportive. Renal replacement therapy is reserved for patients who cannot be stabilized with medical therapy.

Nephrotic Syndrome

Nephrotic syndrome (NS) is characterized by heavy proteinuria (urine protein:creatinine ratio >2 mg:mg), hypoalbuminemia, hypercholesterolemia, and edema. The GFR is usually normal. NS represents a hypercoagulable state and is associated with an increased risk of thromboembolic complications including pulmonary embolism.[7] The risk of these complications is considerably lower in pediatric versus adult patients with NS. NS is divided into primary and secondary causes. A kidney biopsy is reserved for clinically complex cases or patients who fail to respond as expected to standard therapy.

Acute Glomerulonephritis

AGN represents AKI caused by glomerular disorders. It usually presents with gross hematuria and some combination of hypertension, proteinuria, and edema. The diagnosis is confirmed by the presence of red blood cell casts in the urine.[8] This condition has several causes that may be distinguished based on the clinical history, physical examination, and laboratory testing. A kidney biopsy may be necessary to establish the diagnosis and clarify prognosis. Available treatments include corticosteroids, cyclophosphamide, mycophenolate mofetil, rituximab, and plasmapheresis. As in tubular causes of AKI, renal replacement therapy is implemented when conservative medical management fails to stabilize a child.

Syndrome of Inappropriate Antidiuretic Hormone

Under normal conditions, the kidney excretes free water and a dilute urine whenever the serum sodium concentration and osmolality fall below the normal range. In the presence of intravascular volume contraction, the kidney will respond appropriately and retain sodium and water in an effort to restore volume. It prioritizes volume over osmolality and hypo-osmolality may ensue. The diagnosis of syndrome of inappropriate antidiuretic hormone (SIADH) is made in the context of hyponatremia in conjunction with inappropriately concentrated urine in the absence of volume depletion, and thyroid or adrenal insufficiency. Laboratory validation is established by confirming hyponatremia in combination with a urine that is not maximally dilute, a urine sodium concentration greater than 40 mmol/L to exclude intravascular volume contraction, and normal adrenal and thyroid function.[9] SIADH occurs secondary to nonosmotic stimuli to antidiuretic hormone release, including pain, nausea, vomiting, certain medications, and central nervous system disease. It may also occur with pulmonary diseases. The use of the term SIADH in children with pneumonia or other lung diseases who have hyponatremia and a concentrated urine is *not* fully accurate. The pulmonary process may alter the intrathoracic pressure and impair venous return leading to a state of perceived intravascular volume contraction and an "appropriate" renal response. Nonetheless, the term SIADH is used to explain the occurrence of hyponatremia in patients with pulmonary disease. Treatment should focus on the primary lung disease together with restriction of free water.

CONGENITAL ABNORMALITIES OF THE KIDNEY AND URINARY TRACT: OLIGOHYDRAMNIOS, PULMONARY HYPOPLASIA, AND URINOTHORAX

Oligohydramnios and Pulmonary Hypoplasia

CAKUTs are one of the leading anatomic defects to be identified on prenatal ultrasound. CAKUT signifies a broad spectrum of abnormalities, ranging from transient hydronephrosis to bilateral renal agenesis. When kidney function in fetuses with CAKUT is severely affected, urine production is reduced leading to oligohydramnios and impaired lung development.

Lung growth is influenced by physical factors such as the intrauterine space, lung liquid volume and pressure, and fetal breathing movements. During lung development, the main physical force experienced by the lungs is stretching induced by breathing movements and the lung fluid in the airspaces. Physical forces are crucial for regulating fetal lung growth and maturation.[10] The fetus also exhibits episodic fetal breathing movements, which contribute to normal lung development. Lung growth may be compromised by compression of the chest cavity coupled with decreased inspiration of amniotic fluid. The distending pressure created by lung fluid within the airways is the primary physical force stimulating lung development. This highlights the importance of the amniotic fluid in normal lung growth and development.

Amniotic fluid is produced from maternal plasma and secreted from the fetal membranes. Fetal urine contributes to the amniotic fluid as soon as the fetal kidneys start to function and becomes a major contributor to amniotic fluid, at approximately 20 weeks, with production of 300 mL/kg fetal weight per day. Oligohydramnios, defined as less than 500 mL of amniotic fluid, is most often associated with the severest forms of CAKUT, such as posterior urethral valves (PUVs) or bilateral renal agenesis. Oligohydramnios reduces the intrathoracic cavity size, thus disrupting fetal lung growth and leading to pulmonary hypoplasia. Pulmonary hypoplasia, which is induced by maternal oligohydramnios, is associated with decreased lung function in infants. Neonates exposed to oligohydramnios caused by the premature rupture of the amniotic membranes also have an increased risk of acute respiratory morbidity such as pulmonary hypertension and air leaks.

Pulmonary hypoplasia is a substantial cause of death in newborn infants. It also leads to increased risk of pneumothorax after birth. The Potter phenotype develops as a result of severe oligohydramnios. It is therefore associated with high-grade obstruction of the urinary tract, bilateral renal agenesis or severe bilateral renal hypoplasia (see the Beth A. Pletcher and Nelson L. Turcios' article, "Pulmonary Manifestations of Genetic Disorders in Children," elsewhere in this issue). Decreased fetal movement as a result of oligohydramnios and intrauterine constraint of movement causes multiple joint contractures (arthrogryposis) and limb deformities such as talipes equinovarus (club feet). Bilateral renal agenesis is a relatively rare congenital defect and is invariably associated with Potter's sequence, a condition incompatible with life and neonates die shortly after birth.

Urinothorax

This term describes the presence of urine collection in the pleural space, which is a complication of severe forms of CAKUT and obstructive uropathy.[11] It is considered a rare form of pleural effusion, it occurs by the accumulation of urine in the pleural space because of a trauma or blockage of the urinary tract. Urinothorax has been reported secondary to PUVs, nephrolithiasis, blunt renal trauma, ureteral instrumentation, or ureteral surgery. Leakage from the urinary tract may cause a urine collection in the abdominal cavity or retroperitoneal space (urinoma), but the exact mechanism of urine transit from the abdomen into the pleural space has yet to be fully elucidated. The urine may either ascend directly through anatomic defects of the diaphragm, or through diaphragmatic lymphatics due to increased retroperitoneal or intraperitoneal pressure caused by the urinoma.[12]

The diagnosis of urinothorax is based on demonstrating a pleural effusion associated with obstructive or traumatic uropathy. The pleural fluid in urinothorax is a transudate, although the lactic dehydrogenase (LDH) level may be high, causing misclassification as an exudate.

ACUTE KIDNEY INJURY

AKI is commonly found in clinical practice, and it occurs in up to 25% of children and adolescents in the pediatric intensive care unit (ICU) during the first week after ICU admission.

Pediatric AKI presents with a wide spectrum of clinical manifestations ranging from a minimal elevation in serum creatinine to complete anuria. AKI in pediatric patients is classified using the criteria of the pediatric risk, injury, failure, loss and end-stage renal disease (pRIFLE) classification system[13] or the Acute Kidney Injury Network (AKIN) criteria.[14] The pRIFLE staging system stratifies AKI based on urine output and changes in estimated creatinine clearance (eCCl) rather than the absolute serum creatinine (SCr) level (**Table 1**), while the AKIN staging system relies on the absolute SCr concentration. The Kidney Disease Improving Global Outcomes (KDIGO) consortium has put forth modifications to reconcile subtle differences in the adult AKIN and RIFLE criteria[15] (**Table 2**).

Table 1
Pediatric-modified RIFLE criteria and neonatal RIFLE criteria

		Urine Output	
	Estimated CCl	**pRIFLE**	**nRIFLE**
Risk	eCCl decrease by 25%	<0.5 mL/kg/h for 8 h	<1.5 mL/kg/h for 24 h
Injury	eCCl decrease by 50%	<0.5 mL/kg/h for 16 h	<1 mL/kg/h for 24 h
Failure	eCCl decrease by 75% or eCCl <35 mL/min/1.73 m^2	<0.3 mL/kg/h for 24 h or anuria for 12 h	<0.7 mL/kg/ h for 24 h or anuria for 12 h
Loss	Persistent failure >4 wk		
End Stage	Persistent failure >3 mo		

Abbreviations: eCCl, estimated creatinine clearance; nRIFLE, neonatal risk, injury, failure, loss and end-stage renal disease; pRIFLE, pediatric risk, injury, failure, loss and end-stage renal disease.

Data from Akcan-Arikan A, Zappitelli M, Loftis LL, Washburn KK, Jefferson LS, Goldstein SL. Modified RIFLE criteria in critically ill children with acute kidney injury. Kidney international. 2007;71(10):1028-1035 and Ricci Z, Ronco C. Neonatal RIFLE. Nephrology, dialysis, transplantation : official publication of the European Dialysis and Transplant Association - European Renal Association. 2013;28(9):2211-2214.

Although there have been efforts to develop a *neonatal* RIFLE score,[16] the prevailing trend is to use the AKIN criteria based on the changes in eGFR to categorize the severity of AKI.

The most common causes of AKI are volume depletion, infection, and primary renal diseases such as glomerulonephritis and hemolytic uremic syndrome. In hospitalized children, nephrotoxicity is also a frequent etiology with aminoglycoside (AG) and other antibiotics, antifungal agents, diuretics, angiotensin-converting enzyme inhibitors, and nonsteroidal anti-inflammatory drugs being common offending drugs.

Patients with cystic fibrosis (CF) are often treated with multiple courses of AG antibiotics. AKI may develop in up to 30% of noncritically ill children receiving ≥5 consecutive days of an AG medication. The kidney injury during treatment with AG is the result of a direct effect on the renal proximal tubule epithelial cells. Because patients with CF have an accelerated renal clearance and altered pharmacokinetics for AG,[17] high doses of the antibiotics need to be administered to achieve therapeutic concentrations. The kidney injury during treatment with AG antibiotics is the result of a direct

Table 2
Definition and staging of AKI according to the Kidney Disease Improving Global Outcomes modifications of the Acute Kidney Injury Network criteria

Stage	SCr	Urine Output
1	Increase in SCr ≥0.3 mg/dL for 48 h or increase 150%–200% (1.5-fold to 2-fold) from baseline	<0.5 mL/kg/h for 8 h
2	Increase in SCr ≥4 mg/dL or increase of ≥200%–300% from baseline	<0.5 mL/kg/h for 16 h
3	Increase ≥300%, serum creatinine ≥4 mg/dL or dialysis or eCCl <35 mL/min/1.73 m^2 for those <18 year old	<0.3 mL/kg/h for 24 h or anuria for 12 h

Abbreviations: AKI, acute kidney injury; eCCl, estimated creatinine clearance; SCr, serum creatinine.

Data from KDIGO Clinical Practice Guideline for Acute Kidney Injury. Kidney international supplements. 2012;2(1):1-138.

effect on the renal proximal tubule epithelial cells. The proximal tubular damage and acute tubular necrosis result in electrolyte leak, a defect in the urinary concentrating capacity, and increased urinary excretion of tubular proteins and enzymes. Once daily dosing of tobramycin reduces drug accumulation and the risk of nephrotoxicity. Increasing the dosing interval reduces the basal serum AG level and the accumulation of the drug within the kidney, while allowing the high peak serum levels and post-antibiotic effect to potentiate bacterial killing[18] Because the toxicity of AG varies with renal clearance and is dose dependent, serum peak and trough levels should be closely monitored to confirm that levels are within therapeutic and nontoxic ranges.[19,20]

The clinical presentation of AKI varies with the cause and severity of the underlying renal injury, and associated diseases. Most children with mild to moderate AKI are often asymptomatic and are identified solely by laboratory testing. Children with severe cases may be symptomatic and present with respiratory symptoms such as dyspnea and pulmonary edema. Oliguria, anuria, or normal volumes of urine (nonoliguric AKI) are common presentations. Other manifestations of AKI include peripheral edema, listlessness, fatigue, anorexia, nausea, vomiting, and weight gain, development of uremic encephalopathy (expressed by a decline in mental status, asterixis, confusion, or other neurologic symptoms), anemia, or bleeding caused by platelet dysfunction.

The main complications of AKI include volume overload, electrolyte abnormalities including hyperkalemia, metabolic acidosis, hyperphosphatemia, hypocalcemia, and uremia.

Volume overload from AKI, even with preserved cardiac function, has the potential to cause hydrostatic (also known as "cardiogenic") pulmonary edema, sometimes severe enough to lead to respiratory failure. The fluid overload leads to increased pulmonary capillary hydrostatic pressure and transudative edema that responds rapidly to aggressive fluid removal by diuresis or ultrafiltration. However, it is important to keep into consideration that AKI may also induce inflammatory lung injury and nonhydrostatic ("noncardiogenic") pulmonary edema, caused by damage to the capillary membrane, leading to increased capillary permeability and leak of proteinaceous edema fluid. Fluid removal is not as effective for the latter type of pulmonary edema.[21]

The most important management principle for children and adolescents with AKI is prevention. However, once AKI is established, management is primarily supportive, with restoration of intravascular volume, vasopressor support as needed, careful management of fluid and electrolytes, provision of nutrition, avoidance of nephrotoxic drugs, dose adjustment of drugs excreted by the kidney, and timely imitation of renal replacement therapy when required.

NEPHROTIC SYNDROME AND THROMBOEMBOLISM

The hypercoagulable state in NS is multifactorial, attributed to urinary loss of anticoagulants, increased procoagulatory activity, altered fibrinolytic system, thrombocytosis, endothelial dysfunction, and enhanced platelet activation and aggregation.[22] Several other factors may also contribute to an increased risk of thromboembolic complications (TEC) in children with NS including hemoconcentration, increased cholesterol, associated infections, iatrogenic volume depletion due to inappropriate and overuse of diuretics, venipuncture, immobilization (especially in patients with anasarca), and the presence of central venous catheters.

Venous and arterial TEC are relatively infrequent in children compared with adults with NS, but they can cause significant morbidity. Both arterial and venous thromboses have been reported in children with NS, although venous thromboembolism is the predominate form of thromboembolic disease.[23] Deep venous thrombosis is by far the most common TEC.[24] Pulmonary embolism (PE) has been described in patients with NS with or without an evident deep venous thrombosis or renal vein thrombosis,[25] and along with peritonitis is a serious life-threatening complication in children with NS. Pleuritic chest pain, unexplained tachypnea, hypoxemia or persistent, severe cough should alert the physician toward this possibility. Children with PE may even present with sustained hypotension or shock. Signs and symptoms of PE may be subtle and require awareness and prompt recognition to prevent potentially fatal outcomes.

CT pulmonary angiography is the most accurate imaging modality, because it may directly demonstrate thrombi in the pulmonary arteries and branches.

PULMONARY MANIFESTATION OF ACUTE GLOMERULONEPHRITIS

Pulmonary-Renal Syndromes

These are clinical syndromes defined by a combination of diffuse alveolar hemorrhage and glomerulonephritis. Pulmonary-renal syndromes are caused by a distinct spectrum of immune-mediated diseases, including various forms of primary systemic vasculitis namely, granulomatosis with polyangiitis (formerly known as Wegener syndrome) and microscopic polyangiitis, Goodpasture syndrome associated with autoantibodies to the alveolar and glomerular basement membrane, immunoglobulin (Ig)A nephropathy/IgA vasculitis, and systemic lupus erythematosus. Of these disorders, IgA nephropathy (IgAN) is the most common cause of glomerulonephritis worldwide, and it is considered a kidney-limited disease. However, IgAN may present as a systemic vasculitis with a pulmonary-renal syndrome in which pulmonary hemorrhage is a critical feature.[26] These syndromes are covered in detail in the Mary M. Buckley and C. Egla Rabinovich's article, "Pulmonary Manifestations of Rheumatic Diseases in Children"; and Muserref Kasap Cuceoglu and Seza Ozen's article, "Pulmonary Manifestations of Systemic Vasculitis in Children," elsewhere in this issue.

Pulmonary Findings in Acute Glomerulonephritis

Segmental or lobar collapse, consolidation, pulmonary edema, and pleural effusions are some of the lesions encountered in AGN.[27] Fluid overload with pulmonary edema is the most common clinical complication of patients with acute glomerulonephritis. It might require aggressive diuresis or fluid removal with renal replacement therapy.

Diffuse alveolar hemorrhage resulting in hemoptysis is also an unusual clinical manifestation of acute post-streptococcal glomerulonephritis,[28] a common glomerular disease in children.

SLEEP DISORDERS AND KIDNEY DISEASE

This section reviews sleep disorders among patients with end-stage kidney disease (ESKD), including insomnia, excessive sleepiness, sleep apnea, and restless legs syndrome (RLS).

Sleep: General Considerations

An adequate amount and quality of sleep are essential for normal growth and development and overall health of children. Disturbed sleep may adversely affect a child's daytime function, resulting in behavioral and emotional problems as well as decline in daytime alertness and cognitive performance. There is consistent evidence of an increased prevalence of sleep disturbances in children with CKD, and these play a critical role in health-related quality of life (HRQOL). The prevalence of any sleep disorder has been reported in up to 85% in dialysis patients, 30% to 50% in transplanted patients, and 40% to 50% in nondialysis CKD patients.

Sleep disorders are common in patients with ESKD and tend to be underrecognized by health care providers. A systematic review of 17 studies in patients with ESKD indicated that "sleep disturbance" was one of their most common symptoms, with a mean prevalence of 44%.[29] Bedtime resistance, sleep-onset delay, daytime sleepiness, and parasomnia were more commonly reported in hemodialysis-dependent than non–dialysis-dependent children with CKD; both groups had higher scores than the control group. Children with CKD displayed more sleep anxiety and shorter sleep duration than healthy children, with no difference between hemodialysis and non–dialysis-dependent children with CKD.

The diurnal rhythm of melatonin is disturbed in patients with CKD and ESKD. Melatonin, a hormone secreted by the pineal gland, is responsible for the circadian sleep–wake rhythm. It is secreted in small quantities during daytime, but increases during the night, which correlates with the onset of nocturnal sleepiness. Nocturnal melatonin surges are lower in magnitude in patients with ESKD and there also appears to be a lack of circadian rhythm in melatonin secretion. Hemodialysis did not improve melatonin concentrations and there was no improvement following kidney transplantation.

Patients with ESKD have poor sleep architecture. They have short, fragmented sleep with a total sleep time between 260 to 360 minutes and rapid eye movement sleep is decreased. In addition to subjective sleep complaints, there is objective evidence of both sleep loss and sleep disruption among patients with ESKD. Polysomnographic studies have reported lower than normal total sleep time (4.4–6 hours per night), fragmented by a high frequency of arousals (up to 30 per hour), resulting in low sleep efficiency among patients with ESKD.[30]

Insomnia

The inability to fall asleep or stay asleep is characterized by poor sleep quality and poor QOL. Chronic pain is a common problem in patients on dialysis and may be a contributing factor for insomnia in this population. The treatment of insomnia is directed at optimizing renal replacement therapy, as well as using nonpharmacologic interventions such as instituting good sleep hygiene habits, promoting comfortable sleep environment, teaching relaxation modalities and/or a trial of behavioral therapy.

Excessive Daytime Sleepiness

Excessive sleepiness is defined as the inability to stay awake or alert during the day, resulting in unintended lapses into drowsiness or sleep. Excessive daytime sleepiness is manifested by falling asleep involuntarily in either passive (eg, reading, watching television) or active (eg, driving, during conversation) daily activity. Daytime sleepiness is commonly reported among patients with ESKD who are treated with conventional hemodialysis or chronic ambulatory peritoneal dialysis.[29]

Sleep Apnea

Sleep apnea results in repeated hypopnea and apnea episodes during sleep. Characteristics of sleep apnea include loud snoring, breathlessness, waking from sleep, and daytime sleepiness. Sleep apnea among patients with ESKD is due to both destabilization of central ventilatory control and upper-airway obstruction. When reclining overnight, excess fluid shifts from the legs toward the neck ("rostral fluid shift") contributing to collapsibility of the upper airway. This phenomenon also occurs in children with refractory NS.[31]

The prevalence of sleep apnea is similar among patients with ESKD who are treated with peritoneal dialysis or hemodialysis.[32] This suggests that the pathophysiology of sleep apnea in this population is related to kidney failure itself rather than dialysis-related factors. Patients with ESKD may not have the typical manifestations of sleep apnea, and polysomnography may be required to exclude the diagnosis.

Restless Legs Syndrome

RLS is a sensory motor disorder manifested by unpleasant nocturnal sensations in the lower limb, typically in the evening, that is worse during periods of inactivity and transiently relieved by movement. These sensations generally occur deep within the muscle of the leg or the skin, accompanied by an urge to move them. RLS is associated with difficulty initiating sleep, poor sleep quality, and impaired HRQOL.

Factors that exacerbate RLS among patients with ESKD include anemia, iron deficiency, elevated serum calcium, and peripheral and central nervous system abnormalities. Brain iron dysregulation plays a role in RLS, possibly during transport across the blood brain barrier. Because iron is an essential cofactor in the production of dopamine, low iron levels could be related to changes in dopamine metabolism, which occurs in RLS. The syndrome is worsened by iron deficiency and symptoms are improved by iron supplementation. Anemia may result from dialysis, frequent blood tests, and a decrease in levels of erythropoietin. Correcting iron deficiency, which is quite prevalent in individuals on maintenance dialysis, with intravenous iron improves RLS.

PULMONARY COMPLICATIONS OF RENAL REPLACEMENT THERAPIES

The goals of renal replacement therapies (RRT) are to restore fluid, electrolytes, and metabolic balance; remove endogenous or exogenous toxins; allow needed therapy and nutrition; and limit complications. Modalities of RRT include peritoneal dialysis, intermittent hemodialysis, and continuous hemofiltration and dialysis. All these modalities remove solutes and fluid from the blood by different mechanisms that include diffusion, convection, and hydrostatic pressure adjustment across permeable membranes.

PERITONEAL DIALYSIS

Peritoneal dialysis (PD) makes use of the peritoneum as a natural permeable membrane across which water and solutes may equilibrate. PD is the initial dialytic modality for many children with ESKD, because it is less physiologically stressful than hemodialysis, and it does not require vascular access. PD is a relatively easy technique that may be performed at home, which allows patients much greater flexibility. Finally, it may also be associated with enhanced growth, better BP control, and improved QOL.

Pulmonary Complications of Peritoneal Dialysis

Peritonitis and catheter exit site infections are the most common complications of PD. Most other complications relate to an elevation in intra-abdominal pressure after infusion of dialysate. The intra-abdominal pressure may increase from the normal of 0.5 to 2.2 cm of H_2O to as high as 5 cm H_2O with the infusion of 1 L of dialysate fluid. This increase in intra-abdominal pressure then may lead to leakage of peritoneal fluid out of the abdominal cavity and the development of hydrothorax and thoracic, abdominal, and inguinal hernias as well.[33]

Most patients on PD will develop small, chronic pleural effusions secondary to increased movement of fluid from the peritoneal to pleural spaces via the diaphragmatic lymphatics. Hydrothorax secondary to a pleuro-peritoneal communication is an uncommon complication of PD. Signs and symptoms are similar to those of a pleural effusion, with cough or dyspnea, particularly when supine, chest pain, or acute respiratory distress. In addition, the patient might experience weight gain, and decreased dialysis drain volumes. The hydrothorax is usually unilateral and most commonly right-sided, possibly because the heart and pericardium prevent fluid movement across the left hemidiaphragm.

Isotope scanning may identify pleural-peritoneal communication. Video-assisted thoracoscopic surgery may allow direct visualization and surgical obliteration of a pleuroperitoneal communication, if indicated.

The management of hydrothorax starts with the temporary suspension of PD to avoid increasing pleural fluid accumulation and allowing the effusion to regress. Conservative management for pleural leakage in the form of peritoneal rest and intermittent low volume dialysis is rarely successful. Temporary hemodialysis for 2 to 6 weeks is usually required to allow pleuroperitoneal communications to seal. Acute, massive hydrothorax requires the involvement of a thoracic surgeon. High-glucose, low-protein pleural fluid will be found on thoracentesis.

HEMODIALYSIS

In hemodialysis (HD), a patient's blood is circulated under pressure through an extracorporeal circuit with a dialyzer that removes waste and fluid and equilibrates solutes. HD requires vascular access, anticoagulation, and is technically complex. Although critically ill children may require HD to correct life-threatening abnormalities like hyperkalemia, they generally tolerate the procedure poorly. However, it may be successfully used in pediatric patients who require prolonged dialytic treatment before definitive treatment with a kidney transplant.

Pulmonary Complications of Hemodialysis

A variety of pulmonary abnormalities, including pulmonary edema, pleural effusion, acute respiratory distress syndrome, pulmonary fibrosis and calcification, pulmonary hypertension, hemosiderosis, and pleural fibrosis have been documented in adults on chronic HD, but are far less frequent in the pediatric age group with very few reported case reports.

Chest pain may occur while a child is being dialyzed, and it is usually associated with hypotension or dialysis disequilibrium syndrome. Air embolism is a potentially serious cause of chest pain and dyspnea, but it is extraordinarily rare given the presence of air detectors in HD circuits. Acute shortness of breath also may occur while on HD. The dyspnea that occurs before the start of the treatment is usually a result of volume overload, while the dyspnea that starts after the initiation of HD may be secondary to an acute coronary syndrome, bacteremia (related to the access), an allergic reaction to the dialyzer, pericardial effusion with or without tamponade, or pneumonia.

Medications administered with HD may be associated with dyspnea. Intravenous (IV) iron, although rarely, may cause an allergic reaction. Heparin may induce thrombocytopenia, resulting in clotting in the dialyzer and lines with subsequent hypoxemia and capillary leak syndrome.[34] Recurrent episodes of dyspnea occurring on dialysis are most likely to be associated with dialyzer reactions or possibly heparin-associated effects.

The presence of simultaneous symptoms such as cough, fever, chills, and hypotension often help in the identification of the cause of the dyspnea. The timing of onset of dyspnea may also provide clues to its etiology, that is, PE should be considered if dyspnea occurs after declotting (minimally invasive procedures performed to improve or restore blood flow in the fistula and grafts placed in the blood vessels of HD patients).

CONTINUOUS HEMOFILTRATION AND DIALYSIS

Continuous hemofiltration and dialysis (CRRT) is a modality commonly used in the intensive care setting that is technically similar to HD. It is a slower and continuous dialysis technique that is better tolerated than HD by critically ill patients who are hemodynamically unstable. As with HD, it requires vascular access and anticoagulation. CRRT maintains fluid balance for oliguric patients who require high daily input (eg, IV medications, parenteral nutrition).

Pulmonary Complications of Continuous Renal Replacement Therapy

Pulmonary abnormalities of CRRT are unusual, and usually related to fluid management. CRRT is used to reach fluid regulation (balance) in very sick children in the ICU. To achieve fluid balance, it is crucial to understand the differences between machine balance and net patient fluid balance. The balance of anticoagulation, ultrafiltration, and replacement fluid rates will determine the CRRT machine balance.[35] This machine balance may then be added and adjusted to net patient input and output to influence patient fluid balance. It is important to recognize that precise fluid regulation using CRRT needs to consider not only the dynamic changes in machine fluid balance, but also integrate machine fluid balance with dynamic changes in patient fluid balance. For instance, if the physicians considered just the inputs and outputs in the CRRT but did not take into account the various inputs (such as IV fluids) and outputs (such as drain outputs) in the patient, then the balance of fluid therapy would be inadequate and the patient could be at risk for either fluid overload or excessive fluid losses.

PULMONARY COMPLICATIONS AFTER KIDNEY TRANSPLANTATION

Kidney transplantation is the principal treatment option in children with ESKD because it offers the opportunity for complete cure of kidney failure. Infectious complications, including pulmonary infections, are the major cause of morbidity and mortality after pediatric kidney transplantation. They are most often observed in the first 6 months after transplant due to the more intense immunosuppression. For more information, see the Susan E. Pacheco and James M. Stark's article, "Pulmonary Manifestations of Immunodeficiency and Immunosuppressive Diseases other than HIV," elsewhere in this issue.

The risk of pulmonary infection in pediatric kidney transplant patients is determined by their epidemiologic exposures (donor-derived and recipient-derived infections, community and/or nosocomial exposures) and their "net state of immunosuppression."[36] The net state of immunosuppression of the child is a complex function determined by the interactions of several factors such as the intensity of the immunosuppression, underlying diseases, comorbid conditions, neutropenia, and metabolic conditions.[37]

Pulmonary infections may be viral (Epstein–Barr virus, cytomegalovirus), bacterial (atypical mycobacterial pneumonia), or fungal (candidiasis and *Pneumocystis jirovecii*), and all may have a significant negative impact on graft survival.

DISCLOSURE

The authors have nothing to disclose.

REFERENCES

1. Kaplan RE, Springate JE, Feld LG. Screening dipstick urinalysis: a time to change. Pediatrics 1997;100(6):919–21.
2. Lurbe E, Ingelfinger JR. Blood pressure in children and adolescents: current insights. J Hypertens 2016;34(2):176–83.
3. Flynn JT, Kaelber DC, Baker-Smith CM, et al. Subcommittee on screening and management of high blood pressure in children. clinical practice guideline for screening and management of high blood pressure in children and adolescents. Pediatrics 2017;140(3):e20171904.
4. Schwartz GJ, Munoz A, Schneider MF, et al. New equations to estimate GFR in children with CKD. J Am Soc Nephrol 2009;20(3):629–37.
5. Wallace A, Price A, Fleischer E, et al. Estimation of GFR in patients with cystic fibrosis: a cross-sectional study. Can J Kidney Health Dis 2020;7. 2054358119899312.
6. Uber AM, Sutherland SM. Acute kidney injury in hospitalized children: consequences and outcomes. Pediatr Nephrol 2020;35(2):213–20.
7. Downie ML, Gallibois C, Parekh RS, et al. Nephrotic syndrome in infants and children: pathophysiology and management. Paediatr Int Child Health 2017;37(4): 248–58.
8. Madaio MP, Harrington JT. Current concepts. The diagnosis of acute glomerulonephritis. N Engl J Med 1983;309(21):1299–302.
9. Ellison DH, Berl T. Clinical practice. The syndrome of inappropriate antidiuresis. N Engl J Med 2007;356(20):2064–72.
10. Wu CS, Chen CM, Chou HC. Pulmonary hypoplasia induced by oligohydramnios: findings from animal models and a population-based study. Pediatr Neonatol 2017;58(1):3–7.
11. Turcios NL. Pulmonary complications of renal disorders. Paediatr Respir Rev 2012;13(1):44–9.
12. Toubes ME, Lama A, Ferreiro L, et al. Urinothorax: a systematic review. J Thorac Dis 2017;9(5):1209–18.
13. Akcan-Arikan A, Zappitelli M, Loftis LL, et al. Modified RIFLE criteria in critically ill children with acute kidney injury. Kidney Int 2007;71(10):1028–35.
14. Bagga A, Bakkaloglu A, Devarajan P, et al. Improving outcomes from acute kidney injury: report of an initiative. Pediatr Nephrol 2007;22(10):1655–8.
15. KDIGO clinical practice guideline for acute kidney injury. Kidney Int 2012;2(1): 1–138.
16. Ricci Z, Ronco C. Neonatal RIFLE. Nephrol Dial Transplant 2013;28(9):2211–4.
17. Nazareth D, Walshaw M. A review of renal disease in cystic fibrosis. J Cyst Fibros 2013;12(4):309–17.
18. Prayle A, Watson A, Fortnum H, et al. Side effects of aminoglycosides on the kidney, ear and balance in cystic fibrosis. Thorax 2010;65(7):654–8.
19. Smyth A, Lewis S, Bertenshaw C, et al. Case-control study of acute renal failure in patients with cystic fibrosis in the UK. Thorax 2008;63(6):532–5.
20. Smyth A, Tan KH, Hyman-Taylor P, et al. Once versus three-times daily regimens of tobramycin treatment for pulmonary exacerbations of cystic fibrosis–the TOPIC study: a randomised controlled trial. Lancet 2005;365(9459):573–8.
21. Teixeira JP, Ambruso S, Griffin BR, et al. Pulmonary consequences of acute kidney injury. Semin Nephrol 2019;39(1):3–16.
22. Doria A, Gatto M, Iaccarino L, et al. Value and goals of treat-to-target in systemic lupus erythematosus: knowledge and foresight. Lupus 2015;24(4–5):507–15.

23. Zaffanello M, Franchini M. Thromboembolism in childhood nephrotic syndrome: a rare but serious complication. Hematology 2007;12(1):69–73.
24. Kerlin BA, Haworth K, Smoyer WE. Venous thromboembolism in pediatric nephrotic syndrome. Pediatr Nephrol 2014;29(6):989–97.
25. Suri D, Ahluwalia J, Saxena AK, et al. Thromboembolic complications in childhood nephrotic syndrome: a clinical profile. Clin Exp Nephrol 2014;18(5):803–13.
26. Oluwole K, Esuzor L, Adebiyi O, et al. Pulmonary hemorrhage with hematuria: do not forget IgA nephropathy. Clin kidney J 2012;5(5):463–6.
27. Holzel A, Fawcitt J. Pulmonary changes in acute glomerulonephritis in childhood. J Pediatr 1960;57:695–703.
28. Thangaraj Y, Ather I, Chataut H, et al. Diffuse alveolar hemorrhage as a presentation of acute poststreptococcal glomerulonephritis. Am J Med 2014;127(9): e15–7.
29. Nigam G, Camacho M, Chang ET, et al. Exploring sleep disorders in patients with chronic kidney disease. Nat Sci Sleep 2018;10:35–43.
30. Maung SC, El Sara A, Chapman C, et al. Sleep disorders and chronic kidney disease. World J Nephrol 2016;5(3):224–32.
31. Stabouli S, Papadimitriou E, Printza N, et al. Sleep disorders in pediatric chronic kidney disease patients. Pediatr Nephrol 2016;31(8):1221–9.
32. Darwish AH, Abdel-Nabi H. Sleep disorders in children with chronic kidney disease. Int J Pediatr Adolesc Med 2016;3(3):112–8.
33. Hughes GC, Ketchersid TL, Lenzen JM, et al. Thoracic complications of peritoneal dialysis. Ann Thorac Surg 1999;67(5):1518–22.
34. Fletes R, Lazarus JM, Gage J, et al. Suspected iron dextran-related adverse drug events in hemodialysis patients. Am J kidney Dis 2001;37(4):743–9.
35. Davies H, Leslie GD, Morgan D. A retrospective review of fluid balance control in CRRT. Aust Crit Care 2017;30(6):314–9.
36. Fishman JA. Infections in immunocompromised hosts and organ transplant recipients: essentials. Liver Transpl 2011;17(Suppl 3):S34–7.
37. Fishman JA. Infection in organ transplantation. Am J Transplant 2017;17(4): 856–79.

Functional Respiratory Disorders in Children

Manju Hurvitz, MD, Miles Weinberger, MD*

KEYWORDS

• Functional respiratory disease • Habit cough • Vocal cord dysfunction
• Hyperventilation • Dysfunctional breathing

KEY POINTS

- Disorders without medical explanation are functional.
- Functional disorders can create as much disability as those with medical explanation.
- Functional disorders often suffer from iatrogenesis because of being treated with a disorder the physician knows rather than recognizing a disorder as functional.

INTRODUCTION

Functional respiratory disorders (FRDs) are those that are characterized by medically unexplained symptoms (MUSs).[1] That is, they constitute symptoms that have no anatomic or organic etiology. Clinicians caring for children encounter these disorders. Providing appropriate diagnosis and treatment tests the mettle of pediatric health care providers. Failure to diagnose the functional disorder often results in iatrogenesis from unnecessary testing and medication. MUSs in children occur in all systems—gastrointestinal, neurologic, musculoskeletal, and respiratory. This review addresses respiratory MUSs.

The most common MUS involving the respiratory system is the habit cough syndrome. Some less common related variations include habit throat clearing and habit sneezing. Other functional disorders present as dyspnea. These include the various vocal cord dysfunction (VCD) disorders, hyperventilation disorders, functional dyspnea in the absence of any abnormal physiology, and sighing syndrome. The challenge of correctly diagnosing a functional disorder can be complicated by the coexistence of organic disease, such as asthma, which also can cause cough and dyspnea.

Patients with an FRD present to a health care provider with persistent, frequent respiratory symptoms that can be mistaken for organic disease, such as asthma.

Division of Pediatric Respiratory Medicine, Rady Children's Hospital, 3020 Children's Way, MC 5070, San Diego, CA 92123-4282, USA
* Corresponding author. 450 Sandalwood Ct., Encinitas, CA 92024.
E-mail address: miles-weinberger@uiowa.edu

Pediatr Clin N Am 68 (2021) 223–237
https://doi.org/10.1016/j.pcl.2020.09.013

Physicians are prone to diagnose and treat organic disorders they know, such as asthma or infection rather than consider a functional disorder. Failure to consider a functional disorder may result in inappropriate evaluation procedures and delay in effective treatment. Even if a functional disorder is suspected by a physician, reluctance to confirm a functional diagnosis may be the result of discomfort in treating the disorder. Writing a prescription is easier and less time-consuming than providing the behavioral strategies required to treat a functional disorder. Delay of diagnosis contributes, however, to emotional, physical, and social distress for the patient and family in addition to monetary costs from consultations, testing, and medication. The aim of this article is to review the clinical presentation, manifestation, and treatment of FRDs. How health care providers can successfully identify and treat these reversible conditions in the clinical setting is illustrated.

HABIT COUGH AND RELATED DISORDERS

What is a cough? It is readily recognized when heard. The sound of a cough can vary somewhat between individuals and in pitch, volume, and shrillness. What causes that sound? A cough starts with inspiration to fill the lungs, then the glottis closes, subglottic air is compressed, and the sudden opening of the glottis lets out the gust of compressed air. Two physiologic mechanisms of cough can occur. A reflex cough occurs when laryngeal receptors are stimulated by aspiration of foreign material; the inspiratory component then may be more limited. The more usual cough is tracheobronchial, initiated distal to the larynx and can be volitional.[2] The sound occurs from vibration of the large airways and laryngeal structures during turbulent flow of the rapidly expired air from release of the compressed air. Cough is a common symptom that results in a child being brought to a doctor. When cough continues daily for more than 4 weeks, it is considered chronic[3] (8 weeks is used in the adult literature to define a cough as chronic).[4]

Cough is a natural response to various stimuli. It is an important part of the defense mechanism for the lungs. Cough prevents pulmonary aspiration and clears airway debris. The cough reflex readily responds to physical or inflammatory stimuli. A foreign substance anywhere in the airway can stimulate cough. A viral respiratory infection causes inflammation of respiratory mucosa and secretion of mucus, both of which act as a stimulus to cough. Most causes of cough are self-limited. Even the chronic cough of *Bordetella pertussis*, whooping cough, generally runs its course within a hundred days.

There are many causes of chronic cough in children. An algorithmic approach to diagnosis begins with history.[5] That can identify a specific chronic cough, habit cough. The history of habit cough is unique in several ways. Although commonly beginning after an initial ordinary cause of cough, such as an asthma exacerbation or viral bronchitis (chest cold), the cough morphs into having a dry, barking, or honking character. Parents sometimes describe this transition by saying that the child had an ordinary cough for 2 weeks, "and then it changed." The cough becomes repetitive up to several times per minute or repetitive every few minutes for many hours on end. Nonetheless, there is no cough once the child is asleep. The absence once asleep is a sine qua non for diagnosis of the habit cough syndrome.

The pathognomonic nature of this disorder can be seen in a sequence of publications over a 50-year period.[6–13] Each of these 8 articles describes the same type of clinical presentation, a repetitive barking or honking cough that is absent once asleep. With more than 200 children described with these characteristics in multiple clinical reports over many years, this constitutes a well-defined specific syndrome. The child with a repetitive cough, often of a barking or honking character, that is absent once asleep constitutes this syndrome called the habit cough. Although the barking nature of the cough is the classic description, there are variations of the coughing sound. Habit throat clearing essentially is a variation of habit cough.

The name for this syndrome has varied over the years. Habit cough as a diagnostic term for this syndrome began with the first report in 1966 of 6 children seen by a Boston allergist Dr Bernard Berman.[6] Other terms used have included psychogenic cough and tic cough.[7,8] Habit cough was retained as the diagnostic terminology in a 1991 report of 9 children successfully treated by a specific form of suggestion therapy.[9] In 2016, a retrospective study at the University of Iowa from 1995 to 2014 identified 140 children, an average of 7 per year, diagnosed as having habit cough based on the syndromic criteria.[12] Using the same diagnostic criteria, 51 patients were diagnosed over a 6-year period at the Brompton Hospital in London, an average of 9 per year.

Ages of the 140 children with habit cough seen at the University of Iowa ranged from 4 years to 18 years, with a median age of 10 years (**Fig. 1**)[12]; 58% of those children were boys. Duration of cough before the initial visit was a median of 4 months and ranged from less than 1 month to periods of more than 1 year (**Fig. 2**)[12]. The median age of the 51 patients at the Brompton Hospital in London also was 10 years, with the same age range of 4 years to 18 years. The median prior cough duration was 3 months, with a range from 2 months to 3 years.[13]

Children eventually diagnosed with habit cough frequently were subjected to diagnostic procedures that included radiology and tests of lung function. Treatment prior to diagnosis frequently included inhaled albuterol, oral corticosteroids, montelukast, inhaled corticosteroids, various antibiotics, gastric acid suppressants, and cough suppressants, all without benefit. Frequent unscheduled medical care visits were common, and some had been hospitalized for the cough.

Effective treatment of habit cough was first described by Dr Bernard Berman.[6] He reported that cessation of cough was accomplished within a few days or weeks. He stated that "treatment relied on the skills of the physician in being able to convey to the patient the true nature of the disease, providing support and comfort during the period of treatment, and utilizing the art of suggestion."[6] Others subsequently referred to Berman's report and used reassurance and suggestion successfully in 9 children and 3 children, respectively, in 2 publications.[7,8]

Nine patients at the University of Iowa with habit cough were treated by a specific form of suggestion therapy.[9] Symptoms previously had been present for up to 2 years

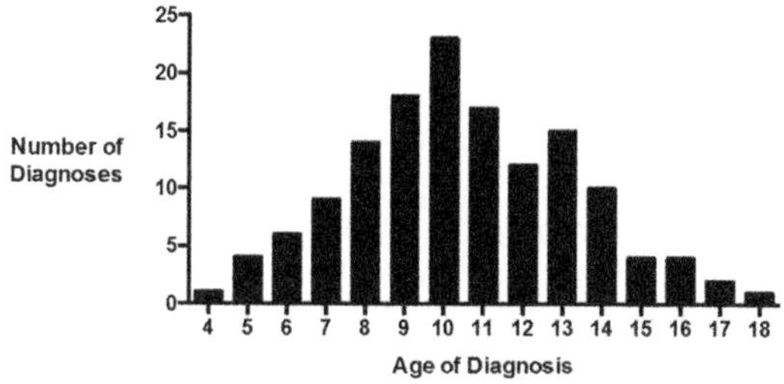

Fig. 1. Distribution of ages among 140 children diagnosed with habit cough from mid-1995 to mid-2014 at the University of Iowa Pediatric Allergy and Pulmonary Clinic. (*From* Weinberger M, Hoegger M. The cough without a cause: the habit cough syndrome. J Allergy Clin Immunol 2016;137:930; with permission.)

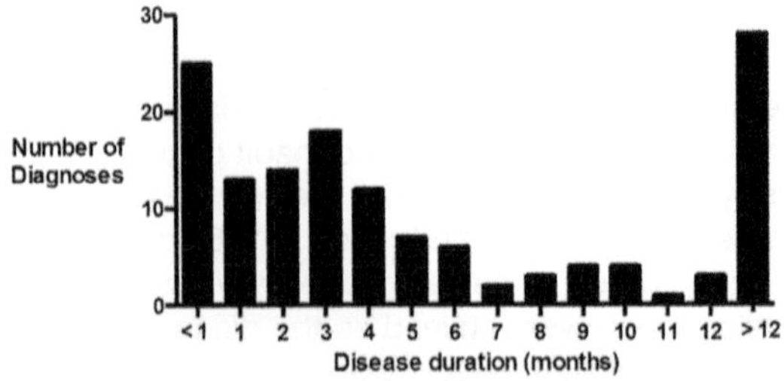

Fig. 2. Duration of repetitive cough prior to a diagnosis of habit cough among 140 children seen from mid-1995 to mid-2014 at the University of Iowa Pediatric Allergy and Pulmonary Clinic. (*From* Weinberger M, Hoegger M. The cough without a cause: the habit cough syndrome. J Allergy Clin Immunol 2016;137:930; with permission.)

(median 2 months). Five of the 9 had been hospitalized for the cough. Evaluation revealed no physiologic or radiologic abnormality. All patients became symptom-free during a single session of suggestion therapy that usually took approximately 15 minutes. During the subsequent week, 1 remained completely asymptomatic and 8 had transient minor relapses that were readily self-controlled by autosuggestion recommendations provided at the initial clinic visit. Seven of the 9 could be contacted for determination of long-term outcome at periods up to 9 years (median 2.2 years) after the session. Six were totally asymptomatic; 1 had occasional minor self-controlled symptoms. A standardized questionnaire assessing psychological symptoms at the time of follow-up revealed no somatization or emotional distress.[12] These data suggested the classic habit cough syndrome is amenable to immediate relief and long-term cure in most cases with a single session of appropriate suggestion therapy.

This conclusion was supported further by the results of 85 children seen during the period 1995 to 2014 who were actively coughing when seen at the University of Iowa[12]; 81 of the 85 had cessation of cough by the end of the clinic visit as a result of a 15-minute to 30-minute session of suggestion therapy performed by the various pediatric pulmonologists seeing patients in the clinic that day.

The principle of suggestion therapy was to ask the child to focus on the examiner and concentrate on being aware of a forthcoming cough. Holding back the cough, if even briefly, was encouraged. During continuous verbal patter, the patient was told that the cough began with some ordinary cough and then a vicious cycle occurred where the original cause of the airway irritation was gone, but now it was the cough causing the cough. The patient was told that each time the cough could be prevented from occurring that it would become easier the next time. An approximation of the script used for suggestion therapy is in **Box 1**. A video providing suggestion therapy to a 12-year-old girl with chronic cough for the previous 3 months is illustrated at www.habitcough.com/ and is reproduced on YouTube (https://www.youtube.com/watch?v=jnQUvD8Qdj0&t=670s).

In performing suggestion therapy, the parents generally were not informed of the diagnosis prior to the suggestion therapy session. Instead, the parents simply were told that the physician would show their child how to stop the coughing. Parents were asked to sit quietly with cell phones silenced and distractions minimized. When the repetitive coughing stops by the end of approximately 15 minutes, the parents were told of the diagnosis, which by then was self-evident.

The subsequent discussion with the patient and parents emphasized that it was not the physician who stopped the cough; it was the child. The child also was told they

Box 1
Major elements of suggestion therapy as a text guide

- Approach the patient with confidence that the coughing will be stopped.
- Explain the cough as a vicious cycle that started with an initial irritant that is now gone.
- Tell the patient that it is the cough itself that is causing irritation and more cough.
- Instruct the patient to concentrate solely on holding back the urge to cough.
- Select an initially brief timed period (eg, 1 min).
- Progressively increase this time period and utilize an alternative behavior, such as sipping lukewarm water to "ease the irritation."
- Tell the patient that each second the cough is delayed makes it easier to suppress further coughing.
- Repeat expressions of confidence that the patient is developing the ability to resist the urge to cough.
- "It's becoming easier to hold back the cough, isn't it" (nodding affirmatively generally results in a similar affirmation movement by the patient).
- When ability to suppress cough is observed (usually by approximately 10 min), ask in a rhetorical manner, "You're beginning to feel that you can resist the urge to cough, aren't you?" (said with an affirmative head nod).
- Discontinue the session when the patient can repeatedly respond positively to the question, "Do you feel that you can now resist the urge to cough on your own?" This question is asked only after the patient has gone 5 minutes without coughing.
- Express confidence that if the urge to cough recurs that the patient can do the same thing at home (autosuggestion[a]).

[a] Autosuggestion involves expressing confidence that 15-minute sessions at home concentrating on holding back the cough using sips of lukewarm water to "ease the irritation causing cough."

From Weinberger M, Lockshin B. When is cough functional, and how should it be treated?; *Reproduced* with permission of the © ERS 2020: Breathe 2017 13: 22-30; DOI: 10.1183/20734735.015216; with permission.

could stop the cough in the future by doing what they had done during the suggestion therapy session with the physician. That comment was important because the stimulus to cough, some children called it their "tickle," would persist for a day or more. The child, therefore, was empowered to control any return of cough. The authors called this autosuggestion, and it was reported by parents that their child utilized the autosuggestion recommendations.

Failure to provide some form of suggestion therapy or self-hypnosis is associated with continued coughing and the disability associated with that disorder, including missed school and decreased quality of life. The course of habit cough diagnosed but not treated beyond informing family of the diagnosis and provision of counseling was examined in a series of 60 children at the Mayo Clinic in Rochester Minnesota, mean age of 10 years. Those children were identified as having no physical cause for their cough; no specific treatment was given.[14] Mean duration of symptoms prior to being diagnosed was 7.6 months. Mean telephone follow-up was 7.9 years. Complete resolution of cough occurred in 44 after a mean duration of 6.1 months; 2 of those subsequently relapsed. Sixteen of the patients were still coughing a mean of 5.9 years after the Mayo Clinic diagnosis.

At the Brompton Hospital in London, treatment was limited to diagnosis and reassurance. Follow-up was possible in 39/55 (71%) children after a median duration of 1.9 years. In 32/39 (82%), the cough had resolved completely, 59% within 4 weeks, including 12% on the day of the clinic visit. Improvement occurred eventually in another 6/39 (15%). In the 29 children of parents who said they believed the diagnosis, there was eventual resolution of the cough in 96%. In the 13 children of parents skeptical or disbelieving of the diagnosis, however, only 54% experienced resolution of the chronic cough during the follow-up period.[13] These experiences at Mayo clinic and the Brompton provide the natural history of habit cough in the absence of specific suggestion therapy.

Habit throat clearing essentially is a variation of the habit cough syndrome. Of 140 children diagnosed with the habit cough syndrome over a 20-year period at the University of Iowa, a repetitive softer throat-clearing sound rather than the more typical barking cough was the presenting symptom in 10% of the patients; 11% exhibited both the barking cough and the softer throat-clearing patterns of coughing.[12] Response to suggestion therapy was as effective in these patients as in those with the harsh barking cough.

Habit sneezing is a much less common disorder than the habit cough syndrome, but there have been several case reports.[15] In the oldest reported case, a 40-year-old lady had repetitive sneezing that eventually was stopped by suggestion therapy.[16] One of the authors of this review (MW) treated an 8-year-old girl who was sneezing several times per minute for a week during waking hours. She had no symptoms when sleeping. The history indicated that the initial trigger was a nasal foreign body, which caused irritation with persistent sneezing that continued after expulsion of the foreign body. Suggestion therapy as used for habit cough stopped the sneezing.

In summary, habit cough is a specific form of chronic cough readily diagnosed by the description of a repetitive persistent cough, often with a barking or honking quality that is totally absent once asleep. Treatment with suggestion therapy has been repeatedly successful for the habit cough and its variations, habit throat clearing and habit sneezing. Diagnosis and treatment with suggestion therapy avoid the morbidity and dysfunction that results from this disorder.

FUNCTIONAL DYSPNEA DISORDERS

Although dyspnea can occur from many physical etiologies, including cardiac, pulmonary, chest wall abnormalities, and muscle disorders, the subjective feeling of dyspnea can be present in the absence of any of these organic or anatomic abnormalities. Functional dyspnea includes VCD and hyperventilation. Hyperventilation often is associated with panic attacks and anxiety. Exercise may be a trigger for both VCD[17] and hyperventilation,[18] both of which also can occur spontaneously or from other stimuli. Functional dyspnea is the feeling of shortness of breath in the absence of physical disease. The dyspnea can be from upper airway obstruction when vocal cords close paradoxically during inspiration and/or expiration. Dyspnea also can occur, however, without any physiologic abnormality of the lungs or physical obstruction to airflow.

Exercise-induced Dyspnea in the Absence of Respiratory, Cardiac, or Neuromuscular Disease

The most common cause of exercise-induced dyspnea in the absence of physical disorders is bronchospasm associated with asthma. Exercise-induced asthma readily is recognized by response to and prevention by an inhaled bronchodilator, such as albuterol. Children with exercise-induced asthma generally have a history of symptoms of asthma beyond simple exercise-induced bronchospasm. When children and adolescents with exercise-induced dyspnea were evaluated systematically with cardiopulmonary exercise testing that reproduced the exercise-induced symptoms, various etiologies, both functional and organic, were identified (**Fig. 3**).[19] The functional disorders included VCDs, exercise-induced hyperventilation, and normal physiologic limitation perceived as pathologic dyspnea. Normal physiological dyspnea occurs after lactic acid is formed during anaerobic metabolism. The metabolic acidosis stimulates respiration at a time when the individual already has reached maximal attainable ventilation. The patient then perceives that they are not getting enough air. Although this is true, it is a function of having reached maximal ventilation.

Vocal Cord Dysfunction

Normally, the vocal cords actively abduct (come apart) to maximize air flow into the lungs during breathing. If the vocal cords adduct (come together), this creates obstruction to air flow. VCD is the abnormal closing (adduction) of vocal cords during inspiration and/or expiration. Patients describe air hunger, dyspnea, and chest or throat tightness. Clinical symptoms include stridor and/or an expiratory stertorious sound, depending on whether the vocal cords are closing on inspiration, or both inspiration and expiration. Videos of those 2 dysfunctional vocal cord movements can be seen at https://www.milesweinberger.com/copy-of-exercise-induced-dyspnea Spirometry corresponding to those videos demonstrates an abnormal inspiratory component of the flow-volume loop for adduction limited to inspiration (**Fig. 4**A) and marked decrease in both components for adduction persisting on both inspiration and expiration (see **Fig. 4**B). The latter is more clinically distressing.

There are 2 distinct phenotypes of VCD. Exercise-induced VCD (EIVCD) is the most common. Spontaneous VCD (SVCD) is more troublesome because it occurs without a specific predictable stimulus like exercise.[17,19] Although exercise, usually vigorous, is

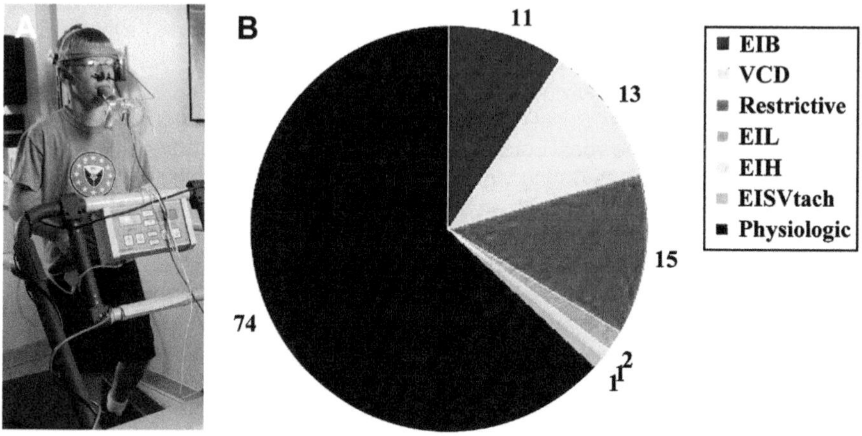

Fig. 3. Treadmill exercise with adolescent equipped for cardiopulmonary measures (*A*). Diagnoses determined by testing with cardiopulmonary physiologic monitoring (*B*). EIB, exercise-induced bronchospasm; EIH, exercise-induced hyperventilation; EISVTach, exercise-induced supraventricular tachycardia; Physiologic, physiologic limitation without other abnormality; Restrictive, apparent restriction of chest wall movement. (*From* Weinberger M, Abu-Hasan M. Pseudo-asthma: when cough, wheezing, and dyspnea are not asthma. Pediatrics 2007;120(4):862; with permission.)

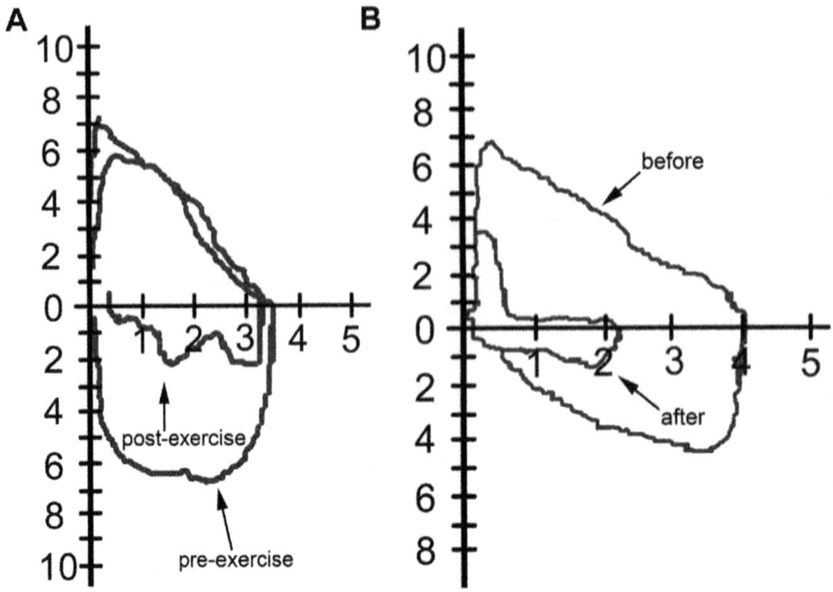

Fig. 4. Flow-volume recordings of 2 patterns of VCD: (*A*) paradoxical movement where exercise-induced adduction rather than abduction occurs on inspiration with relaxation of the cords on expiration; (*B*) spontaneous adduction on both inspiration and expiration. (*From* Weinberger M. Doshi D. Vocal Cord Dysfunction: A Functional Cause of Respiratory Distress. Breathe 2017;13:15-21; with permission.)

the precipitant for EIVCD, the precipitating factors for SVCD are variable and often unpredictable. The primary symptom of VCD is dyspnea. Diagnosis of EIVCD requires reproducing symptoms during exercise.[20] Although a treadmill is most appropriate for reproducing exercise-induced dyspnea for runners or with sports, such as basketball or soccer, an alternative device has been reported for monitoring symptoms in swimmers while they are swimming.[21]

Treatment of VCD classically has been reported to involve instruction from a speech therapist to take voluntary control of the vocal cords.[22] Patients learn to stop the inappropriate adduction of the vocal cords from continuing with this technique. Performing speech therapy techniques during vigorous and competitive exercise, however, can be difficult. Based on the vagal innervation of the vocal cords,[23–25] a rationale has been made for an inhaled anticholinergic aerosol for prevention of EIVCD by blocking the afferent pharyngeal vagal receptors. An ipratropium metered dose inhaler (Atrovent), used prior to planned exercise, has been observed to prevent EIVCD. A placebo-controlled clinical trial is needed to confirm those clinical observations.[17,26] The question has been raised as to whether a long-acting anticholinergic aerosol, such as tiotropium, would be effective as daily maintenance to prevent SVCD. Published experience regarding this approach for controlling SVCD has not yet been described, but there is a rationale for blocking the vagal effect.

The natural history of VCD was described among 28 patients identified with VCD. When contacted a median of 5 months (range of 1 week to 5 years) after the initial evaluation and diagnosis, 15 of 17 were asymptomatic; only 2 with EIVCD reported still using the ipratropium metered dose inhaler prior to exercise. All 11 SVCD patients no longer had VCD symptoms.[18] Based on those data, there appears to be a high rate of spontaneous resolution of VCD.

An imitator of EIVCD is exercise-induced laryngomalacia (EIL).[27] In some cases, this may be a residual of congenital laryngomalacia.[28] Inspiratory stridor does not occur from laryngomalacia until vigorous exercise results in sufficient air movement to invaginate the arytenoids or the epiglottis, depending on the specific anatomy.[29] When exercise testing identifies upper airway obstruction, as illustrated in **Fig. 4**A, visualization is necessary to distinguish EIVCD from the much less common EIL. The treatment of EIL, if needed, is supraglottoplasty.[30,31]

In summary, VCD can be limited to occurring only with exercise, EIVCD, or can occur spontaneously, SVCD. Although these often are distinct phenotypes, some patients manifest both SVCD and EIVCD. Speech therapy is the recommended treatment of SVCD, which can provide the patient with the ability to stop VCD when it occurs. Pre-exercise treatment with an anticholinergic appears to be an effective prevention for EIVCD. A high rate of natural resolution occurs for VCD.

Hyperventilation Syndrome

Acute hyperventilation syndrome (HVS) consists of inappropriate rapid and deep breathing triggered by anxiety or stressful events. It sometimes is part of a panic attack, characterized by intense fear or discomfort, palpitations, and a racing heartbeat.[32] Panic attacks can last minutes to hours.

Patients with HVS often present with nonrespiratory symptoms. The physiologic result of hyperventilation is an increase in alveolar ventilation in excess of metabolic needs. The arterial P_{CO_2} decreases and the arterial pH increases, resulting in respiratory alkalosis.[33] The increase in pH causes protein binding of free calcium that decreases free calcium levels. That may result in symptoms of lightheadedness and numbness or tingling in the fingers, face, or feet. Muscle twitching, carpopedal spasm, and even tetany can occur. Palpitations and anxiety frequently occur. Confusion and progression to stupor or coma can occur if hyperventilation and increased pH progress. Although the subject may feel they are not getting sufficient air into the lungs, it is the symptoms resulting from the metabolic effects of hyperventilation that often are most prominent.

In a review of 44 children seen at Duke University Medical Center with diagnoses of HVS, the chief complaint was related to respiration in only 18 (43%). Although the increased depth and rate of ventilation may be apparent to the examiner, the symptoms often are not dyspnea and air hunger. Dizziness, blackout spells, fainting, shakiness, palpitations, weakness, and numbness of the hands were prominent symptoms. Spells or attacks were described frequently.[34] Ages ranged from 5 years to 16 years, with those aged 12 years to 13 years demonstrating the highest prevalence (**Fig. 5**). Similar symptoms were described in a review of experience at the Children's Hospital of Alabama where 74 children, ages 11 years to 17 years, received a diagnosis of HVS.[35] The mean age there was 13.6 years; 74% were between ages 12 years and 16 years. A history of those nonrespiratory symptoms is sufficient to suspect that the episode described involved hyperventilation.

Diagnosis of hyperventilation requires distinguishing the symptoms from other causes. Observing the deep rapid breathing can make both patient and observer suspect respiratory distress as from asthma.[36] Patients with a history of asthma may have difficulty distinguishing the dyspnea associated with asthma from the symptoms associated with hyperventilation. A study of 120 adolescents with asthma found that HVS was 10 times more common in subjects with asthma (25%) than in those without asthma (2.5%), with a higher predilection in female adolescents.[37]

Because the acute episode may not be present when a physician is evaluating the patient, diagnosing the cause of the episodes depends primarily on obtaining a history

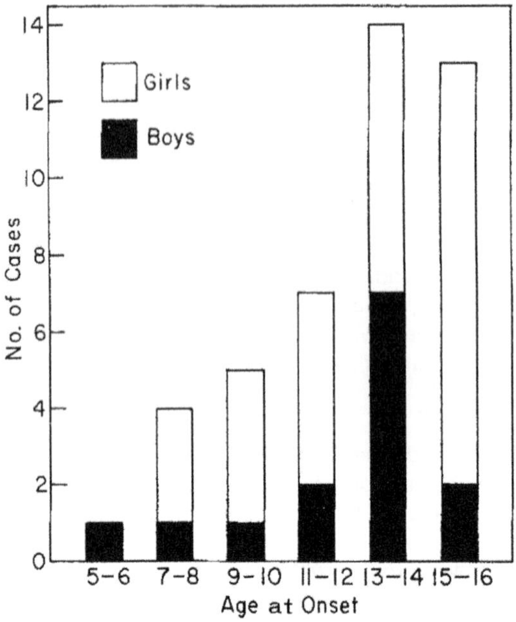

Fig. 5. Gender and age of 44 children and adolescents seen at Mayo Clinic with hyperventilation syndrome. (*From* Enzer NB, Walker PA. Hyperventilation syndrome in childhood: a review of 44 cases. J Pediatr 1967;70:523; with permission.)

of the symptoms. Confirmation of a suspicion obtained from the history can be obtained by having the patient voluntarily hyperventilate. Reproduction of the symptoms described by the patient during previous episodes confirms the suspicion determined from the history.[34]

Children with severe asthma seen during residential treatment have been observed using voluntary hyperventilation to initiate wheezing with active asthma (personal observation of MW at the National Jewish Hospital in Denver, Colorado). HVS in children often is misdiagnosed as an acute asthma exacerbation resulting in inappropriate and ineffective interventions.

During an acute episode, children and adolescents often appear anxious or distressed with deep breathing that can use accessory muscles of respiration. Lower airway sounds usually are clear with absence of the polyphonic wheezes that characterize asthma. Some patients may have diaphoresis and tachycardia but, overall, the physical examination is normal in the absence of concomitant cardiopulmonary disease.

Treatment of an acute episode includes rebreathing into a bag combined with reassurance. A caution against rebreathing into a bag has been published by UpToDate,[38] based on a study of 14 adult volunteers who deliberately hyperventilated.[39] Nonetheless, in a report of 44 children and adolescents from Duke University, a rebreathing bag was reported as employed with universal success in all with symptoms at the time of examination.[34] The use of a rebreathing bag gradually raises the P_{CO_2}, which lowers the pH, thereby eliminating the physiologic cause of most of the physical symptoms. Any makeshift rebreathing bag, paper or plastic, works. Once the symptoms from the respiratory alkalosis are relieved, the rebreathing bag should be discontinued, and verbal reassurance then is more likely to be effective.[34]

For a child with asthma who has difficulty distinguishing hyperventilation from respiratory distress of asthma, a device, such as a peak flow meter or a hand-held portable spirometer, can be provided for the patient to use when dyspneic. If a child with asthma presents for urgent care with respiratory distress, a normal oxygen saturation by a pulse oximeter warrants consideration for a blood gas. If the P_{CO_2} is low and the pH high, hyperventilation is diagnosed, although coexistent asthma is not excluded.

The long-term outcome of children and adolescents who experience recurrent episodes of hyperventilation has been examined at the Mayo Clinic (Rochester, Minnesota).[40] Those 18 years old and younger seen at the Mayo Clinic between 1970 and 1975 diagnosed with HVS were sent a questionnaire. Thirty responses (88%) were received, providing follow-up of 2 years to 28 years. Symptoms at time of follow-up found a substantial frequency of anxiety, hyperventilation, and depression (**Table 1**).[38]

In summary, hyperventilation attacks cause a variety of symptoms other than respiratory for many children. The peak age is early adolescence, but symptoms of hyperventilation can occur throughout childhood. The most severe symptoms are those with panic attacks. Relief of acute symptoms can be obtained by use of a rebreathing bag,[34] which results in elimination of the respiratory alkaloses by increasing the P_{CO_2}, and then providing reassurance. Children and adolescents with recurring hyperventilation attacks appear to continue being troubled by anxiety and hyperventilation attacks at follow-up.

Functional Dyspnea without Hyperventilation

Functional dyspnea without hyperventilation is characterized by subjective air hunger without abnormal minute ventilation or hypoxemia. There appears to be overlap between functional dyspnea without hyperventilation and psychogenic or somatoform respiratory disorders.[41] Patients typically complain of feeling short of breath. Anxiety usually is present as the cause of the subject's dyspnea. Physical examination is

Table 1
Frequency of symptoms at the time of follow-up among the 30 children and adolescents 6–18 y of age seen at the Mayo Clinic from 1950 to 1975 with hyperventilation syndrome

Anxiety	53%
Hyperventilation	40%
Depression	35%
Cold sweats	33%
Headaches	33%
Nail biting	33%
Gastrointestinal disorders	27%
Light-headedness	27%
Dry mouth	23%
Chest pain	20%
Fear of crowds	17%
Fear of dead bodies	17%
Palpitations	13%
Paresthesias	13%

Data from Herman SP, Stickleter GB, Lucas AR. Hyperventilation syndrome in children and adolescents: long-term follow-up. Pediatrics 1981;67:183-187.

grossly normal and devoid of adventitious breath sounds. If tachypnea is present, tidal volume is likely to be low so that minute ventilatory rate is normal. Confirmation of a clinical suspicion includes demonstrating normal pulse oximetry, blood gas pH, and Pco_2.

Treatment consists of reassurance and providing evidence of normal cardiopulmonary testing and vitals during subjective air hunger. Pharmacotherapy is not indicated unless prescribed because of continuing anxiety not relieved by counseling.

Sigh Syndrome, also known as Habit Sighing

Sighing is a normal organic act described as a deep, audible prolonged breath. Although the physiologic function of sighing is not understood completely, it appears to have a role in varying tidal volume and preventing alveolar collapse.[42] Although interactions between the respiratory center and central nervous system can produce voluntary sighing, the sigh syndrome is characterized by an unusual frequency of involuntary sighing for an extended period. Sigh syndrome typically presents as an involuntary intermittent deep inspiration followed by protracted expiration. Accessory muscles of respiration may be involved; however, there is no change in oxygen saturation or ongoing respiratory rate. Sighing may be the result of emotional distress, weariness, or just an acquired habit for unapparent reasons. When asked, patients may report that they felt a need for more air.

Sigh syndrome originally was described in 1929 by White and Hahn as a rare symptom due to "nervous excitability."[43] Various terms have been used to define this entity, including sigh syndrome, sighing dyspnea, and anxiety dyspnea. For purposes of this text, the authors prefer the term, sigh syndrome or habit sighing, because it is not always apparent that afflicted patients have accompanying dyspnea or anxiety.

Episodes often occur during quiet times, with a frequency of sighing several times a minute. This pattern is absent during sleep. A study by Wong and colleagues[44] demonstrated that there was little difference in the anxiety profiles of children with sigh syndrome compared with those without sigh syndrome. There are no specific physiologic tests that distinguish sigh syndrome. Unless there is concomitant organic illness, serum electrolytes and blood gas are normal. Chest radiograph findings are negative and nonspecific in sigh syndrome. Pulmonary function findings in sigh syndrome are normal.[45]

Sigh syndrome appears to be a benign and self-limited disorder that disturbs primarily the parents observing the child but not the child with the repeated sighing. Neither school nor usual activities are affected by the sighing, which appears more common during periods of quiet activity, such as watching TV. A study of 40 patients with sigh syndrome found that none reported clinical symptoms at an 18-month follow-up period.[46] Treatment consists largely of providing reassurance to the parents. It is important to validate patient symptoms and discuss that sigh syndrome is a real, albeit benign, diagnosis. With correct diagnosis and reassurance, the prognosis appears to be good for eventual spontaneous cessation.

Functional Component of Asthma

Asthma is the most common chronic disease of childhood, affecting millions of children annually in the United States alone.[47] Children with asthma can demonstrate a functional component that can complicate or confound treatment. A study of 206 children with persistent asthma found that 5% reported dysfunctional breathing despite normal pulmonary function.[48] A functional component of asthma was more common in girls compared with boys, and these patients also experienced poorer asthma control.

A functional component of asthma in a child should be considered when complaints of dyspnea or hyperventilation are present in the absence of physiologic abnormalities of asthma, demonstrable by measuring pulmonary function. Treatment should be aimed at educating the patient and family regarding asthma symptoms and management. Objective self-assessments with a peak flow meter or portable spirometer can provide the patient and caregivers with a means to distinguish anxiety-induced dyspnea from actual asthma.

SUMMARY OF FUNCTIONAL RESPIRATORY DISORDERS

FRDs can be as troublesome as physical disorders. A chronic cough may occur from multiple causes. The repetitive nature and absence once asleep distinguish the habit cough syndrome from organic disorders. The functional causes of dyspnea may occur in the presence or absence of physiologic causes. Dysfunctional breathing can confound and complicate diagnosis and treatment of asthma. Those caring for children with respiratory disease need to be as familiar with these functional disorders as they are with organic disease.

CLINICAL CARE POINTS

- Morbidity from functional disorders can match or exceed organic disorders.
- Functional disorders have clinical characteristics that enable identification - they are not diagnoses of exclusion.
- Recognize when symptoms encountered are different from organic diseases with which you are familiar.
- When unusual symptoms are encountered, do not just treat what you know; search the literature for what you don't know.
- Recognizing that a disorder is functional requires skillful application of the art of medicine.
- Make the correct diagnosis before beginning treatment.

DISCLOSURE

The authors have nothing to disclose.

REFERENCES

1. Isaac ML, Paauw DS. Medically unexplained symptoms. Med Clin North Am 2014;98:663–72.
2. Chang AB. The physiology of cough. Paediatr Respir Rev 2006;7:2–8.
3. O'Grady KF, Drescher BJ, Goyal V, et al. Chronic cough postacute respiratory illness in children: a cohort study. Arch Dis Child 2017;102:1044–8.
4. Gibson PG. Management of Cough. J Allergy Clin Immunol Pract 2019;7:1724–9.
5. Weinberger M, Fischer A. Differential diagnosis of chronic cough in children. Allergy Asthma Proc 2014;35:95–103.
6. Berman BA. Habit cough in adolescent children. Ann Allergy 1966;24:43–6.
7. Kravitz H, Gomberg RM, Burnstine RC, et al. Psychogenic cough tic in children and adolescents. Nine case histories illustrate the need for re-evaluation of this common but frequently unrecognized problem. Clin Pediatr (Phila) 1969;8:580–3.
8. Weinberg EG. "Honking": psychogenic cough tic in children. S Afr Med J 1980; 57:198–200.
9. Lokshin B, Lindgren S, Weinberger M, et al. Outcome of habit cough in children treated with a brief session of suggestion therapy. Ann Allergy 1991;67:579–82.

10. Cohlan SQ, Stone SM. The cough and the bedsheet. Pediatrics 1984;74:11–5.
11. Anbar RD, Hall HR. Childhood habit cough treated with self-hypnosis. J Pediatr 2004;144:213–7.
12. Weinberger M, Hoegger M. The cough without a cause: habit cough syndrome. J Allergy Clin Immunol 2016;137:930–1.
13. Wright MFA, Balfour-Lynn IM. Habit-tic cough: presentation and outcome with simple reassurance. Pediatr Pulmonol 2018;53:512–6.
14. Rojas AR, Sachs MI, Yunginger JW, et al. Childhood involuntary cough syndrome: a long-term follow-up study [abstract]. Ann Allergy 1991;66:106.
15. Lin TJ, Maccia CA, Turnier CG. Psychogenic intractable sneezing: case reports and a review of treatment options. Ann Allergy Asthma Immunol 2003;91:575–8.
16. Shilkret HH. Psychogenic sneezing and yawning. Psychosom Med 1949;11: 127–8.
17. Doshi D, Weinberger M. Long-term outcome of vocal cord dysfunction. Ann Allergy Asthma Immunol 2006;96:794–9.
18. Hammo AH, Weinberger M. Exercise induced hyperventilation: a pseudoasthma syndrome. Ann Allergy Asthma Immunol 1999;82:574–8.
19. O'Connell M. Vocal cord dysfunction: ready for prime-time? Ann Allergy Asthma Immunol 2006;96:762–3.
20. Bhatia R, Abu-Hasan M, Weinberger M. Exercise-induced dyspnea in children and adolescents: Differential diagnosis. Ann Allergy 2019;48:e121–7.
21. Walsted ES, Swanton LL, van van Someren K, et al. Laryngoscopy during swimming: A novel diagnostic technique to characterize swimming- induced laryngeal obstruction. Laryngoscope 2017;27:2298–301.
22. Christopher KL, Wood RP II, Eckert RC, et al. Vocal-cord dysfunction presenting as asthma. N Engl J Med 1983;308:1566–70.
23. Nishino G. Physiological and pathophysiological implications of upper airway reflexes in humans. Jpn J Physiol 2000;50:3–14.
24. Zalvan C, Sulica L, Wolf S, et al. Laryngopharyngeal dysfunction from the implant vagal nerve stimulator. Laryngoscope 2003;113:221–5.
25. Ardesch JJ, Sikken JR, Veltink PH, et al. Vagus nerve stimulation for epilepsy activates the vocal folds maximally at therapeutic levels. Epilepsy Res 2010;89: 227–31.
26. Weinberger M, Doshi D. Vocal cord dysfunction: A functional cause of respiratory distress. Breathe (Sheff) 2017;13:15–21.
27. Arora R, Gal TJ, Hagan LL. An unusual case of laryngomalacia presenting as asthma refractory to therapy. Ann Allergy Asthma Immunol 2005;95:607–11.
28. Hilland M, Roksund OD, Sandvik L, et al. Congenital laryngomalacia is related to exercise-induced laryngeal obstruction in adolescence. Arch Dis Child 2016;101: 443–8.
29. Smith RH, Kramer M, Bauman NM, et al. Exercise-induced laryngomalacia. Ann Otol Rhinol Laryngol 1995;104:537–41.
30. Bent JP 3rd, Miller DA, Kim JW, et al. Pediatric exercise-induced laryngomalacia. Ann Otol Rhinol Laryngol 1996;105:169–75.
31. Heimdal JH, Maat R, Nordang L. Surgical Intervention for Exercise-Induced Laryngeal Obstruction. Immunol Allergy Clin North Am 2018;38:317–24.
32. Kinkead R, Tenorioc L, Drolet G, et al. Respiratory manifestations of panic disorder in animals and humans: A unique opportunity to understand how supramedullary structures regulate breathing. Respir Physiol Neurobiol 2014;204:3–13.
33. Gardner WN. The pathophysiology of hyperventilation disorders. Chest 1996;109: 516–34.

34. Enzer NB, Walker PA. Hyperventilation syndrome in childhood: a review of 44 cases. J Pediatr 1967;70:521–32.
35. Hodgens JB, Famurik D, Hanna DE. Adolescent hyperventilation syndrome. Ala J Med Sci 1988;25:423–6.
36. Niggermann B. Functional symptoms confused with allergic disorders in children and adolescents. Pediatr Allergy Immunol 2002;13:312–8.
37. D'Alba I, Carloni I, Ferrante AL, et al. Hyperventilation syndrome in adolescents with and without asthma. Pediatr Pulmonol 2015;50:1184–90.
38. Schwartzstein RM, Richards J, Edlow JA, et al. Hyperventilation syndrome in adults. UpToDate. Waltham, MA: UpToDate Inc. https://www.uptodate.com/contents/hyperventilation-syndrome-in-adults. Accessed September 30, 2020.
39. Callaham M. Hypoxic hazards of traditional paper bag rebreathing in hyperventilating patients. Ann Emerg Med 1989;18:622.
40. Herman SP, Stickleter GB, Lucas AR. Hyperventilation syndrome in children and adolescents: long-term follow-up. Pediatrics 1981;67:183–7.
41. Gruber C, Lehmann C, Weiss C, et al. Somatoform respiratory disorders in children and adolescents – Proposals for a practical approach to definition and classification. Pediatr Pulmonol 2012;47:199–205.
42. Ramirez JM. The integrative role of the sigh in psychology, physiology, pathology and neurobiology. Prog Brain Res 2014;209:91–129.
43. White PD, Hahn RG. The symptom of sighing in cardiovascular diagnosis with spirographic observations. Am J Med Sci 1929;177:179.
44. Wong KS, Huang YS, Huang YH, et al. Personality profiles and pulmonary function of children with sighing dyspnoea. J Paediatr Child Health 2007;43:280–3.
45. Aljadeff G, Molho M, Katz I, et al. Pattern of lung volumes in patients with sighing dyspnea. Thorax 1993;48:809–11.
46. Sody AM, Kiderman A, Biton A, et al. Sigh syndrome: is it a sign of trouble. J Fam Pract 2008;57:E1–5.
47. National Survey of Children's Health. Child and Adolescent Health Measurement Initiative (CAHMI), "2011-2012 NSCH: Child Health Indicator and Subgroups SAS Codebook, Version 1.0" 2013, Data Resource Center for Child and Adolescent Health, sponsored by the Maternal and Child Health Bureau. Available at: www.childhealthdata.org. Accessed February 14, 2020.
48. De Groot EP. Dysfunctional breathing in children with asthma: a rare but relevant comorbidity. Eur Respir J 2013;41:1068–73.

Pulmonary Implications of Pediatric Spinal Deformities

Diane Dudas Sheehan, ND, APRN, FNP-BC[a,b,*], John Grayhack, MD, MS[a,c]

KEYWORDS

• Spinal deformities • Consequential pulmonary implications • Scoliosis
• Pediatric spinal deformities • Kyphosis

KEY POINTS

- Scoliosis and kyphosis in childhood rarely cause functional difficulties or respiratory symptoms.
- The progression of thoracic scoliosis may lead to deterioration of pulmonary function, along with increased incidence and severity of back pain and deformity.
- The aim of early identification, orthopedic referral, and treatment in spinal deformities is to halt curve progression before skeletal maturity, to avoid the issues above described and consequent surgery.
- Surgical indications and goals in patients with severe curvature are to avoid further progression, improve spinal deformity, and achieve and maintain spinal balance and alignment in order to mitigate the long-term natural history outcomes and prevent respiratory morbidity and mortality.

INTRODUCTION

Clinical screening of children and adolescents for spinal deformities (SD) involves evaluation of spinal alignment in both the coronal and the sagittal planes by visualization, palpation, and with movement including the Adams forward bend test (FBT). Assessment of SD comprises recognition of accompanying disorders, which may be the cause or impact the subsequent natural history of such deformities. Definitive diagnosis most commonly includes radiographs, which allow for evaluation of underlying congenital or developmental anomalies, the skeletal growth remaining, overall alignment and balance, and magnitude of the deformity, as defined by measurement of the "Cobb angle" (CA).

[a] Division of Orthopaedic Surgery and Sports Medicine, Ann & Robert H. Lurie Children's Hospital of Chicago, 225 East Chicago Avenue, Box 69, Chicago, IL 60611, USA; [b] Department of Physical Medicine and Rehabilitation, Feinberg School of Medicine of Northwestern University, Chicago, IL, USA; [c] Department of Orthopaedic Surgery, Feinberg School of Medicine of Northwestern University, Chicago, IL, USA
* Corresponding author.
E-mail address: dsheehan@luriechildrens.org

Pediatr Clin N Am 68 (2021) 239–259
https://doi.org/10.1016/j.pcl.2020.09.012
pediatric.theclinics.com

Early identification and referral to an appropriate specialist would most often allow for elucidation and discussion of the cause, assessment for accompanying disorders or issues, discussion of the natural history of the SD, and review of treatment options with the patient and family. In particular, children with early onset of progressive SD are at greater risk for associated thoracic cage deformity, subsequent short-term and long-term pulmonary functional impairment, and physiologic issues associated with this.

Current treatment options are directed toward mitigating long-term issues, including but not limited to, back pain, arthritis, cosmetic deformity, and pulmonary complications. A discussion of the indications, goals, and risk/benefit of the different treatment options, including the choice of surgical intervention, allows for shared decision making with the patient and family. Review of the evidence for each along with the outcomes and complication rates allows for appropriate discussion and decision making.

SPINAL DEFORMITIES: DEFINITIONS/CATEGORIES/INCIDENCE

Scoliosis is characterized by a lateral curvature of the spine of greater or equal to 10° with vertebral rotation.[1,2] In the most common deformity, idiopathic scoliosis (IS), this presents as a 3-dimensional rotational deformity presenting as a lateral curvature and thoracic hypokyphosis/lordosis, with resulting asymmetric posterior rib prominence.[3,4]

Scoliosis is found in 1% to 3% of the population, occurs more often in girls, and is categorized according to underlying cause or associated disorder.[1,2] IS is a diagnosis of exclusion with *no* identifiable cause for the curvature. IS most commonly presents as dextroscoliosis of the thoracic spine and levoscoliosis of the lumbar spine, resulting in an S-shaped curvature, but may present with other patterns. IS, which accounts for 85% of cases, is further subdivided by age of onset: infantile (IIS), juvenile (JIS), and adolescent (AIS).[5,6]

Congenital scoliosis (CS) results from abnormal development of the vertebrae during embryogenesis (weeks 4–6 of gestation), such as failure of segmentation of the vertebra (resulting in a "bar") and/or failure of formation of a portion or all of the vertebra (hemivertebra, butterfly vertebra, or "tripedicular "vertebra). Such anomalies may result in minimal or very significant SD depending on their combination and severity. CS is often accompanied by other congenital anomalies and represents 1 component of a multiorgan syndrome; thus, a thorough evaluation is warranted.[7]

Scoliosis may be associated with neurologic and muscular disorders both central and peripheral.[3] Neuromuscular (NM) curves are more commonly long, sweeping C-shaped curves, impacting alignment, function, balance, care, and quality of life (QOL). Syndromic scoliosis may be associated with a plethora of conditions; these patients may warrant more consistent spinal screening (**Fig. 1**). Any scoliosis identified before the age of 5 is considered "early onset scoliosis" (EOS) and may have an increased risk of progression and/or issues secondary to growth remaining.[8]

KYPHOSIS

Kyphosis is a normal aspect of the sagittal alignment of the thoracic spine but may be exaggerated beyond the normal range of 20° to 45° in children and adolescents.[9] The varying causes of hyperkyphosis are associated with differing natural histories and implications. Exaggerated kyphosis with normal vertebral development may occur as a postural variant or from NM disorders. Congenital kyphosis results from developmental vertebral anomalies, which may result in wedging of the vertebra. Scheuermann is an idiopathic structural sagittal plane deformity that develops during

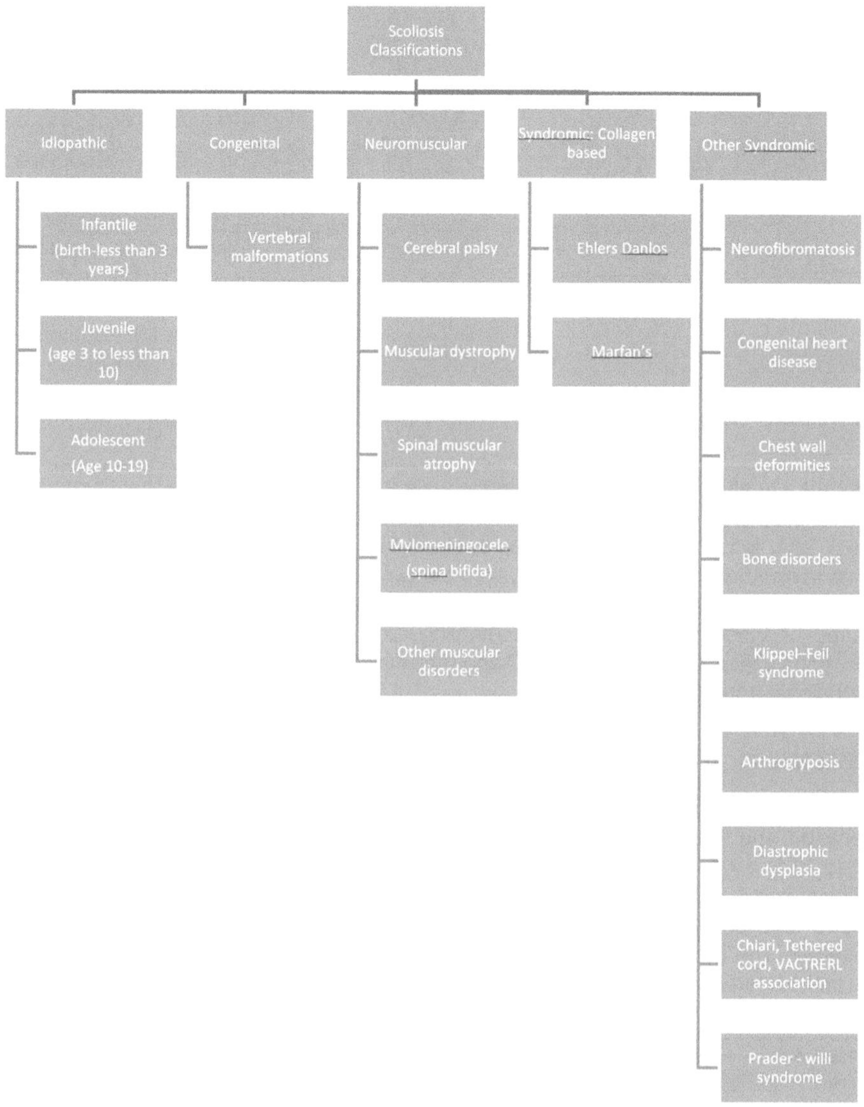

Fig. 1. Classification of scoliosis.

adolescence and has 3 or more consecutive wedged vertebrae, most commonly with irregularity of vertebral endplates and loss of disc space height.[10] Certain syndromes, such as achondroplasia, may show an associated thoracic or thoracolumbar kyphosis[11] (**Fig. 2**).

NATURE OF SPINAL DEFORMITIES

Commonly, pediatric SD have few symptoms and limited signs. Most of these patients demonstrate normal function with no evidence of increased pain, neurologic issue, or pulmonary complaints when compared with the general population. An estimated 33% of healthy children has generalized back pain complaints, in which half of these

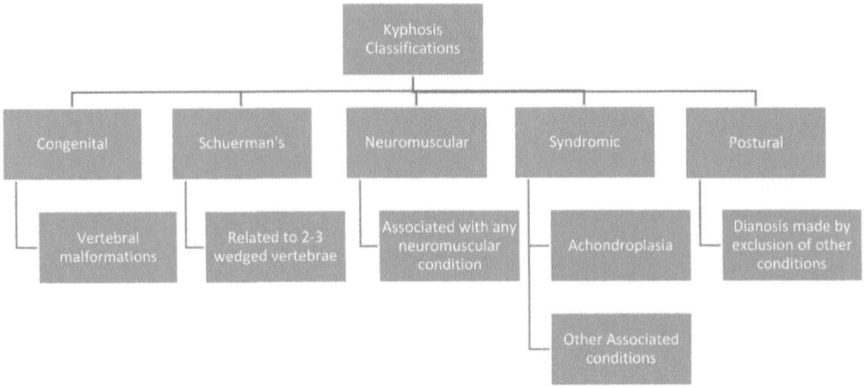

Fig. 2. Kyphosis classification.

prompt a health care visit.[12] Some individuals and families recognize the asymmetry, round back posture, or posterior prominence, which leads to evaluation (**Table 1**). Back pain is ordinarily muscular or postural in nature and typically improves with core strengthening activities or physical therapy). Significant back pain, which interrupts a child's or adolescent's daily activities or sleep, unrelenting symptoms, or associated neurologic signs (numbness/tingling, bowel or bladder control issues) and functional difficulties, is rare with SD and may warrant further evaluation for underlying pathologic condition.[6,9]

ASSESSMENT

Clinical screening for SD, scoliosis or kyphosis, may be performed on all pediatric patients but should be a part of the standard examination for girls aged 10 to 12 and boys aged 12 to 14. Inspection for presence of SD or asymmetry should include the FBT. Clinical screening should be performed in a standing position with feet at shoulder width, legs straight, bending to 90° at the waist with arms dangling and palms together. The provider assesses for significant rotational prominence, usually using an inclinometer centered along the spine from the upper thoracic to the lumbosacral

Table 1
Presenting signs for scoliosis and kyphosis

Presenting Asymmetric Signs for Scoliosis	Presenting Signs for Kyphosis
Head tilt	Head and neck in front of trunk/body
Uneven shoulders	Rounded/anteriorly forward shoulders
Prominence on 1 side of the back	Prominence of C7/T1 junction
Pronounced, uneven, or a winged scapula	Hunchback/rounded back appearance
Amplified concave flank region	Slouching when sitting
Waist asymmetry	Stooped posture
One hip appearing higher than the other	
Overall imbalance, trunk shift, or leaning toward 1 side	
Associated rib prominence or asymmetry of chest wall	
Chest wall rotation relative to the pelvis	

region. An asymmetry or angle of trunk rotation (ATR) measurement of 5° to 7° or greater may detect a significant scoliosis meriting radiographic examination and/or orthopedic referral.[13]

Appreciation of increased round-back sagittal alignment while standing and any gibbus deformity (sharp angulation appreciated during forward flexion) raises the suspicion of significant kyphosis. Aside from assessing the cosmetic magnitude of the curve, clinical examination includes evaluation of the flexibility. Evaluation of the flexibility can be assessed by extension in an upright standing or seated position, in a prone position with the patient arching on elbows, or in a supine position over a bolster at the apex. Abnormalities of spinal alignment necessitating a vigilant comprehensive examination evaluates for other conditions (such as heritable collagen diseases, neurologic conditions, or skeletal dysplasia)[9,13] (**Box 1**).

Clinical examination of children with special needs, nonambulatory patients, and those with NM conditions may be challenging because of cognitive, communicative, and/or physical limitations. The FBT may be unobtainable or nonreproducible. Seated and supine evaluation includes asymmetry of the pelvis and the presence of windswept hips as it relates to spinal alignment[14] (**Box 2**).

IMAGING/TESTING

Posterior-anterior (PA) and lateral radiographs of the full spine should be obtained with the patient in the most reproducible upright position (standing, seated, supine). The vertebra should be assessed for normal development. Each curve may be described with an apex (the vertebra with the greatest lateral distance from the center of the spine), and the angle defined by 2 vertebrae at the ends of the curve (the upper- and lower-end vertebrae). The magnitude of the curves is a measured angle/ CA defined by the endplates of these superior and inferior end vertebrae. Coronal balance on the PA film is defined by relative displacement of a plumb line dropped from C7 to the center sacral vertical line, with normal being within 2 cm[5] (**Figs. 3–5**). Lateral radiograph assessment includes vertebrae size and shape, any evidence of anomaly or wedging, abnormal sagittal alignment such as hypokyphosis (flattening of the thoracic spine), hyperlordosis, or hyperkyphosis. In a similar fashion, a CA measurement of the sagittal curves (kyphosis and lordosis) and the overall sagittal alignment/balance may be determined from this lateral view.

Children with NM disorders may require imaging in a supine or seated position. Images obtained while recumbent (eliminating the impact of gravity) produce important differences in curve magnitude and characteristics which must be considered (**Fig. 6**).

The rate and magnitude of thoracic spinal growth are associated with the increase in thoracic cage volume (predicted to double during the peak growth velocity from age 10 to 14/16 years)[15] and the risk of curve progression and scoliosis. In patients with IS, the peak height velocity is most commonly before menarche and before Risser 1. Skeletal age, and therefore growth remaining, may be assessed by chronologic age, onset of menarche, and radiographic signs, that is, Risser sign, triradiate cartilage closure, and bone age (Sanders classification).[2] Interventions are directed at minimizing curve progression during this rapid growth period.

Advanced imaging, such as MRI or computed tomographic scan, may be necessary in patients with atypical curves, congenital or developmental deformities of the spine, neurologic signs or symptoms, significant persistent pain, or certain syndromes.[6]

Pulmonary function tests (PFTs) may be indicated for major thoracic deformities to determine associated lung function compromise, preoperative baseline assessment and postoperative pulmonary changes, and estimation of long-term outcomes.[15]

Box 1
Comprehensive physical examination components to diagnose spinal deformities

General: sex, age, height, weight, body mass index (BMI), growth percentiles, plot on growth chart

Endocrine: Tanner staging

Integument: café-au-lait spots, midline sacral cutaneous anomalies (dimple, tuft of hair)

Alignment: assess overall posture in coronal and sagittal planes; head/torso imbalance, rib rotation, shoulder scapulae, waist for asymmetry

Chest deformity, asymmetric rib prominence
- Pectus excavatum = abnormal ribs/sternum, sunken in appearance
- Pectus carinatum = chest protrudes over the sternum, birdlike appearance

Respiratory: assess lung sounds, quality of breathing, symmetric/asymmetric chest expansion

Musculoskeletal: Lower-extremity range of motion (ROM): hip motion, popliteal angles, pelvic asymmetry, joint hypermobility

Extremities: Assess for leg length discrepancy (LLD). If concern, measure each leg length from anterior superior iliac spine to the medial malleolus to determine if different

Muscle strength testing: extensor hallux longus, flexor hallux longus, gastrocnemius, tendon Achilles quadriceps, hamstrings, hip flexors, hip abductors, and adductors

Spine: assess bony prominence, palpate for paraspinal pain or tenderness, assess flexibility, ROM side bending, flexion, extension, assess for hypokyphosis/kyphosis (sagittal plane)

ADAM forward bend test to obtain *ATR*: measured in degrees with an inclinometer

Neurologic: Sensation: sensory distribution to light touch

Reflexes: umbilical, deep tendon reflexes at knees and ankles, clonus/Babinski reflex

Gait pattern

Adapted from Sheehan, D.D. & Grayhack, J. (2017) Scoliosis in Pediatrics: Identification, Categories, Treatment Options and Surgical Management, Ann & Robert H. Lurie Children's of Chicago Child's Doctor: Online CME Rounds: January 2017. https://www2.luriechildrens.org/ce/online/article.aspx?articleID=370]; with permission.

ASSOCIATED CHEST DEFORMITIES

Vertebral rotation of the thoracic spine in scoliosis creates the chest wall deformity by rotating the ribs posteriorly and cephalad on the convex side and anteriorly on the concave side.[16] Radiographic parameters seen in the thoracic cage of patients with scoliosis that were statistically correlated to restrictive ventilatory disorder include main thoracic large CA, main thoracic rib hump, apical vertebral translation, and thoracic hypokyphosis.[15,17–19] This 3-dimensional chest deformity in severe thoracic scoliosis and the appearance of restrictive lung disease are caused by a mechanical alteration (torsion) of the diaphragm and altered chest wall compliance (distensibility), compression of the lung parenchyma with progressive decrease in lung volumes, and force-generating capacities.[16] The risk of *thoracic insufficiency syndrome* is especially recognized in EOS, which may result from progressive SD, rib abnormalities, decreased thoracic height, and/or early fusion, which limits the growth potential of the spine and therefore the chest.[8,18] In the very young child, severe scoliosis may result in diminished lung growth and alveolar development.[20]

Box 2
Supplemental physical examination considerations for special needs children

General appearance: alertness, cognition (ability to follow directions), communication abilities: verbal, use of signs or expressions

Height (%), weight (%) (gain or loss since last visit?), BMI; compare growth pattern expectations on specific chart, growth chart for children with cerebral palsy

Endocrine: Tanner staging (signs of early puberty)

Integument: skin lesions, surgical scars, vigilant skin assessment for signs of pressure injury or skin breakdown

Cardiovascular: pulses: pedal, capillary refill time, extremities cool or warm to touch

Frontal alignment/chest deformity: chest wall configuration, asymmetric rib prominence

Respiratory: assess quality of breathing (noise, presence of secretions in throat/upper airway) breath support for talking, if an abdominal breather, symmetric/asymmetric chest expansion, ability to perform deep breath on command

Musculoskeletal: muscle strength testing (if cooperative and reliable)

Joint hypermobility or restrictions

Upper extremities: ability to use (reaching/grip patterns), presence of atrophy/muscle wasting, typical positioning/posturing, limitations in passive range of joint motion, presence of contractures

Lower extremities: active movements, limitations in passive ROM, or presence of contractures

Supine hip and leg alignment: windswept appearance: abduction of 1 hip with external rotation of the leg; adduction of contralateral hip with internal rotation of the leg

Hips ROM: abduction, flexion, extension, internal, and external rotation. Knees: extension, flexion, and popliteal angles. Ankles: dorsiflexion, plantar flexion, foot position

Assess for LLD: Galeazzi test to assess for hip dislocation, Allis sign for lower-leg discrepancy. If concern for LLD, measure each leg length from anterior superior iliac spine to the medial malleolus to determine difference

Pelvis: pelvic obliquity, asymmetry, rotation, increased lordosis

Spine alignment/signs of asymmetry: assess trunk posture in various positions; supine, ability to sit upright with and without support (quality and endurance), leaning to 1 side, and standing posture (need for support)

Palpate paraspinal pain or tenderness, assess bony prominence, flexibility, ROM side bending, flexion and extension, assess hypokyphosis/kyphosis (sagittal plane)

ATR-modified: try forward bend test with support, leaning forward in wheelchair or over a parent's lap, *measurement should be reproducible to be useful*

Neurologic: sensation: sensory distribution to light touch

Reflexes: Deep tendon reflexes at knees and ankles, presence of clonus with ankle dorsiflexion, negative/positive Babinski, appreciation of spasticity (brisk movement of the limbs, appreciating a catch vs slow sustained end ROM)

Gait pattern: if able to walk or take reciprocal steps, quality, assess for crouching, hip/knee flexion, foot placement, need for assistance, with or without additional use of equipment (braces), quantify distance and speed

Gross Motor Functional Classification System (I–V)

Adapted from Sheehan, D.D. & Grayhack, J. (2017) Scoliosis in Pediatrics: Identification, Categories, Treatment Options and Surgical Management, Ann & Robert H. Lurie Children's of Chicago Child's Doctor: Online CME Rounds: January 2017. https://www2.luriechildrens.org/ce/online/article.aspx?articleID=370]; with permission.

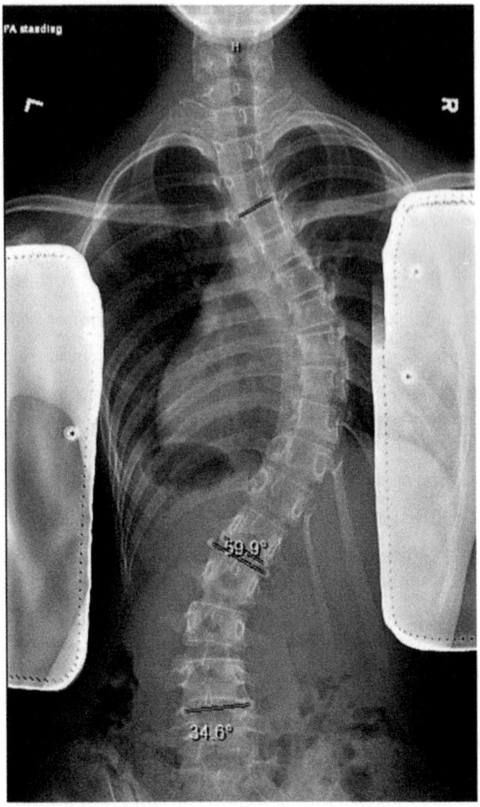

Fig. 3. AIS PA view. Standing PA image of a teenager with AIS reveals a 60° right thoracic curve from T4 to L1 and a compensatory 35° left lumbar curve from L1 to L4.

CORRELATING PULMONARY COMPROMISE

Spirometry currently represents the standard of reference to evaluate pulmonary function; it may provide a good estimate of the restrictive defect because the decrease in forced vital capacity (FVC) is proportional to the decrease in total lung capacity (TLC). However, generating reliable spirometric data depends on patient compliance.[21] The volume changes and negative correlation with lung function through PFTs evaluate dynamic breathing parameters involving the movement of the chest and rib cage, such as deep expiration and inspiration.[17] Absolute spirometric values are normalized as a percentage of predicted based on arm spans or length of specific bones (eg, ulnar length), because height is directly influenced by spine curvature.

Generally, mild to moderate scoliosis (CA <60°) produces very few respiratory signs and symptoms, although exercise capacity may be decreased with dyspnea on exertion as one of the first manifestations.[4,22] Obstructive lung disease is defined by a low forced expiratory volume in the first second divided by the FVC during a maximal expiratory flow maneuver (FEV_1)/FVC. A reduced FEV_1/FVC ratio less than the 95% confidence interval for age, sex, race, and height reflecting narrowing, constriction, or compression of intrathoracic airways was seen in 34% of AIS with associated higher CA; retested after bronchodilator administration, 73% persisted, consistent with irreversible airway obstruction.[23] Multicenter studies of preoperative AIS patients

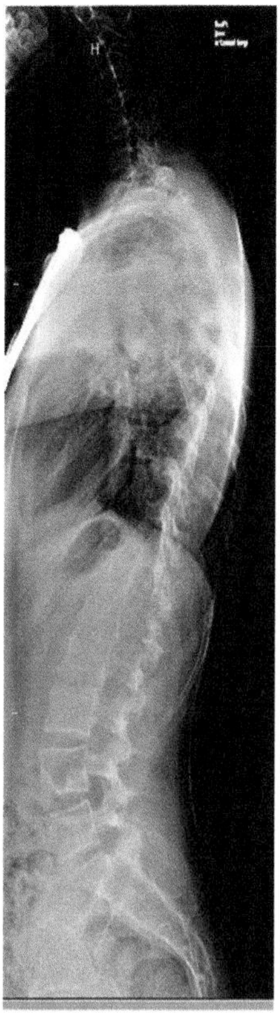

Fig. 4. AIS lateral view. The same adolescent's lateral view shows thoracic hypokyphosis and rib rotation.

revealed 20% to 25% had clinically relevant degree of respiratory impairment (FEV_1/FVC <65%) with thoracic curves with CA 60° to 70°.[18,21] Extrinsic mechanisms, such as compression and gas trapping or intrinsic mechanisms, including hypersecretions, are suggested causes.[15] Therefore, restrictive lung disease (with measurable decrease in FEV_1/FVC) is likely to occur with thoracic curves greater than 70°. CA of greater than 90° significantly predisposes to cardiorespiratory failure.

PFT results varied between patients with different causes. JIS patients had lower predicted FEV_1 associated with more significant midthoracic curves and hypokyphosis compared with AIS patients.[18] Significantly worse pulmonary function was found in patients with CS compared with age- and CA-matched patients, thought to be associated with lung hypoplasia, owing to thoracic deformity during the period of very rapid lung growth and development.[20] Compared with IS patients, more rib cage and chest wall deformity in CS patients may be another factor, which may lead to decreased chest wall compliance and thus worse respiratory function. Patients with CS and fused rib had lower PFTs than those without rib anomalies.[24]

NATURAL HISTORY OF SPINE ABNORMALITIES

Functional difficulties are uncommon in otherwise healthy pediatric patients with SD. However, self-esteem and psychological well-being may be negatively affected. If the

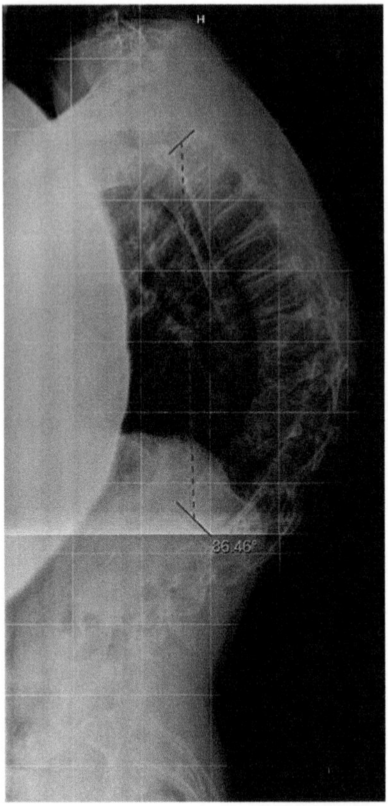

Fig. 5. Hyperkyphosis lateral view. Adolescent with exaggerated postural kyphosis measuring 86°.

SD is of sufficient magnitude (generally CA >50°), one may expect continued progression even after skeletal maturity, resulting in further altered spinal alignment, decreased spine flexibility, and eventual degenerative changes leading to pain and loss of function over the patient's lifetime.[3] Neurologic disability is extremely rare. Kyphosis is associated with a modest increased risk of back pain and possibly a negative impact on body image.[1,2]

Reviewing the natural history of AIS (retrospective and then prospective studies), two-thirds of the untreated AIS population progressed after skeletal maturity; curves less than 30° tended not to progress, and curves between 50° and 75° at maturity, particularly thoracic curves, progressed the most. Having a CA of 50° at adulthood is a significant predictor of decreased pulmonary function; patients with curves greater than 80° had greater odds of shortness of breath; however, mortalities were the same as the general population. Adult AIS patients had more chronic back pain and more acute pain of greater intensity and duration than their peers, yet ability to work and perform activities of daily living was similar to the control group. Employment, marriage rates, reproductive experiences, and mortalities are comparable (AIS and matched peers).[2]

The natural history of IIS is linked to likelihood of curve progression, which in turn is associated with magnitude at presentation (if >25°), phase 2 rib alignment (overlap of

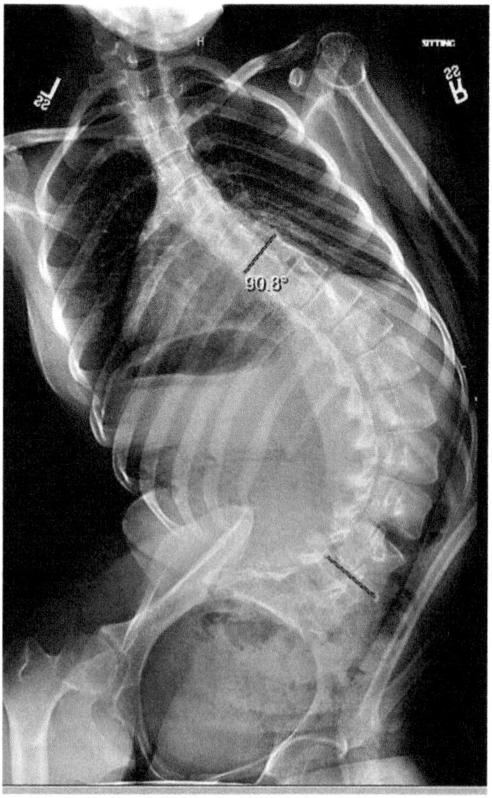

Fig. 6. NM scoliosis sitting PA view. Teen with CP, NM scoliosis, PA view validates a long C-shaped 91° right thoracolumbar curvature from T10 to L4 and a pelvic obliquity.

the rib heads and vertebral body at the apex of the curve), and increased rib vertebral angle difference of greater than 20° (tilt of the ribs at the apex). Persistent curve progression in the absence of treatment results in increasing chest wall deformity, rib rotation, and subsequent restrictive pulmonary disease. The earlier appearance of SD produces chest wall rotation, limiting the space available for the development, growth, and function of the lungs. This limitation of the ability for the lungs to grow may be associated with earlier death in untreated IIS children.[8]

THERAPEUTIC OPTIONS

Approximately two-thirds of patients with AIS experience curve progression before skeletal maturity; thus, therapeutic options are considered to mitigate the longer-term issues accompanying this.[1] The main goals of these treatments are to prevent further worsening of the curve and to restore trunk asymmetry and balance, while minimizing morbidity and pain, and improving long-term outcomes. Treatment considerations are dependent on the magnitude and location of the curvature, growth remaining, truncal balance, general health, level of function and satisfaction, and patient's and parent's treatment goals.[3]

Orthosis (brace) treatment has been proven efficacious and therefore is recommended in AIS patients who have curves of 25° to 45° and spinal growth remaining.

Children with significant growth remaining have the greatest potential for curve progression, and therefore, the focus of treatment strategies to reduce the risk of progression, altering the natural history/issues and avoiding surgical intervention. A customized brace provides external forces with the aim of achieving maximum correction of the pathologic curve.[3] Multicenter studies have shown that bracing is effective for many AIS patients when worn 13 to 18 hours per day to significantly reduce the risk of curve progression and subsequent surgery without significant short-term harms but may have a significant negative impact on the QOL of children and adolescents.[1–3,25] Although bracing is commonly used in JIS, IIS, neuromuscular scoliosis, and syndromic scoliosis, there is more limited evidence for the efficacy in altering the natural course in these settings. In NMS, an orthosis may improve posture during activities, social interactions, and care, alleviate pressure and soreness, and assist in therapeutic goals.

Thoracic Scheuermann kyphosis bracing typically requires a brace with clavicle or cervical extension while there is growth remaining. The orthosis may provide some correction of the kyphosis; however, partial loss of this improvement may occur after brace discontinuation.[10]

Other nonsurgical therapeutic options for SD include spinal manipulation, chiropractic care, and physiotherapeutic specific exercises (PSE), that is, "Schroth" methods. These exercises have limited evidence of efficacy. Core strengthening, spinal alignment education, and proprioception training if consistently used may positively influence postural kyphosis and symptoms.[1,26–30] General fitness (yoga, Pilates, tai chi, swimming, martial arts), sports, and physical education class participation are generally encouraged following the diagnosis of SD, although there is little or no evidence of impact on risk of progression or long-term natural history with these. Combining bracing with PSE may increase treatment efficacy.[3,25] Serial casting of the trunk is an option typically reserved for IIS and sometimes younger JIS patients for uncontrollable curves, sometimes attempted in conjunction with eventual bracing used to delay surgical intervention.[8]

SURGICAL TREATMENT

Surgery is generally reserved for children and teens with scoliosis curves greater than 45° to 50°, or more rarely, for those with significant imbalance or symptoms (up to 0.1% of AIS patients will eventually require surgery).[3] Surgical intervention for kyphosis is less commonly undertaken, but may be an option for patients who have curves of significant magnitude, sharp deformities of a lesser degree with the potential of neurologic compromise, or unacceptable cosmetics. Surgical approach is selected in patients addressing numerous factors, including cause, curve magnitude, spinal balance, growth remaining, surgeon preferences, surgical center's experiences, and patient/family cosmetic concerns.

Surgical advances have been made in procedural safeguards, surgical techniques, and instrumentation to improve patient outcomes. Although technological advances have evolved over decades, the goals of the surgery remain largely unchanged: prevent the progression of the curvature with subsequent decreasing of the risk of long-term pain and arthritis, functional disability, deterioration in pulmonary function caused by progressive thoracic deformity, and most often improving alignment and overall balance. Surgical goals include achieving adequate and balanced thoracic kyphosis and lumbar lordosis, or in "selective thoracic fusion" (fixation of the primary thoracic curve only), spontaneous coronal and sagittal correction of the unfused lumbar curve. Ideally, fusing the lowest number of mobile segments and properly correcting the existing deformity may help maintain lung volume after spine fusion, with a focus on limiting the potential for additional interventions or surgeries throughout the child's lifetime.[5,17] Spinal fusion intervention includes instrumentation (combination of rods, with hooks, cables, wires, and pedicle screw fixation systems as anchors to the spine) and bone graft (autograft, allograft, and bone substitutes) to create bone fusion of the vertebrae to achieve long-term stability and alignment[3] (**Figs. 7** and **8**).

Posterior spinal fusion (PSF) is the most common approach; however, alternatively, anterior thoracic techniques, such as thoracotomy with instrumentation and thoracoscopic instrumentation, are options. A systematic review of the literature reported with thoracoscopic anterior instrumentation and fusion had similar curve correction, fewer instrumented levels, improved cosmetics, reduced morbidity, and less blood loss, although had longer operative time and greater incidence of perioperative pulmonary complications. Despite initial decrease in PFTs values, FVC and TLC recovered to baseline levels without significant difference.[31]

Surgical alternatives, such as in situ fusion, "growing constructs" (sliding or motorized rods, which allow for or encourage spinal growth), or those addressing accompanying chest wall deformity, such as Vertical Expandable Prosthetic Titanium Rib), may be indicated for specific pathologic condition (such as CS, JIS, IIS, and rib anomalies).[8,20] Developing technologies include vertebral stapling or tension tethering to exploit spinal growth for limitation or even correction of curves are in their nascent

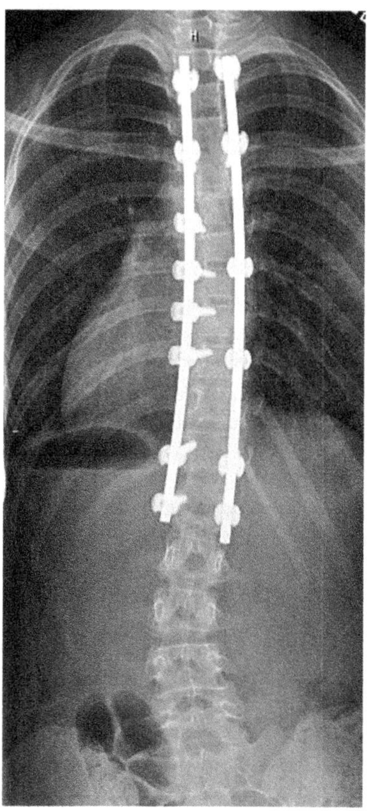

Fig. 7. AIS PSF PA view. Same teen with AIS status postsurgical fusion.

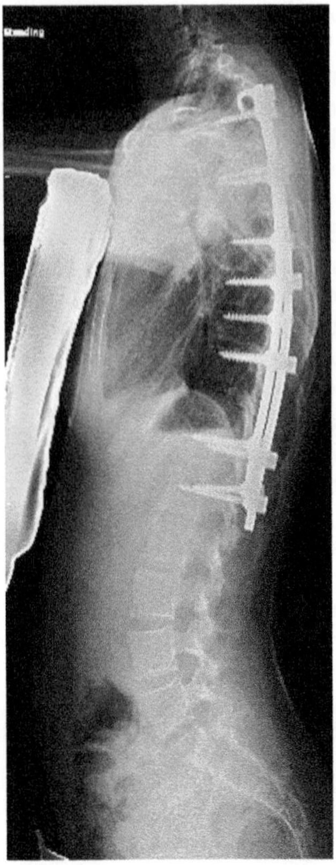

Fig. 8. AIS PSF. Same teen with AIS status postsurgical fusion; lateral view.

phase. In theory, these allow for greater spine flexibility than rigid constructs, yet there remains concern regarding the longevity of these fusionless surgeries.[32] Although the risks of spine surgery include infection, blood loss with need for transfusion, failure of instrumentation or fusion, and rarely, respiratory or neurologic compromise, these complications are relatively uncommon in the pediatric population.[33] The shared decision to undertake surgical intervention is based on the patient's and family's determination of the potential long-term benefits to alter the natural history and avoid the issues that accompany this, such as pain, cosmetic deformity, functional difficulty, and pulmonary implications, weighed against the extensive effort of surgery, postoperative recovery with limitations imposed, and the potential for related postsurgical complications.

Surgical treatment decisions for patients with NMS may be more multifaceted, as both the natural history and the response to treatment are quite heterogeneous. The underlying neurologic cause and disease course without such intervention are highly variable; thus, long-term outcomes are less predictable. The risk of curve progression is influenced by the disease itself, the magnitude and rigidity of the curve, and balance of the spine. Furthermore, because of muscular imbalance, scoliosis may progress after the child has reached skeletal maturity. Surgical intervention for NMS most often entails instrumentation to the lower lumbar spine or to the pelvis to positively affect balance and sitting tolerance, comfort, and care.

Decision making in collaboration with the patient and family for spinal surgery weighs the potential benefits against the possible risks (prolonged anesthesia, increased blood loss, higher risk of infection and other complications based on underlying NM disease severity, comorbidities, past medical/surgical history, overall patient health, including long-term survival and respiratory function after scoliosis surgery).[34–36] In certain cases, surgical intervention is determined by the parents' perspective on the child's behalf, with health-related QOL measures. The validated tool, Caregiver Priorities and Child Health Index of Life with Disability (CPCHILD), considers the following domains: personal care and activities of daily living; transferring, mobility, comfort; communication and social interaction, general health, overall QOL. A recent therapeutic study (n = 69) demonstrated a significant improvement in CPCHILD scores, with benefits maintained even 5 years after surgery[37] (**Figs. 9** and **10**).

POSTSURGICAL CONSIDERATIONS

Postsurgical management includes monitoring the patient's status: vital signs, neurologic examination, gastrointestinal/gentitourinary function, respiratory function, pain, and surgical site for signs of infection. IS patients are typically ambulating on the first postoperative day and discharged within 4 days. The postoperative care for NM,

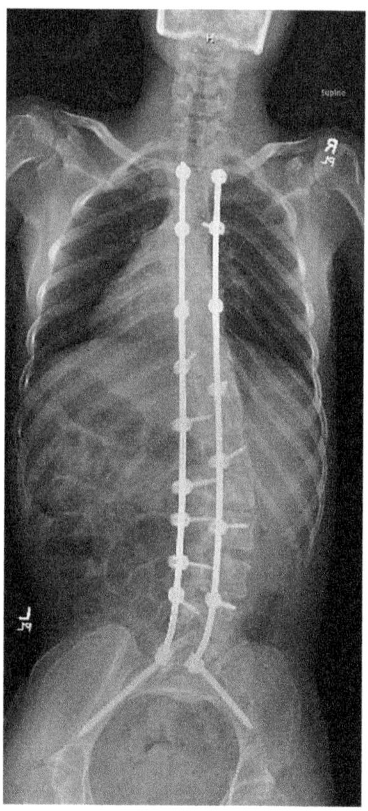

Fig. 9. NM PSF supine AP view. Teen with CP and NM scoliosis with PSF instrumentation from T2 extended to the ilia for pelvic balance.

syndromic, and congenital patients is more variable, but early return to preoperative functional levels is similarly rapid in most patients. Return to preoperative activity levels is commonly limited for 3 to 9 months as bone fusion occurs, yet most patients return to prior levels of activities/sports.

SURGICAL OUTCOMES/COMPLICATIONS REPORTED

The Scoliosis Research Society tracks statistical complication rates for all SD surgeries, including pulmonary, neurologic deficit, and wound infection rates. The reported studies of operative treatment in pediatric SD and incidence of complication rates differed based on scoliosis cause, including IS, NMS, and CS. The reported overall complication rates ranged from 4.4% to 15.4%, 17.9% to 48.1%, and 8.3% to 31%, respectively, with the highest rates in the NM population. Pulmonary complications, although a significant cause of morbidity and mortality in the immediate postoperative period, were relatively low: 0.6% for IS, 1.9% for NMS, and 1.1% for CS.[38,39] These complications are associated with both preoperative and intraoperative factors resulting in issues including atelectasis, pneumonia, pulmonary edema, pulmonary fat emboli, and respiratory failure.

Comparing outcomes of nonambulatory cerebral palsy (CP) patients treated with PSF and cared for using an accelerated discharge (AD) pathway versus a more traditional discharge pathway, a trend toward fewer pulmonary complications in the AD group was noted (21% vs 38%); these included aspiration, pleural effusion, pneumonia, and acute respiratory failure requiring reintubation postoperatively.[40]

Recent metaanalysis of mid- to long-term outcomes demonstrated decreased, and very low, rates of pseudoarthrosis, neurologic deficit and revision surgery, and lower infection rates in AIS patients with pedicle screw constructs (1.18%) after 5 years when compared with higher rates with earlier forms of instrumentation (ie, Harrington rods); however, follow-up of the latter was greater than 27 years.[41]

PULMONARY FUNCTION AFTER SURGERY

Surgical correction with PSF with instrumentation resulted in decreased curve measurement (CA) and stable or small to moderate increases in pulmonary function/increased postoperative thoracic volume in AIS patients.[17,42–44] Pulmonary function and lung volume after surgery may be dependent on fusion length (more restricted as the fusion length increases). Generally, exercise capacity and oxygen consumption (Vo_{2max}) testing in AIS patients were within normal range before and after spinal fusion ($n = 37$).[45] Thoracic deformity is responsible for poor pulmonary function many years after PSF in AIS.[46] PFTs declined 5 years postoperatively for anterior instrumented cases (which used intrathoracic approaches and instrumentation) compared with stable PFTs in the posterior cases (with or without anterior release).[47] Generally, pulmonary volumes normally decline during adulthood (in the mid fourth decade); thus, more long-term follow-up for postsurgical patients is necessary.

FUTURE DIRECTIONS

Evidence-based long-term outcome studies are needed of SD patients with comparisons between surgical intervention (subgroups with variable instrumentation and techniques) versus those conservatively managed. In addition, randomized clinical research trials are required to either validate the current philosophy of pediatric SD treatment decisions or possibly guide alternative strategies for care.

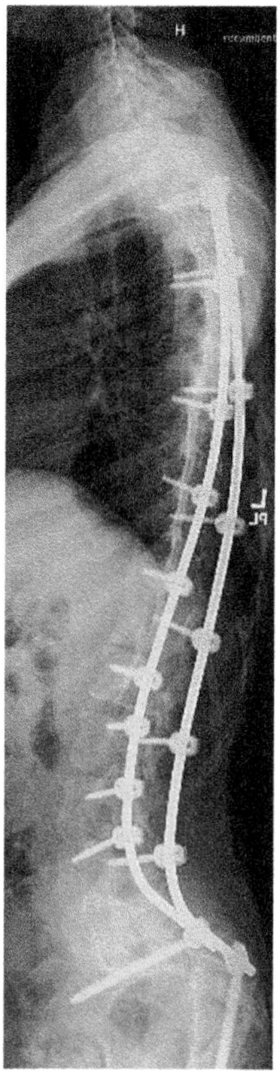

Fig. 10. NM PSF supine lateral view. Same teen with CP and NM scoliosis and PSF, instrumentation, and sagittal balance.

SUMMARY

For children and adolescents with significant scoliosis or kyphosis, patients and families are encouraged to consider the long-term issues involved in the complex decision making regarding intervention with bracing or surgery. The use of a brace has the most proven efficacy to prevent the progression of AIS in skeletally immature patients, yet may have less effect for EOS IIS, JIS NM scoliosis patients, and kyphosis management. Current long-term outcome data support spine fusion treatment in children and adolescents who are surgical candidates, with excellent healing rates (bone fusion) and minimal complication rates. Long-term pulmonary issues are associated with scoliosis, may persist with treatment, and are not necessarily improved with surgery yet fare better than those without intervention (compared with natural history reports).

CLINICAL CARE POINTS

- The forward bend test should be reproducible and reliable in detecting spinal asymmetry. For patients with neuromuscular conditions a modified FBT can be attempted, yet may be less reliable and without evidence based relevance. Thus a comprehensive physical exam can determine the issues (commonly long sweeping C-shaped curves; impacting alignment, function, balance, care and quality of life) associated with scoliosis in this particular population.

- Early identification of idiopathic scoliosis in an adolescent with growth remaining provides a opportunity to utilize a thoracolumbar brace which has been proven to mitigate curve progression.
- Decreased exercise capacity, dyspnea on exertion, and detectable restrictive lung disease are likely to occur with thoracic curves greater than 70 degrees.
- Spinal fusion surgery, which has been performed for decades, combines instrumentation and bone graft to create bone fusion of the vertebrae for long term stability and alignment. In the idiopathic scoliosis population this has been demonstrated to improve long term outcomes including pain and disability when compared to the untreated natural history. In neuromuscular patients, studies have demonstrated sustained improvement in care, comfort and quality of life.
- The surgeon and the family make a shared decision to undertake spinal surgical intervention based upon potential long term benefits to alter the natural history of scoliosis or kyphosis weighed against the risks of complications (anesthesia, blood loss with need for transfusion, infection, failure of instrumentation or fusion and rarely respiratory or neurologic compromise).

DISCLOSURE

The authors have nothing to disclose.

REFERENCES

1. Dunn J, Henrikson NB, Morrison CC, et al. Screening for adolescent idiopathic scoliosis: evidence report and systematic review for the US Preventive Services Task Force. JAMA 2018;319(2):173–87.
2. Weinstein SL. The natural history of adolescent idiopathic scoliosis. J Pediatr Orthop 2019;39(6):44–6.
3. Bettany-Saltikov J, Weiss HR, Chockalingam N, et al. Surgical versus non-surgical interventions in people with adolescent idiopathic scoliosis. Cochrane Database Syst Rev 2015;(4):CD010663.
4. Abdelaal A Kafy E, Elayat M, Sabbahi M, et al. Changes in pulmonary function and functional capacity in adolescents with mild idiopathic scoliosis: observational cohort study. J Int Med Res 2018;46(1):381–91.
5. Eardley-Harris N, Munn Z, Cundy PJ, et al. The effectiveness of selective thoracic fusion for treating adolescent idiopathic scoliosis: a systematic review protocol. JBI Database Syst Rev Implement Rep 2015;13(11):4–16.
6. Hresko MT. Clinical practice. Idiopathic scoliosis in adolescents. N Engl J Med 2013;368(9):834–41.
7. Pahys JM, Guille JT. What's new in congenital scoliosis? J Pediatr Orthop 2018; 38(3):e172–9.
8. Karol LA. The natural history of early-onset scoliosis. J Pediatr Orthop 2019;39(6 Suppl 1):S38–43.
9. Sarwark J, LaBella C. Spinal deformities: idiopathic scoliosis. Pediatric orthopaedics and sports injuries: a quick reference guide. 2nd edition. Elk Grove (IL): American Academy of Pediatrics; 2014. p. 123–36.
10. Etemadifar M, Jamalaldini M, Layeghi R. Successful brace treatment of Scheuermann's kyphosis with different angles. J Craniovertebr Junction Spine 2017;8(2):

136. Available at: https://link-gale-com.turing.library.northwestern.edu/apps/doc/A496317167/AONE?u=northwestern&sid=AONE&xid=d2cda847.
11. Ahmed M, ElMakhy M, Grevittt M. The natural history of thoracolumbar kyphosis in achondroplasia. Eur Spine J 2019;28:2602–7.
12. Fabricant PD, Heath MR, Schachne JM, et al. The epidemiology of back pain in American children and adolescents. Spine (Phila Pa 1976) 2019;1–18. https://doi.org/10.1097/BRS.0000000000003461.
13. Hresko TM, Talwalkar VR, Schwend RM. Position statement - screening for the early detection for idiopathic scoliosis in adolescents. SRS/POSNA/AAOS/AAP Position Statement. 2015. Available at: https://www.srs.org/about-srs/news-and-announcements/position-statement—screening-for-the-early-detection-for-idiopathic-scoliosis-in-adolescents. Accessed March 28, 2020.
14. Brooks JT, Sponseller PD. What's new in the management of neuromuscular scoliosis? J Pediatr Orthop 2016;36(6):627–33.
15. Bouloussa H, Pietton R, Vergari C, et al. Biplanar stereoradiography predicts pulmonary function tests in adolescent idiopathic scoliosis: a cross-sectional study. Eur Spine J 2019;28:1962–9. Available at: https://doi-org.ezproxy.galter.northwestern.edu/10.1007/s00586-019-05940-3.
16. Alexandre AS, Sperandio EF, Yi LC, et al. Photogrammetry: a proposal of objective assessment of chest wall in adolescent idiopathic scoliosis. Rev Paul Pediatr 2019;37(2):225–33.
17. Fujita N, Yagi M, Michikawa T, et al. Impact of fusion for adolescent idiopathic scoliosis on lung volume measured with computed tomography. Eur Spine J 2019;28(9):2034–41.
18. Johnston CE, Richards B, Sucato DJ, et al. Spinal Deformity Study Group. Correlation of preoperative deformity magnitude and pulmonary function tests in AIS. Spine (Phila Pa 1976) 2011;36(14):1096–102.
19. Wang Y, Yang F, Wang D, et al. Correlation analysis between pulmonary function test and the radiological parameters of the main right thoracic curve in AIS. J Orthop Surg Res 2019;14:443.
20. Campbell R, Smith M. Thoracic insufficiency syndrome and exotic scoliosis. J Bone Joint Surg Am 2007;89(Suppl 1):108–22.
21. Dreimann M, Hoffmann M, Kossow K, et al. Scoliosis and chest cage deformity measures predicting impairments in pulmonary function: a cross-sectional study of 492 patients with scoliosis to improve the early identification of patients at risk. Spine (Phila Pa 1976) 2014;39(24):2024–33.
22. Tsiligiannis T, Grivas T. Pulmonary function in children with idiopathic scoliosis. Scoliosis 2012;7:7. Available at: https://link-gale-com.turing.library.northwestern.edu/apps/doc/A298403263/AONE?u=northwestern&sid=AONE&xid=dd35bec1.
23. McPhail GL, Ehsan Z, Howells SA, et al. Obstructive lung disease in children with idiopathic scoliosis. J Pediatr 2015;166(4):1018–21. ISSN 0022-3476.
24. Xue X, Shen J, Zhang J, et al. An analysis of thoracic cage deformities and pulmonary function tests in congenital scoliosis. Eur Spine J 2015;24:1415–21. Available at: https://doi-org.ezproxy.galter.northwestern.edu/10.1007/s00586-014-3327-6.
25. Negrini S, Donzelli S, Lusini M, et al. The effectiveness of combined bracing and exercise in adolescent idiopathic scoliosis based on SRS and SOSORT criteria: a prospective study. BMC Musculoskelet Disord 2014;15:263. Available at: http://www.biomedcentral.com/1471-2474/15/263.

26. Romano M, Negrini A, Parzini S, et al. SEAS (Scientific Exercises Approach to Scoliosis): a modern and effective evidence based approach to physiotherapic specific scoliosis exercises. Scoliosis 2015;10:3.
27. Kuru T, Yeldan I, Dereli EE, et al. The efficacy of three-dimensional Schroth exercises in adolescent idiopathic scoliosis: a randomised controlled clinical trial. Clin Rehabil 2016;30(2):181–90.
28. Fishman LM, Groessl EJ, Sherman KJ. Serial case reporting yoga for idiopathic and degenerative scoliosis. Glob Adv Health Med 2014;3:5.
29. Amaricai E, Suciu O, Onofrei RR, et al. Respiratory function, functional capacity, and physical activity behaviours in children and adolescents with scoliosis. J Int Med Res 2019. [Epub ahead of print].
30. Romano M, Minozzi S, Bettany-Saltikov J, et al. Exercises for adolescent idiopathic scoliosis. Cochrane Database Syst Rev 2012;(8):CD007837.
31. Padhye K, Soroceanu A, Russell D, et al. Thoracoscopic anterior instrumentation and fusion as a treatment for adolescent idiopathic scoliosis: a systematic review of the literature. Spine Deform 2018;6:384–90.
32. Lavelle WF, Moldavsky M, Cai Y, et al. An initial biomechanical investigation of fusionless anterior tether constructs for controlled scoliosis correction. Spine J 2016;16:408–13.
33. Farley FA, Ying L, Jong N, et al. Congenital scoliosis SRS-22 outcomes in children treated with observation, surgery and VEPTR. Spine (Phila Pa 1976) 2014;39(22): 1868–74.
34. Whitaker AT, Sharkey M, Diab M. Spinal fusion in patients with globally involved cerebral palsy. J Bone Joint Surg Am 2015;97:782–7.
35. Cheuk DKL, Wong V, Wraige E, et al. Surgery for scoliosis in Duchenne muscular dystrophy. Cochrane Database Syst Rev 2015;(10):CD005375.
36. Simon B, Roberts SB, Tsirikos AI. Factors influencing the evaluation and management of neuromuscular scoliosis: a review of the literature. J Back Musculoskelet Rehabil 2016;29:613–23.
37. Miyanji F, Nasto LA, Sponseller PD, et al. Assessing the risk-benefit ratio of scoliosis surgery in cerebral palsy: surgery is worth it. J Bone Joint Surg Am 2018; 100(7):556–63.
38. Smith JS, Kasliwal MK, Crawford A, et al. Scoliosis Research Society outcomes, expectations, and complications overview for the surgical treatment of adult and pediatric spinal deformity. Spine Deformity 2012;1(1):4–14.
39. Reames DL, Smith JS, Fu K-MG, et al. Complications in the surgical treatment of 19,360 cases of pediatric scoliosis. A review of the Scoliosis Research Society morbidity and mortality database. Spine (Phila Pa 1976) 2011;36(18):1484–91.
40. Bellaire LL, Bruce RW, Ward LL, et al. Use of an accelerated discharge pathway in patients with severe cerebral palsy undergoing posterior spinal fusion for neuromuscular scoliosis. Spine Deform 2019;7:804–11.
41. Lykissas M, Jain V, Nathan S, et al. Mid- to long-term outcome in adolescent idiopathic scoliosis after instrumented posterior spinal fusion: a meta-analysis. Spine (Phila Pa 1976) 2013;38(2):113-9.
42. Kato S, Murray JC, Ganau M, et al. Does posterior scoliosis correction improve respiratory function in AIS? A systematic review and meta-analysis. Glob Spine J 2019;9(8):866–73.
43. Wozniczka JK, Ledonio CGT, Polly DW, et al. Adolescent idiopathic scoliosis thoracic volume modeling: the effect of surgical correction. J Pediatr Orthop 2017;37(8):e512–8.

44. Duray C, Ferrero E, Julien-Marsollier F, et al. Pulmonary function after convex thoracoplasty in adolescent idiopathic scoliosis patients treated by posteromedial translation. Spine Deform 2019;7(5):734–40.
45. Jeans KA, Lovejoy JF. How is pulmonary function and exercise tolerance affected in patients with AIS who have undergone spinal fusion? Spine Deform 2017;5:416–23.
46. Akazawa T, Kuroya S, Iinuma M, et al. Pulmonary function and thoracic deformities in adolescent idiopathic scoliosis 27 years or longer after spinal fusion with Harrington instrument. J Orthop Sci 2018;23:45–50.
47. Yaszay B, Jankowski PP, Bastrom TP, et al. Progressive decline in pulmonary function 5 years post-operatively in patients who underwent anterior instrumentation for surgical correction of AIS. Eur Spine J 2019;28:1322–30.

Pulmonary Manifestations of Skin Disorders in Children

Bernard A. Cohen, MD[a,*], Nelson L. Turcios, MD[b]

KEYWORDS

• Systemic • Cutaneous • Pulmonary • Genetic

KEY POINTS

- Cutaneous lesions may be associated with lung manifestations.
- Identify pulmonary features of systemic diseases that also affect the skin.
- Recognize the prognostic significance of cutaneous and pulmonary complications of systemic diseases.

INTRODUCTION

Systemic diseases often manifest with cutaneous findings. Many pediatric conditions with prominent skin findings also have significant pulmonary manifestations. These conditions include both inherited multisystem genetic disorders such as yellow nail syndrome (YNS), neurofibromatosis type 1 (NF1), tuberous sclerosis complex (TSC), hereditary hemorrhagic telangiectasia (HHT), Klippel–Trénaunay–Weber (KTW) syndrome, cutis laxa, Ehlers–Danlos syndrome (EDS), dyskeratosis congenita (DKC), reactive processes such as mastocytosis, and aquagenic wrinkling of the palms. This overview discusses the pulmonary manifestations of skin disorders.

YELLOW NAIL SYNDROME

YNS is mostly a disease of early middle age, affecting women more commonly than men by 1.6:1.0[1]; however, neonatal chylothorax has been described in association with YNS. It has also been reported in a male infant born with congenital lymphedema, who developed bilateral pleural effusions and a pericardial effusion at 6 months of age.[1]

The classic clinical presentation includes yellowish nail discoloration and dystrophy (89%), lymphedema (80%), and pleuropulmonary disease (63%).[2] Two of the 3 clinical manifestations are required for the diagnosis. The cause of this syndrome remains unknown, although a few cases seemed to follow episodes of pneumonia. Many cases

[a] Division of Pediatric Dermatology, Johns Hopkins Medical Institutions, 200 N. Wolfe Street, Baltimore, MD 21287, USA; [b] Hackensack Meridian School of Medicine, Nutley, NJ 07110, USA
* Corresponding author.
E-mail address: bcohena@jhmi.edu

Pediatr Clin N Am 68 (2021) 261–276
https://doi.org/10.1016/j.pcl.2020.09.009 pediatric.theclinics.com

have been attributed to congenital lymphatic hypoplasia, similar to that occurring in primary lymphedema.[2] YNS has been associated with numerous malignancies and immunodeficiencies.[1]

YNS is characterized by thickened yellow to green nails resulting from significantly decreased linear nail growth with prominent transverse and longitudinal nail thickening and reduction of cuticle.[3] Nail changes are insidious in onset, bilateral, and affect both hands and feet (**Fig. 1**).

The pleuropulmonary manifestations include pleural effusions and bronchiectasis.[1] Pleural effusion may precede the onset of nail changes by several years. Pleural effusions range from small, unilateral, and asymptomatic to large, bilateral, and recurrent. The fluid may be an exudate or transudate.[2] The pleural effusion may be due to defective lymphatic drainage rather than excess production of pleural fluid. Electron microscopy has revealed the presence of dilated lymphatic capillaries in the visceral pleura, suggesting an obstruction to the lymph drainage.[1] There is also an increased incidence of sinusitis and lower respiratory tract infections in patients with YNS, possibly related to an inherent immunodeficiency.[4] Bronchiectasis affects mostly the upper lobes and the cause is unknown.[1] YNS associated with bilateral cystic lung disease was reported in a 4-year-old girl, which suggests that normal lymphatic drainage is essential for normal lung development.[5]

Other features that have been described in YNS include Raynaud's phenomenon (discoloration of the fingers and/or the toes after exposure to changes in temperature [cold or hot] or emotional events caused by spasm of the blood vessels that diminished blood supply to the local tissues), eyelid lymphedema, fetal hydrops, nephrotic syndrome, pericardial effusions, chylous ascites, intestinal lymphangiectasia, and selective antibody deficiency.[4,6,7] Several cases of YNS in association with cancer of breast, lung, and larynx have been reported. The nail changes are related to lymphatic obstruction, which is caused by the underlying malignancy.

Large, recurrent pleural effusions may require repeated thoracentesis, pleuroperitoneal shunting, chemical or surgical pleurodesis, or pleurectomy.[8] Chylous effusions are more difficult to treat and may require dietary restriction of fat and supplements of medium chain triglycerides.[9] Treatment of the pulmonary disease or malignancy has resulted in resolution of nail changes.

NEUROFIBROMATOSIS TYPE 1

NF1, also called von Recklinghausen's disease or peripheral NF, is a common, autosomal-dominant neurocutaneous disorder. Virtually every organ system may be

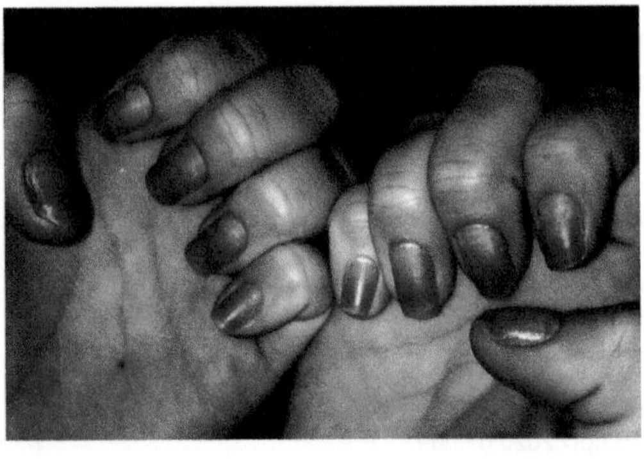

Fig. 1. YNS.

affected. These protean features may be present at birth or in early childhood, but complications are generally delayed for years.[10] Diagnosis is based on established clinical criteria as outlined in **Box 1**.[11]

NF1 occurs in 1:3000 individuals; there is no ethnic or gender predilection. NF1 has a high spontaneous mutation rate (50%) and variable expression with penetrance approaching 100% by age 20.[12] Details of genetic and molecular mechanisms leading to clinical manifestation of NF has been extensively investigated and are readily available (**Fig. 2**).

Pulmonary involvement resulting from NF1 is uncommon and may manifest later in childhood or early adulthood. Pulmonary manifestations include diffuse pulmonary fibrosis, bullous lung disease, pulmonary hypertension, endobronchial neurofibromas, and mediastinal masses.[13–16] When mediastinal lesions are located in the posterior mediastinum, they may present as dumbbell tumors with intraspinal extension. MRI of the involved spinal area is helpful in assessing the anatomic relationships of such tumors. Primary pulmonary neurofibromas are rare. Affected patients typically present with dyspnea on exertion.[16]

Chest radiographs and chest computed tomography scan reveal reticulonodular infiltrates in the bases and bullous lesions in the apices.[17,18] Histologically, alveolar septal fibrosis and alveolitis lead to a mixed obstructive and restrictive lung dysfunction. In 5% of patients with NF1, the neurofibromas, regardless of their location, may undergo malignant degeneration and commonly metastasize to the lungs.[17] Scar cancer of the lung may complicate longstanding NF1 pulmonary involvement.

THE TUBEROUS SCLEROSIS COMPLEX

Tuberous sclerosis is characterized by focal seizures, mental retardation, and characteristic skin findings, such as congenital hypomelanotic macules and facial angiofibromas. Historically, this disease was thought to consist of facial angiofibromas and disabling neurologic disorders, including epilepsy, mental retardation, and autism, but it is now acknowledged to affect many organ systems including the eyes, kidneys, heart, and lungs. Its incidence is approximately 1 in 6000.[19]

TSC is a disorder of cellular differentiation and proliferation that is inherited as an autosomal-dominant trait with variable expression and a high spontaneous mutation rate.[20] Molecular genetic analysis has implicated 2 causal mutations in the genesis of TSC: TSC1 on chromosome 9q34, which encodes hamartin; and TSC2, on chromosome 16p13, which encodes tuberin.[21] Younger patients generally present with neurologic manifestations, whereas pulmonary manifestations are more common in later life.

Box 1
Diagnostic criteria for neurofibromatosis

The patient should have 2 or more of the following:
1. Six or more café-au-lait macules larger than 5 mm in greatest diameter in prepubertal individuals and larger than 15 mm in greatest diameter in postpubertal individuals
2. Axillary or inguinal freckling
3. Two or more iris Lisch nodules
4. Two or more neurofibromas or one plexiform neurofibromas
5. Dysplasia of the sphenoid: dysplasia or thinning of long bone cortex
6. Optic pathway gliomas
7. A first-degree relative with NF1 whose diagnosis was based on aforementioned criteria

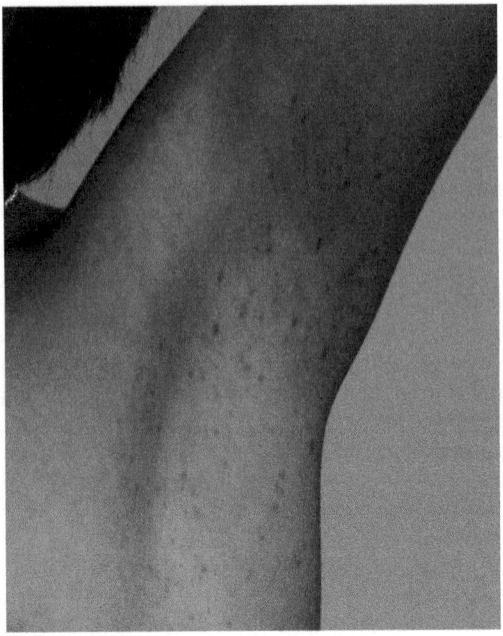

Fig. 2. Axillary freckling.

Pulmonary involvement in TSC is uncommon, typically occurring in adolescent girls or women. Respiratory symptoms include chronic cough, progressive dyspnea, hemoptysis, and recurrent pneumothoraces.[21] Pulmonary involvement is rare in males or children. Pulmonary involvement is extremely rare in males or children. Unilateral lung cysts and a large pneumothorax were described in a 7-year-old boy with TSC.[22] Recurrent acute respiratory distress syndrome secondary to TSC was reported in a 4-year-old boy.[23]

Histopathologically, 2 patterns of lung involvement have been described: lymphangiomyomatosis, also called lymphangioleiomyomatosis, and micronodular pneumocyte hyperplasia/multifocal alveolar hyperplasia. Lymphangiomyomatosis occurs exclusively in women of childbearing age and is characterized by widespread proliferation of abnormal smooth muscle cells surrounding lymphatic and blood vessels and small airways.[24]

Angiomyolipomas may produce generalized cystic or fibrotic changes in the lung and lead to spontaneous pneumothorax. Lymphatic obstruction may cause chylous effusion, and venous obstruction may lead to alveolar hemorrhage and hemoptysis. Bronchiolar obstruction results in air trapping and later lung cyst formation.

Radiographic evidence indicates that the incidence of lymphangiomyomatosis among women with TSC may be up to around 40%.[25] Chest radiographs may be normal or reveal diffuse interstitial lung disease or multifocal cysts. Thoracic computed tomography scan may show variable thin-walled cysts scattered in all parts of the lungs interspersed between normal appearing lung tissue.

Treatment for TSC is symptomatic. Many physical findings are generally stable and nonprogressive such as the pigmentary and connective tissue changes in the skin. Other findings, such as cardiac rhabdomyomas, frequently recede spontaneously.

Therapy for pulmonary TSC is similar to that for lymphangiomyomatosis, which some consider a *forme fruste* of TSC.[24] Hormonal factors may play a role in the pathogenesis of lymphangiomyomatosis and TSC, which is consistent with the typical presentation in premenopausal females and is a potential therapeutic target. Medroxyprogesterone has been recommended when the disease becomes symptomatic or shows deterioration on pulmonary function testing. Oophorectomy, radiotherapy, or a combination of these therapies has shown benefit. Cyclophosphamide has also shown some benefit. Tamoxifen has yielded mixed results to date, and corticosteroids are ineffective. Surgery has a role in pulmonary tuberous sclerosis to obtain a lung biopsy specimen for diagnosis, and to treat complications such as pneumothorax, to excise bullae, and to perform pleurodesis.

Because tumor cells from patients with TSC activate mammalian target of rapamycin, sirolimus—a mammalian target of rapamycin inhibitor—has been identified as a potential therapeutic agent. The results of a clinical trial of sirolimus in patients with TSC and in patients with lymphangiomyomatosis revealed that lymphangiomyomatosis regressed during sirolimus therapy but tended to increase in volume after therapy was stopped. Suppression of mammalian target of rapamycin signaling might constitute an ameliorative treatment in patients with the TSC or sporadic lymphangioleiomyomatosis.[21]

The prognosis for patients with pulmonary TSC is generally one of progressive decline as a result of lymphatic obstruction, alveolar hyperplasia, pleural thickening, and cysts formation. In severe cases, progressive respiratory insufficiency and death may occur.

HEREDITARY HEMORRHAGIC TELANGIECTASIA

HHT, also known as Osler–Weber–Rendu syndrome, is an autosomal dominantly inherited condition with late onset penetrance and variable phenotype, characterized by skin, mucous membranes, and visceral telangiectasias, which represent arteriovenous malformations (AVMs). Recurrent epistaxis is often the presenting symptom and gastrointestinal and genitourinary hemorrhage may present later in life manifesting as iron deficiency anemia. Angiomas of the skin, oral, nasal, and conjunctival mucosa become evident in the second or third decade of life.[26,27] They are bright red, punctate, or linear, and blanch with pressure. See Beth A. Pletcher and Nelson L. Turcios' article, "Pulmonary Manifestations of Genetic Disorders in Children," in this issue.

HHT is the most common cause of pulmonary AVMs. Pulmonary AVMs occur in approximately 30% of affected individuals and may remain asymptomatic for many years.[28] Fistulous vascular communications in the lungs may be large and localized, or smaller, multiple, and diffuse. They are frequently bilateral and have a predilection for the lower lobes.[28] The usual communication is between the pulmonary artery and pulmonary vein; direct communication between the pulmonary artery and the left atrium is extremely rare. Desaturated blood in the pulmonary artery is shunted through the fistula into the pulmonary veins, bypassing the lungs, and entering the left side of the heart. This shunt may result in systemic arterial oxygen desaturation and cyanosis. The shunt across the fistula is of low pressure and resistance so that pulmonary artery pressure is normal; cardiomegaly is not present. The electrocardiogram is normal.

The severity of pulmonary manifestations depends on the magnitude of the right-to-left shunting. Patients may present with dyspnea, exercise intolerance, and polycythemia. Hemoptysis is rare in children, but is the most common presenting symptom in adults. Physical findings may include cyanosis, a systolic or continuous bruit over the site of the fistula, and digital clubbing. Features of HHT occur in about 50% of patients or other family members and include recurrent epistaxis and gastrointestinal tract bleeding.[28] Recurrent epistaxis secondary to telangiectasia of the nasal septa and turbinates is the presenting sign in more than 50% of patients and occurs in 95% at some point during the course of illness. Nosebleeds in patients with HHT, typically spontaneous and often nocturnal, have a mean age of onset of 12 years and a mean frequency of 18 episodes per month.[29] **Box 2** outlines the criteria to establish the diagnosis of HHT.

Chest radiographs may show oval or round, homogenous, nodular opacities from a few millimeters to several centimeters in diameter owing to large fistulas. Pulmonary angiography with contrast usually reveals an artery entering the fistula and a vein leaving it.[28]

Multiple fistulas may be visualized by fluoroscopy as abnormal pulsations, or magnetic resonance with contrast. Selective pulmonary arteriography may be required to confirm site, extent, and distribution of fistulas and may establish the diagnosis in virtually all cases (**Fig. 3**).

In addition to pulmonary complications, patients with HHT may have AVMs of the brain. Brain and systemic abscesses are potentially serious complications in patients with HHT. Brain abscess may be the initial presentation in a patient with previously asymptomatic pulmonary AVM. Forty percent of patients with pulmonary AVMs may present with central nervous system manifestations, such as transient dizziness, diplopia, aphasia, motor weakness, and seizures. These findings may result from cerebral thrombosis, abscess, or paradoxic embolic events.[28] AVMs also may manifest in the gastrointestinal tract, but are more typically seen in the liver. Hepatic AVMs, possibly more common in female patients, can lead to complications including hemorrhage, portal hypertension, and cirrhosis.

Pulmonary hypertension in association with HHT may involve the ALK-1 mutation, resulting in vascular dilatation and occlusion of small pulmonary arteries more typical of idiopathic pulmonary arterial hypertension. External manifestations, including perioral and intraoral telangiectasia, as well as facial and hand involvement, generally occur during the third or fourth decades. Abnormal nailfold capillaries also may be seen. Other complications include high-output congestive heart failure and portosystemic encephalopathy from hepatic AVMs. Disseminated intravascular coagulopathy has been reported in 50% of patients with documented HHT.

Current treatment includes pulmonary artery embolization using coils and other intravascular devices.[30] Multiple embolizations may be necessary in some patients because new fistulas may occur after successful treatment of earlier ones. Although embolization is the initial treatment of choice, large, solitary, or localized pulmonary AVMs may require lobectomy or wedge resection, which usually results in complete resolution of the symptoms.[30] In most instances, fistulas are widespread such that surgery is not possible. If there is a communication between the pulmonary artery and the left atrium, it may be obliterated by division and suture.

Box 2
Diagnostic criteria of HHT

HHT is diagnosed in an individual who meets 3 or more of the following criteria:
- Spontaneous, recurrent epistaxis; nocturnal nosebleeds heighten concern
- Mucocutaneous telangiectasias (tongue, lips, oral cavity, fingers, and nose)
- Internal AVMs (pulmonary, cerebral, hepatic, gastrointestinal, spinal)
- First-degree relative with HHT according to these criteria

A diagnosis is possible or suspected when 2 are present and unlikely when less than 2.

Data from Unger PD, Geller SA, and Anderson PJ. Pulmonary lesions in patients with neurofibromatosis Arch. Pathol. Lab. Med.1984; 108: 654-657.

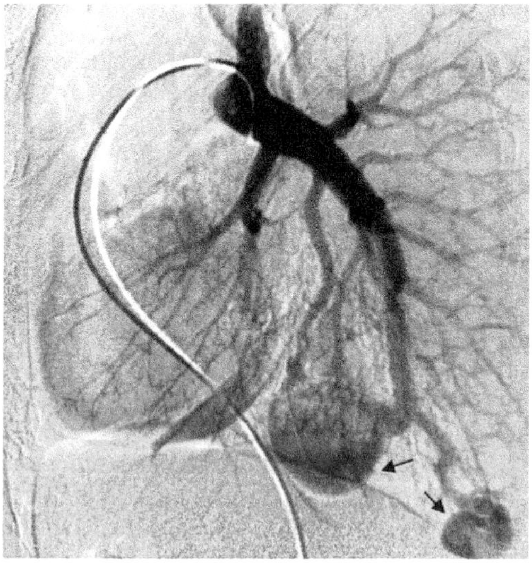

Fig. 3. Pulmonary angiography shows 2 PAVMs with a common feeding artery (*arrows*).

KLIPPEL–TRÉNAUNAY–WEBER SYNDROME

KTW syndrome, or angioosteodystrophy, is a noninheritable disorder that is characterized by extremity capillary–lymphatic malformation, or capillary–lymphatic–venous malformation accompanied by hypertrophy of affected limb. It consists of the triad of cutaneous vascular malformation, venous varicosities, and bony or soft tissue overgrowth. The cause of KTW is unknown, and diagnosis is based on clinical features. Affected patients typically present with a unilateral, lower extremity, extensive "geographic" capillary malformation (port wine stain) at birth that may or may not be associated with congenital ipsilateral extremity overgrowth. Thick-walled venous varicosities typically become apparent ipsilateral to the vascular malformation after the child begins to ambulate. The deep venous system may be absent, hypoplastic, or obstructed resulting in lymphedema. Lymphedema and osteohypertrophy tend to occur later, resulting in limb length and/or girth asymmetry. Pain can result from associated chronic venous insufficiency, cellulitis, superficial thrombophlebitis, and deep venous thrombosis.[31]

Pulmonary involvement is rare; however, recurrent pulmonary thromboembolic events are well-described and may occur in up to 25% of affected patients. Pulmonary embolism in the setting of KTW has been reported in children, but its mechanism is unclear.[32] Recurrent disease may be complicated by chronic thromboembolic pulmonary hypertension and small vessel pulmonary arterial hypertension.[33]

Consideration should be given to estrogen avoidance, aggressive deep vein thrombosis prophylaxis in patients undergoing surgical procedures, and anticoagulation where appropriate. In high-risk patients, venographic evaluation of the pelvic and abdominal venous anatomy may be warranted, and suprarenal filter placement considered.[34]

Surgical correction or palliation is often difficult. Leg length differences should be treated with orthotic devices to prevent the development of spinal deformities. One avenue of research investigation into KTW has focused on the role of vasoactive factors. The angiogenic factor VG5Q has been recently described in KTW patients and may relate to the pulmonary–vascular complications associated with KTW.[35]

CUTIS LAXA (GENERALIZED ELASTOLYSIS)

Congenital cutis laxa is a rare disorder of generalized elastolysis characterized by inelastic, hyperextensible loose, hanging skin with decreased resilience and elasticity, leading to the appearance of loose, prematurely aged skin most prominently in flexural areas.[36] The extracutaneous manifestations include pulmonary emphysema, bladder diverticula, and pulmonary artery stenosis. The disease is inherited most commonly in a severe autosomal recessive form, or as a relatively benign, autosomal dominant form. There is often systemic organ involvement in patients with the autosomal recessive form. Cardiopulmonary abnormalities are common and mainly determine the prognosis and life expectancy.

Pulmonary emphysema owing to a loss of elastic tissue in the lungs is very common.[37] Cor pulmonale and right-sided heart failure generally caused by the pulmonary hypertension are often seen in infancy. Other pulmonary complications reported include pneumothorax, pulmonary fibrosis, recurrent pulmonary infections, bronchiectasis, and tracheobronchomegaly. Various cardiovascular abnormalities including aortic aneurysm, hypoplasia and stenosis of the pulmonary arteries, and pulmonary valve stenosis have been reported in patients with this form of congenital cutis laxa. Several studies suggest a biochemical defect in elastin in cutis laxa.

EHLERS–DANLOS SYNDROME

EDS is a heterogeneous group of inherited disorders characterized by abnormalities in connective tissue. Affected children seem to be normal at birth, but soon they develop skin hyperelasticity, fragility of the skin and blood vessels, and joint hypermobility. Variable clinical presentations may be explained by tissue-specific distribution and different composition of extracellular matrix, including collagen I, III, and V and tenascin-X. as well as enzymes involved in the post-translational modification of collagen; however, the basic defect is a quantitative deficiency of collagen.[38] EDS have historically been classified up to 11 distinct subtypes (types I–XI) based on clinical and molecular features, but it has been recently reclassified in an attempt to simplify the taxonomy. Pulmonary complications have been described in patients with classic subtype EDS (formally known as type I EDS) including spontaneous pneumothorax from bullous lung disease and severe panacinar emphysema, but the vast majority of cases reported in the literature are associated with vascular subtype EDS.[39] EDS-related weakness of the pulmonary arterial wall has resulted in rupture and hemoptysis, and spontaneous dissection of the aorta may occur. Tracheobronchomegaly similar to that in Mounier–Kuhn syndrome, has been reported in a child with EDS.[40] An unusual pulmonary manifestation of EDS consisting of parenchymal cysts and fibrous and fibro-osseous nodules has also been described.[41] These manifestations may be related to an abnormal attempt at repair of parenchymal or vascular tears. Recurrent congenital diaphragmatic hernia in young children has also been reported.[42]

The treatment of EDS-related pulmonary disease includes standard management of pneumothoraces with thoracotomy tubes, pleurodesis, and bullectomy where indicated.[43] Although no good data exist on the lung mechanics of this patient population, if mechanical ventilatory support is required, excessive tidal volumes or ventilatory rates may predispose toward pneumothorax and should be avoided. Patients with vascular subtype EDS tend to succumb prematurely owing to complications associated with arterial rupture.

HERMANSKY–PUDLAK SYNDROME

HPS is an autosomal recessive inherited disorder characterized by oculocutaneous albinism, platelet dysfunction with prolonged bleeding times, and lysosomal accumulation of ceroid-like lipofuscin in the reticuloendothelial system, resulting in granulomatous colitis and pulmonary fibrosis in some cases. In northwestern Puerto Rico, the prevalence is 1 in 1800, with 1 in 22 being carriers of the mutation. See Susan E. Pacheco and James M. Stark's article, "Pulmonary Manifestations of Immunodeficiency and Immunosuppressive Diseases other than HIV," in this issue. There are several subtypes of HPS and affected patients can exhibit a range of cutaneous pigmentary dilution from frank albinism resembling oculocutaneous albinism type I to a pale tan hue with lentigines and freckling.[44] Pulmonary disease, which is common in patients with HPS, usually begins in the third or fourth decades of life and presents with chronic nonproductive cough and progressive dyspnea.[45] It follows a functional restrictive lung disease process quite similar to idiopathic pulmonary fibrosis. The incidence of pulmonary disease is twice as high in women as in men. See Susan E. Pacheco and James M. Stark's article, "Pulmonary Manifestations of Immunodeficiency and Immunosuppressive Diseases other than HIV," in this issue.

Findings on chest radiographs include a reticulonodular interstitial pattern, perihilar fibrosis, and pleural thickening. High-resolution computed tomography scan reveals septal thickening, ground glass opacities, and peribronchovascular thickening.[45] Age older than 30 years and the presence of HPS-1 mutations portend more severe pulmonary involvement, and high-resolution computed tomography findings correlate well with decreasing percentage of forced vital capacity.

Because the associated pulmonary fibrosis is an irreversible, progressive process, symptomatic treatment is the only option. No therapeutic interventions are currently approved by the US Food and Drug Administration for the treatment of HPS and HPS with pulmonary fibrosis. However, 2 antifibrotic drugs, pirfenidone and nintedanib, appear to slow the progression of pulmonary fibrosis in patients with HPS who have significant residual lung function.[46] Intravenous or intramuscular desmopressin injections have improved platelet aggregation in some patients with this syndrome. Patient's response to desmopressin should be evaluated before elective surgical procedures. The report of a child with the characteristic findings of HPS, which often goes unrecognized because of the discrete nature of the cutaneous and hemorrhagic manifestations, highlights the importance of considering this diagnosis because of the risk not only of hemorrhagic, but also of granulomatous colitis and long-term pulmonary fibrosis.[47]

Management of HPS requires lifelong UV light protection, treatment of associated visual impairment, and treatment of any systemic complications arising from end-organ damage. Patients with HPS should wear a medical alert bracelet owing to associated bleeding diathesis. These patients should also avoid the use of nonsteroidal anti-inflammatory drugs or aspirin. Childhood vaccinations should still be given according to the guidelines set forth by the American Academy of Pediatrics. Oral and hormonal contraceptives should be considered to decrease bleeding associated with menstruation.

ERYTHEMA MULTIFORME

Erythema multiforme is a confusing term that has come to encompass a spectrum of disorders ranging from the typically benign, localized erythema multiforme minor, generally confined to the skin, to the more severe Stevens–Johnson syndrome (SJS) and toxic epidermal necrolysis (TEN).

SJS/TEN is a multisystem inflammatory dermatosis that most commonly results from a hypersensitivity response to a medication. Medications associated with SJS/TEN include sulfonamides, penicillin antibiotics, antiseizure medications (phenytoin), and nonsteroidal anti-inflammatory agents such as ibuprofen, pyrazolones, piroxicam, and salicylates. Less commonly SJS/TEN may be associated with infections owing to herpes simplex virus or *Mycoplasma pneumoniae*.

Pulmonary complications are atypical in SJS/TEN.[48] One prospective evaluation found that early pulmonary complications occurred in 27% of cases and usually involved bronchial mucosal sloughing. Other respiratory complications described have included hemoptysis and expectoration of bronchial mucosal casts, pulmonary edema, patchy pneumonic infiltrates, and bronchiolitis obliterans.[49]

Clinical respiratory manifestations include cough, hoarseness, hemoptysis, and dyspnea. Interstitial infiltrates on chest radiograph and diffuse loss of bronchial epithelium in the proximal airways may be seen on bronchoscopy. Bronchial biopsies reveal epithelial necrosis with a mixed mononuclear inflammatory infiltrate. In a recent study, 90% of patients with early pulmonary complications ultimately required ventilatory support and 40% died of complications associated with respiratory failure.[50]

Treatment of SJS/TEN is controversial. Immediate cessation of suspected medications and treatment of potential infectious triggers and supportive therapy are the mainstays. The role of systemic corticosteroids and/or intravenous immunoglobulin is unclear. A number of recent reports have supported the use of intravenous immunoglobulin in adults and children with evolving SJS/TEN if started early in the course of the disease in the absence of renal risk factors.[50]

MASTOCYTOSIS

Mastocytosis is a disorder of mast cells and may develop at any age, but usually occurs in the first weeks to months of life.[51] The cause is unknown. In young children, the disease involves increased mast cells in the skin but rarely other organs. In older children (age at diagnosis >10 years) and adults, it is more likely to be a systemic disease. The most common types in children are solitary mastocytomas, urticaria pigmentosa, and diffuse cutaneous mastocytosis.[51]

With the exception of diffuse cutaneous mastocytosis, pulmonary involvement in any of these forms of mastocytosis is generally not seen. Pulmonary complications have been rarely reported in patients with urticaria pigmentosa and systemic mastocytosis.[52] Radiographic evidence of lung involvement in diffuse cutaneous mastocytosis occurs in 16% to 43% and may include reticulonodular opacities, nodules, and cysts (**Fig. 4**).[53]

Treatment includes avoiding triggers of histamine release when possible. These include sudden weather changes, hot beverages, hot baths, insect stings, mechanical irritation, and certain infections. Drugs known to induce symptoms include but are not limited to alcohol, nonsteroidal anti-inflammatory agents, aspirin, polymyxin B, vancomycin, morphine, codeine, and some local and general anesthetics. Anesthesiologists should be informed of the condition before any surgical procedures to avoid histamine-releasing agents. In addition, a nonsedating H1 blocker may be used for systemic symptoms. More severe symptoms may require a classic (sedating) H1 blocker and/or H2 blockers (good for gastrointestinal symptoms). There is some evidence that treatment with high-potency topical steroids can decrease the reactivity of mastocytomas. If they are causing significant systemic symptoms, solitary mastocytomas may be surgically excised. EpiPens are recommended for patients with

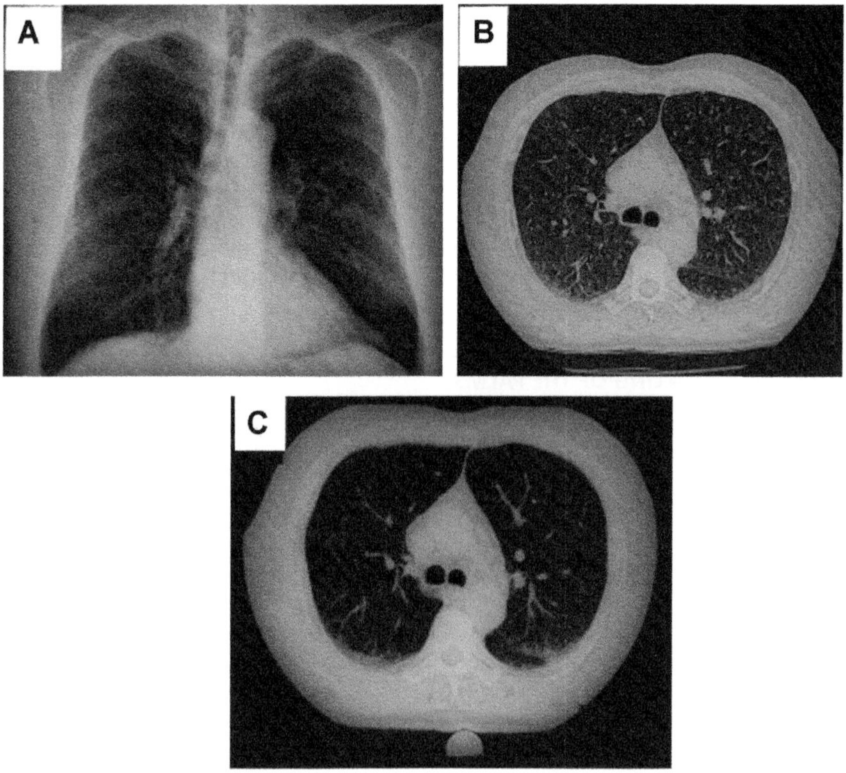

Fig. 4. Chest radiograph on a patient with systemic mastocytosis, (*A*) showing diffuse fine reticular interstitial infiltration pattern of both lungs. Computed tomography (CT) scan of thorax (*B*) shows faint cystic and nodular lesions of lung interstitium as well as mediastinal adenopathy at the time before IFN-α treatment. After 6 months of treatment with IFN-α interstitial lesions of the lung had markedly improved (*C*). (*Adapted from* Kelly AM, Kazerooni EA. HRCT appearance of systemic mastocytosis involving the lungs. J Thorax Imaging 2004;19(1):52-55; with permission.)

extensive disease, although all patients and their parents should be counseled about this possible complication.

DYSKERATOSIS CONGENITA

DKC is a rare inherited condition with multiple systemic manifestations characterized by cutaneous reticulated hyperpigmentation, nail dystrophy, premalignant oral mucosa leukoplakia, and pancytopenia. The inheritance pattern in most cases of DKC is X-linked recessive (caused by mutations in the *DKC1* gene on chromosome Xq28), but autosomal dominant (typically lack classical skin findings) and recessive patterns have been reported. It is also associated with idiopathic pulmonary fibrosis and cryptogenic fibrosing alveolitis.

The mucocutaneous features of DKC typically develop between 5 and 15 years of age. Abnormal skin pigmentation with tan-to-gray hyperpigmented or hypopigmented macules and patches with typical distribution is on sun exposed areas, including the upper trunk, neck, and face. Mucosal leukoplakia occurs on the buccal mucosa and can affect the tongue and oropharynx. There is an increased incidence of malignant neoplasms, namely, squamous cell carcinoma of the skin, mouth, nasopharynx, esophagus, rectum, vagina, and cervix.

Pulmonary disease is present in up to 20% of patients with DKC. Affected patients had a decreased carbon monoxide diffusing capacity and/or a restrictive defect on pulmonary function testing.[54] Pulmonary complications are the second most common cause of death in patients with DKC, about one-half occurring in patients who undergo bone marrow transplant. The prognosis of adults with usual interstitial pneumonia is poor, the majority of patients succumbing within 5 years of diagnosis.[55] Children given a diagnosis of idiopathic pulmonary fibrosis or cryptogenic fibrosing alveolitis often live much longer and have a nonprogressive course, suggesting that they do not have usual interstitial pneumonia.

AQUAGENIC WRINKLING OF THE PALMS

Aquagenic wrinkling of the palms (also known as aquagenic palmoplantar keratoderma) is a rare disorder characterized by exaggerated transient wrinkling of the palms after exposure to water. This condition is commonly found in patients with cystic fibrosis (CF), but may also occur in mutation carriers of the CF gene and has been linked to the p.F508del mutation of the CFTR gene.[56] Other associated conditions have been described including marasmus, atopic dermatitis, hyperhidrosis, and medication related (including selective cyclooxygenase-2 inhibitors, angiotensin-converting enzyme inhibitors, angiotensin-receptor blockers, and nonsteroidal anti-inflammatory drugs).[56] Although the exact pathophysiology of this entity is unknown, it has been associated with a salt imbalance in the skin leading to increased transepidermal water loss.[57]

The cutaneous features of aquagenic wrinkling are characterized by edematous translucent papules often coalescing into plaques that occurs after approximately

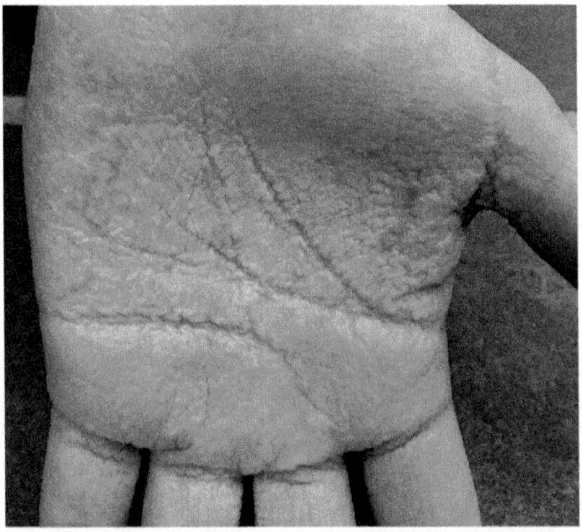

Fig. 5. Mild thickening of the central palms. After immersion of her hands in water for 3 minutes, numerous white translucent papules and marked wrinkling of both palms appeared in an adolescent girl with a longstanding history of transient excessive wrinkling of her palms after brief exposure to water and sweating. She reported some uncomfortable tightness of the skin during these episodes. She was otherwise well and has no significant past medical history. (*Adapted from* Huang AH and Cohen BA. Girl's hands shrivel when exposed to water. Contemporary Pediatrics 2018;35(12):39-40; with permission.)

7 minutes of exposure to water or longer in mutation carriers of the CF gene as compared with 2 to 3 minutes among homozygotes.[58] Lesions may be pruritic or have burning sensation and typically resolve within 10 to 60 minutes of drying.

The diagnosis is often clinical and may be confirmed by immersing hands in water for 2 to 3 minutes, after which the cutaneous findings discussed elsewhere in this article are observed, known as the hand-in-bucket sign. Biopsy is typically not necessary, but when performed may demonstrate orthokeratosis, dilated acrosyringia, and dilated eccrine ostia. Because the diagnosis of CF broadens to include patients with a mild disease phenotype, aquagenic palmar wrinkling may be the initial presenting sign among otherwise healthy patients.

Although no treatments are available that have been approved by the US Food and Drug Administration, previously tried therapies include antiperspirants such as 20% aluminum chloride, botulinum injections, and oral antihistamines to reduce associated symptoms. Patient are advised to avoid exposure to water and humidity (**Fig. 5**).

CLINICS CARE POINTS

- Healthy patient with yellow/green nails should be evaluated for occult pulmonary disease. However, some primary dermatologic disorders and nail infection can present with similar findings.
- Legius syndrome as well as other genetic dermatoses not associated with pulmonary findings should be considered in patients with cafe au lait macules who do not satisfy clinical markers for NF1.
- Erythema multiforme, SJS/TEN, particularly SJS/TEN may be causes by several triggers, and treatment is primarily supportive. However, there is evidence suggesting that TNF-alpha inhibitors may shut down the inflammatory process if administered early in the course.
- Don't forget to demonstrate a Darier sign in a patient with skin lesions suspicious for mast cell disease.
- Aquagenic wrinkling may be a marker for cystic fibrosis or carrier status, buy it may be seen in some primary dermatologic disorders not associated with pulmonary disease.

ACKNOWLEDGMENTS

The authors are deeply grateful to Dr Deepa Patel (JHMI-Medicine) for her outstanding assistance with the literature search, article review, and editing suggestions.

DISCLOSURE

The authors have nothing to disclose.

REFERENCES

1. Vignes S, Baran R. Yellow nail syndrome: a review. Orphanet J Rare Dis 2017; 12:42.
2. Wang M, Colegio OR. Nail changes, lymphedema, and respiratory symptoms. JAAD Case Rep 2019;5(9):773–5.
3. Cecchini M, Doumit J, Konigsberg N. Atypical presentation of congenital yellow nail syndrome in a 2-year-old female. J Cutan Med Surg 2013;17(1):66–8.
4. Bokszczanin A, Levinson AI. Coexistent yellow nail syndrome and selective antibody deficiency. Ann Allergy Asthma Immunol 2003;91:496–500.

5. Sacco O, Fregonese B, Marino CE, et al. Yellow-nail syndrome and bilateral cystic lung disease. Pediatr Pulmonol 1998;26:429–33.
6. El Alami J, Galicier L, Huynh S, et al. Congenital yellow nail syndrome presenting with eyelid lymphedema and fetal hydrops. JAAD Case Rep 2019;5(11):1010–2.
7. Nanda A, Al-Essa FH, El-Shafei WM, et al. Congenital yellow nail syndrome: a case report and its relationship to nonimmune fetal hydrops. Pediatr Dermatol 2010;27(5):533–4.
8. Brofman JD, Hall JB, Scott W, et al. Yellow nails, lymphedema and pleural effusion: treatment of chronic pleural effusion with pleuroperitoneal shunting. Chest 1990;97:743–5.
9. Tan WC. Dietary treatment of chylous ascites in yellow nail syndrome. Gut 1989; 30:1622–3.
10. Gutmann DH, Aylsworth A, Carey JC, et al. The diagnostic evaluation and multidisciplinary management of neurofibromatosis 1 and neurofibromatosis 2. JAMA 1997;278(1):51–7.
11. Alves Júnior SF, Zanetti G, Alves de Melo AS, et al. Neurofibromatosis type 1: state-of-the-art review with emphasis on pulmonary involvement. Respir Med 2019;149:9–15.
12. Ward BA, Gutmann DH. Neurofibromatosis 1: from lab bench to clinic. Pediatr Neurol 2005;32(4):221–8.
13. Trisolini R, Livi V, Lazzari Agli L, et al. Diffuse lung disease in neurofibromatosis. Lung 2012;190(2):249–50.
14. Montani D, Coulet F, Girerd B, et al. Pulmonary hypertension in patients with neurofibromatosis type I. Medicine (Baltimore) 2011;90(3):201–11.
15. Malviya A, Mishra S, Kothari SS. Type neurofibromatosis and Pulmonary hypertension: a report of two cases and a review. Heart Asia 2012;4(1):27–30.
16. Unger PD, Geller SA, Anderson PJ. Pulmonary lesions in patients with neurofibromatosis. Arch Pathol Lab Med 1984;108:654–7.
17. Webb WR, Goodman PC. Fibrosing alveolitis in patients with neurofibromatosis. Radiology 1977;122:289–93.
18. Aughenbaugh GL. Thoracic manifestations of neurocutaneous disease. Radiol Clin North Am 1984;22:741–56.
19. Kliegman RM, St. Geme J, editors. Nelson's textbook of pediatrics. 21th edition. Philadelphia: Elsevier; 2019.
20. Gupta N, Henske E. Pulmonary manifestations in tuberous sclerosis complex. Am J Med Genet C Semin Med Genet 2018;178(3):326–37.
21. Bissler JJ, McCormack FX, Young LR, et al. Sirolimus for angiomyolipoma in tuberous sclerosis complex or lymphangioleiomyomatosis. N Engl J Med 2008; 358:140–51.
22. Bowen J, Beasley SW. Rare pulmonary manifestations of tuberous sclerosis in children. Pediatr Pulmonol 1997;23:114–6.
23. Vicente MP, Pons M, Medina M. Pulmonary involvement in Tuberous Sclerosis. Pediatr Pulmonol 2004;37:178–80.
24. Ryu JH, Moss J, Beck GJ, et al. the NHLBI lymphangiomyomatosis registry: characteristics of 230 patients at enrollment. Am J Respir Crit Care Med 2006;173: 105–11.
25. Franz DN, Brody A, Meter C, et al. Mutational and radiographic analysis of pulmonary disease consistent with lymphangioleiomyomatosis and microdular pneumocyte hyperplasia in women with tuberous sclerosis. Am J Respir Crit Care Med 2001;164:661–8.

26. Westermann CJ, Rosina AF, De Vries V, et al. The prevalence and manifestations of hereditary hemorrhagic telangiectasia in the Afro-Caribbean population of the Netherlands Antilles: a family screening. Am J Med Genet 2003;116A:324–8.
27. Letteboer TG, Mager JJ, Snijder RJ, et al. Genotype-phenotype relationship in hereditary hemorrhagic telangiectasia. J Med Genet 2006;43(4):371–7.
28. Schotland H, Denstaedt S. Hereditary hemorrhagic telangiectasia. N Engl J Med 2019;381:2552.
29. Assar A, Friedman CM, White RI Jr. The natural history of epistaxis in hereditary hemorrhagic telangiectasia. Laryngoscope 1991;101:977–80.
30. Guttmacher AE, Marchuk DA, White RI Jr. Hereditary hemorrhagic telangiectasia. N Engl J Med 1995;333(14):918–24.
31. Lee A, Driscoll D, Gloviczki P, et al. Evaluation and management of pain in patients with Klippel-Trenaunay syndrome: a review. Pediatrics 2005;115(3):744–9.
32. Huiras EE, Barnes CJ, Eichenfield LF, et al. Pulmonary thromboembolism associated with Klippel-Trenaunay syndrome. Pediatrics 2005;116(4):e596–600.
33. Ulrich S, Fischler M, Welder B, et al. Klippel-Trenaunay syndrome with small vessel pulmonary arterial hypertension. Thorax 2005;60(11):971–3.
34. Klippel-Trenaunay Syndrome - Genetics Home Reference - NIH. U.S. National Library of Medicine, National Institutes of Health. 2020. Available at: ghr.nlm.nih.gov/condition/klippel-trenaunay-syndrome. Accessed June 28, 2020.
35. Tian XL, Kadaba R, Sun-Ah Y, et al. Identification of an angiogenic factor that when mutated causes susceptibility of KT syndrome. Nature 2004;427(6975):640–6457.
36. Gara S, Litaiem N. Cutis Laxa (Elastolysis). In: StatPearls [Internet]. Treasure Island (FL): StatPearls Publishing; 2020. Available at: https://www.ncbi.nlm.nih.gov/books/NBK532944/.
37. Hatake K, Morimura Y, Kudo R, et al. Respiratory complications of Ehlers-Danlos syndrome type IV. Leg Med (Tokyo) 2013;15(1):23–7.
38. Harris JG, Khiani SJ, Lowe SA, et al. Respiratory symptoms in children with Ehlers-Danlos syndrome. J Allergy Clin Immunol Pract 2013;1(6):684–6.
39. Dowton SB, Pincott S, Demmer L. Respiratory complications of Ehlers-Danlos syndrome Type IV. Clin Genet 1996;50(6):510–4.
40. Cavanaugh MJ, Cooper DM. Chronic pulmonary disease in a child with the Ehlers-Danlos syndrome. Acta Paediatr Scand 1976;65:679–84.
41. Murray RA, Poulton TB, Saltarelli MG, et al. Rare pulmonary manifestation of Ehlers-Danlos syndrome. J Thorac Imaging 1995;10(2):138–41.
42. Lin IC, Ko SF, Shieh CS, et al. Recurrent congenital diaphragmatic hernia in Ehlers-Danlos syndrome. Cardiovasc Intervent Radiol 2006;29(5):920–3.
43. Safdar Z, O'Sullivan M, Shapiro JM. Emergency bullectomy for acute respiratory failure in Ehlers-Danlos syndrome. J Intensive Care Med 2004;19(6):349–51.
44. Loredana Asztalos M, Schafernak KT, Gray J, et al. Hermansky-Pudlak syndrome: report of two patients with updated genetic classification and management recommendations. Pediatr Dermatol 2017;34(6):638–46.
45. Avila NA, Brantly M, Premkumar A, et al. Hermansky-Pudlak syndrome: radiography and CT of the chest compared with pulmonary function tests and genetic studies. Am J Roentgenol 2002;179(4):887–92.
46. Vicary GW, Vergne Y,A, Santiago-Cornier A, et al. Pulmonary fibrosis in Hermansky-Pudlak syndrome. Ann Am Thorac Soc 2016;13(10):1839–46.
47. Hengst M, Naehrlich L, Mahavadi P, et al. Hermansky-Pudlak syndrome type 2 manifests with fibrosing lung disease early in childhood. Orphanet J Rare Dis 2018;13(1):42.

48. Lee HY, Walsh SA, Creamer D. Long-term complications of Stevens-Johnson syndrome/toxic epidermal necrolysis (SJS/TEN): the spectrum of chronic problems in patients who survive an episode of SJS/TEN necessitates multidisciplinary follow-up. Br J Dermatol 2017;177(4):924–35.
49. Seccombe EL, Ardern-Jones M, Walker W, et al. Bronchiolitis obliterans as a long-term sequela of Stevens-Johnson syndrome and toxic epidermal necrolysis in children. Clin Exp Dermatol 2019;44(8):897–902.
50. Metry DW, Jung P, Levy M. Use of intravenous immunoglobulin in children with Stevens Johnson syndrome and toxic epidermal necrolysis: seven cases and review of the literature. Pediatrics 2003;112(6 Pt 1):1430–6.
51. Wilcock A, Bahri R, Bulfone-Paus S, et al. Mast cell disorders: from infancy to maturity. Allergy 2019;74(1):53–63.
52. Schmidt M, Dercken C, Loke O, et al. Pulmonary manifestations of systemic mast cell disease. Eur Respir J 2000;15(3):623–5.
53. Kelly AM, Kazerooni EA. HRCT appearance of systemic mastocytosis involving the lungs. J Thorax Imaging 2004;19(1):52–5.
54. Khincha PP, Bertuch AA, Agarwal S, et al. Pulmonary arteriovenous malformations: an uncharacterised phenotype of dyskeratosis congenita and related telomere biology disorders. Eur Respir J 2017;49(1). https://doi.org/10.1183/13993003.
55. Utz JP, Ryu JH, Myers JL, et al. Usual interstitial pneumonia complicating dyskeratosis congenita. Mayo Clin Proc 2005;80(6):817–21.
56. Berk DR, Ciliberto HM, Sweet SC, et al. Aquagenic wrinkling of the palms in cystic fibrosis: comparison with controls and genotype-phenotype correlations. Arch Dermatol 2009;145(11):1296–9.
57. Arkin LM, Flory JH, Shin DB, et al. High prevalence of aquagenic wrinkling of the palms in patients with cystic fibrosis and association with measurable increases in transepidermal water loss. Pediatr Dermatol 2012;29(5):560–6.
58. Huang AH, Cohen BA. Girl's hands shrivel when exposed to water. Contemp Pediatrics 2018;35(12):39–40.

Adverse Environmental Exposure and Respiratory Health in Children

Peter D. Sly, AO, MBBS, MD, DSc

KEYWORDS

- Pollution • Household air pollution • Ambient air pollution
- Traffic-related air pollution • Children

KEY POINTS

- Pollution, especially air pollution, is a major cause of childhood morbidity and mortality.
- Due to their different physiology and the way they interact with their environment, children receive a higher relative dose of toxicants in any given environment.
- Two-way interactions exist between ambient air pollution and climate change and these contribute to adverse health outcomes for children.

INTRODUCTION

As reported in the recent *Lancet* Commission on Pollution and Health, pollution killed more people in 2016 than the acquired immunodeficiency syndrome, tuberculosis, and malaria combined.[1] The burden imposed by pollution falls more on those living in low-income and middle-income countries (LMICs) and affects children more than adults. Children are more susceptible to pollution due to their different physiology. Relative to their body weight, children breathe more air (L/kg/d), drink more water (mL/kg/d), and eat more food (calories/kg/d) than do adults.[2,3] They also have a higher surface area–to–body weight ratio than adults. The younger the child, the more pronounced the physiologic differences. As such, children receive a higher dose of toxicant in any polluted environment than do adults. In addition, young children are less likely to be able to detoxify xenobiotics due to immature enzyme systems.[4] Thus, in addition to receiving a higher dose, children are more likely to suffer adverse consequences from the dose they receive.

Children interact with their environment differently from how adults do. This is related to their developmental stage. Infants and young children are likely to spend more time on the floor. The so-called hand-to-mouth behavior, which describes the

Children's Health and Environment Program, Child Health Research Centre, The University of Queensland, Level 7, 62 Graham Street, South Brisbane, Queensland 4101, Australia
E-mail address: p.sly@uq.edu.au

Pediatr Clin N Am 68 (2021) 277–291
https://doi.org/10.1016/j.pcl.2020.09.018 pediatric.theclinics.com

tendency for young children to put their hands, feet, and almost any object they can into their mouth, is not as common for older children or adults.[2,3] The placenta does not provide a barrier to protect the developing fetus from maternal exposures, as once thought. In essence, almost anything the mother is exposed to may cross the placenta and pose a risk to the fetus.[5,6] Many chemicals, especially lipophilic compounds, enter breast milk and expose the breastfeeding infant.[7] These factors result in exposure pathways that differ between children and adults. Children's exposure pathways are shown in **Fig. 1**.

Most air pollution results from incomplete combustion and consists of a mixture of particulate matter (PM) and gases.[2,8] The pollution composition is influenced by many factors, including what is burnt, the temperature and efficiency of the combustion process, and the combustion source (ie, what is doing the burning).[9]

PM generally has a carbonaceous core with various chemicals, metals, or other toxicants adsorbed to the surface. These adsorbed components generally are thought to determine the toxicity of the particles, although black carbon per se may contribute to toxicity.[10] PM is classified by size, determined by measuring the mass median aerodynamic diameter (MMAD). Coarse particles are those with an MMAD greater that 10 μM. These particles generally do not reach the lungs, being filtered out in the nose and upper airway. Particles with MMAD less than 10 μM are referred to as PM_{10} and are mainstream of most air quality monitoring. Respirable particles, that is, those that easily enter the lungs, are those with MMAD less than 5 μM to 8 μM. Fine particles have an MMAD less than 2.5 μM and are referred to as $PM_{2.5}$. Other particle sizes of interest are ultrafine particles (MMAD <1 μM [$PM_{1.0}$]) and nanoparticles (MMAD <0.1 μM [$PM_{0.1}$]). The ability of particles to penetrate into the airway is determined, partly, by their size.

Air pollution also contains gases, such as carbon monoxide (CO), oxides of nitrogen (NOx), sulfur dioxide (SO_2), and volatile organic compounds (VOCs). Ozone (O_3) is a secondary pollutant, formed as a photoreaction between NOx and VOCs (benzene, toluene, and metal traces), in the presence of sunlight. The ability of gases to penetrate the respiratory system is influenced markedly by their solubility, with high water-

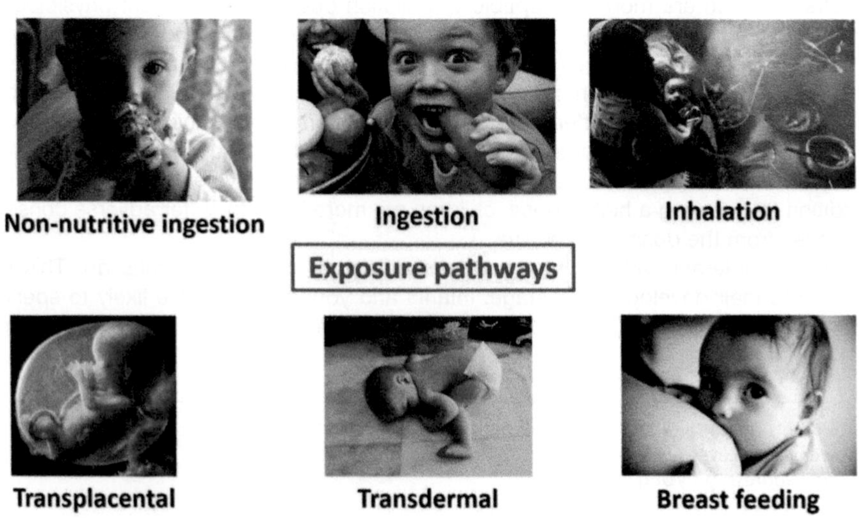

Fig. 1. Schematic representation of pathway by which children are exposed to environmental toxicants.

soluble gases (eg, SO_2) mainly having an impact on mucous membranes in the eyes and nose, whereas gases of lower solubility (eg, NO_2) penetrate deeper into the airway tree. Surface-level O_3 is a toxic pollutant and should not be confused with stratospheric O_3, which provides protection from the sun's UV radiation.

Epidemiologic links between air pollution and adverse health effects are strong; however, the precise mechanisms involved are not clear. The exposure pathways and mechanisms involved in adverse health effects have been reviewed recently[2,8] and are thought to include oxidative stress (OS), a term used when oxidant stimuli overwhelm the antioxidant defenses and cause tissue damage and inflammation.

A relatively recently described combustion product, environmental-persistent free radicals (EPFRs),[11] induces OS and may provide an important link between pollution exposure and adverse health effects.[12] Free radicals are considered to be short-lived, oxidizing whatever they contact within seconds. EPFRs persist, however, in both the environment and biological systems for prolonged periods. EPFRs are found in $PM_{2.5}$ generated from traffic or industrial sources.[13,14] The effects of EPFRs in vitro may be mitigated by antioxidants, providing both information about their mechanism of action and a potential therapeutic approach.

EXPOSURE TO AIR POLLUTION INSIDE THE HOME

The term, *household air pollution (HAP)*, refers to exposure to air toxicants inside the home. The type of toxicants and the adverse health effects, however, depend on the type and location of the housing. The exposure experienced in poor houses in low-income countries is different than those experienced in more affluent housing in high-income countries (**Fig. 2**). By recent convention, the term, HAP, refers to exposures seen in low-income countries, predominantly due to burning unclean, solid, or

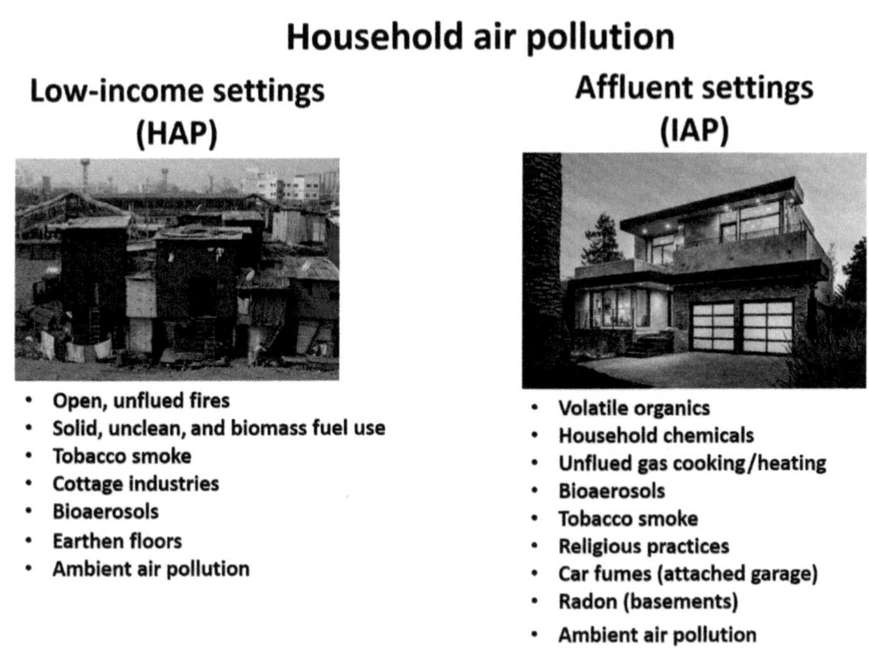

Household air pollution
Low-income settings (HAP)
Affluent settings (IAP)
Open, unflued fires
Solid, unclean, and biomass fuel use
Tobacco smoke
Cottage industries
Bioaerosols
Earthen floors
Ambient air pollution
Volatile organics
Household chemicals
Unflued gas cooking/heating
Bioaerosols
Tobacco smoke
Religious practices
Car fumes (attached garage)
Radon (basements)
Ambient air pollution

Fig. 2. HAP differs with the type and location of housing.

biomass fuels. Air pollution inside more affluent homes in higher-income countries generally is referred to in the literature as indoor air pollution (IAP).

Household Air Pollution

The World Health Organization (WHO) estimates that approximately 3 billion people are reliant on unclean, solid, and biomass fuels for cooking, lighting, and heating. The global distribution of the type of fuel used is not even; those in high-income countries generally use clean fuel, whereas those in LMICs make do with unclean, solid, and biomass fuels (**Fig. 3**). HAP is responsible for 4 million excess deaths per annum from noncommunicable disease and for 50% of pneumonia deaths in children under 5 years of age (**Box 1**). The global distribution of the burden of disease is uneven, with most disability-adjusted life years (DALYS) in children under 5 years of age occurring in LMICs (**Fig. 4**).

Although the primary exposure pathway from HAP is inhalation during the cooking process (see **Fig. 1**), soot and other combustion products also may contaminate food stored within the house. **Fig. 5** shows a house in Central America, where food stored in the rafters to keep it away from vermin is contaminated by soot produced by burning biomass fuel for cooking on an open fire inside the house. Children living in such homes may be exposed to HAP by nutritive and non-nutritive ingestion.

Burning biomass releases PM of various sizes, a variety of gases, including CO, CO_2, methane (CH_4), VOCs, aldehyde, organic acids, and inorganic elements. Factors influencing emission composition include fire temperature—less complete combustion is likely to result in more toxic emissions,[9] in a manner similar to cigarette smoke[15]; types of fuel burnt—burning crop residue results in emissions containing dioxins and furans[16]; moisture content of the fuel; and atmospheric conditions inside the house. Infants and young children are exposed along with their mother, especially during cooking meals. Depending on cultural practices, female children are likely to be exposed to an older age because they stay inside to help with household duties, whereas male children more likely are occupied with outdoor chores.

The adverse health consequences of HAP are vast, affecting the developing fetus, the respiratory system, the cardiovascular/circulatory system, and the brain. Anemia

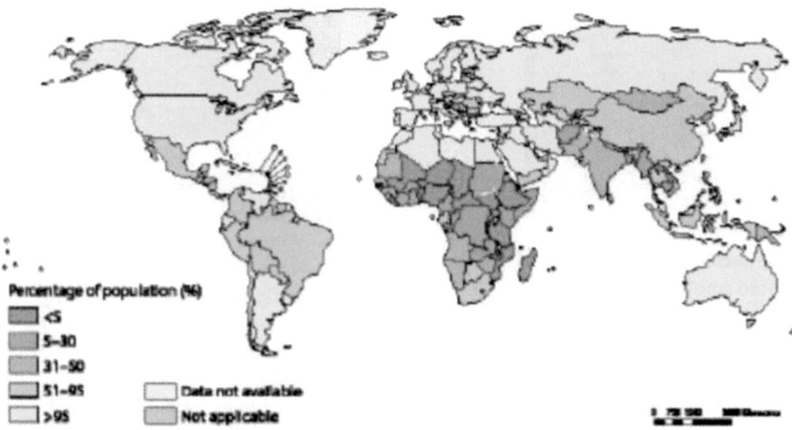

Fig. 3. Percentage of population with access to clean fuel and technology at the household level. (*From* Inheriting a Sustainable World? Atlas on Children's Health and the Environment. Geneva: World Health Organization; 2017 with permission.)

Box 1
Extracts from the World Health Organization fact sheet on household air pollution

HAP and health: WHO fact sheet

Approximately 3 billion people cook on open fires/stoves burning kerosene, biomass, or coal

4 million excess deaths annually attributable to HAP from noncommunicable diseases (stroke, cardiovascular disease, chronic obstructive pulmonary disease, lung cancer) or childhood pneumonia

Approximately 50% of pneumonia <5 y deaths attributable to HAP

From https://www.who.int/news-room/fact-sheets/detail/household-air-pollution-and-health. Accessed 03/19/2020; with permission.

during pregnancy and childhood is more common and more severe in those exposed to biomass emissions[17] (**Fig. 6**). Although the adverse effects on other organ systems are beyond the scope of this article, the effects relevant to children's respiratory health[1,2,8,17–26] are summarized in **Table 1**.

Indoor Air Pollution

As defined previously, exposure to air toxicants inside modern homes in middle-income and higher-income countries generally is referred to as IAP. The sources and toxicants vary from those seen with HAP (see **Fig. 1**). PM, toxic gases, and VOCs are common components of IAP. In many parts of the world, tobacco smoke also is a common component of IAP. In particular, NO_2 from gas cooking and formaldehyde (HCHO) from particle board furniture, glues, and preservatives commonly are found in IAP.[2,8,27] Incense burning, especially as part of home-based religious practices, adds to IAP, with PM and HCHO among the emissions.[28]

The extent to which pollutants from external sources, such as industry[29] or traffic, contribute to IAP is not well characterized. Certainly, children in La Plata, Argentina, living near major petrochemical production facilities were exposed to higher levels of VOCs inside their home.[29] On first principles, it would be expected that penetration

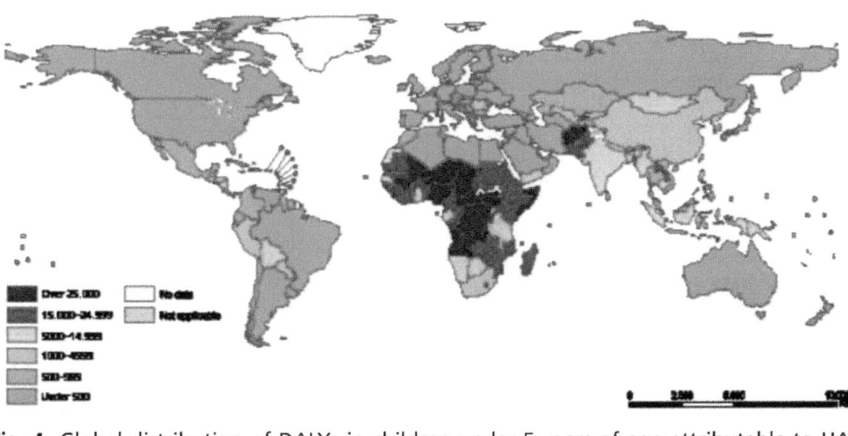

Fig. 4. Global distribution of DALYs in children under 5 years of age attributable to HAP. (*From* World Health Organization. Inheriting a Sustainable World? Atlas on Children's Health and the Environment. Geneva: World Health Organization; 2017, with permission.)

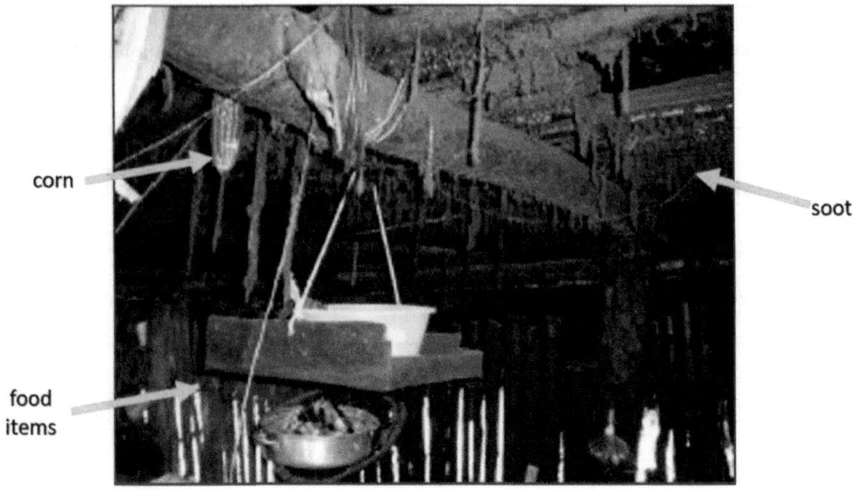

Fig. 5. Contamination of food stored in the rafters by soot from burning biomass fuel for cooking on an open fire. (*Courtesy of* Professor F. Diaz Barriga, MA, PhD, San Luis Potosí, Mexico.)

of outdoor pollutants into homes to be greater in summer and where windows are regularly open and lower in winter and where air conditioners are used.[27]

The exposure pathways, mechanisms involved, and adverse health consequences of IAP are qualitatively similar to those associated with HAP. There is more literature examining associations between IAP and asthma inception and exacerbation than with HAP.[2,8,27,30] Exposure to tobacco smoke inside the home increases the rate of allergic sensitization[31] and the risk and severity of childhood asthma.[32,33] The literature relating IAP to wheeze and adverse respiratory outcomes in children is inconsistent, with not all studies finding strong associations.[34] Some of this may relate to the individual child's antioxidant defense capacity because those with null mutations in

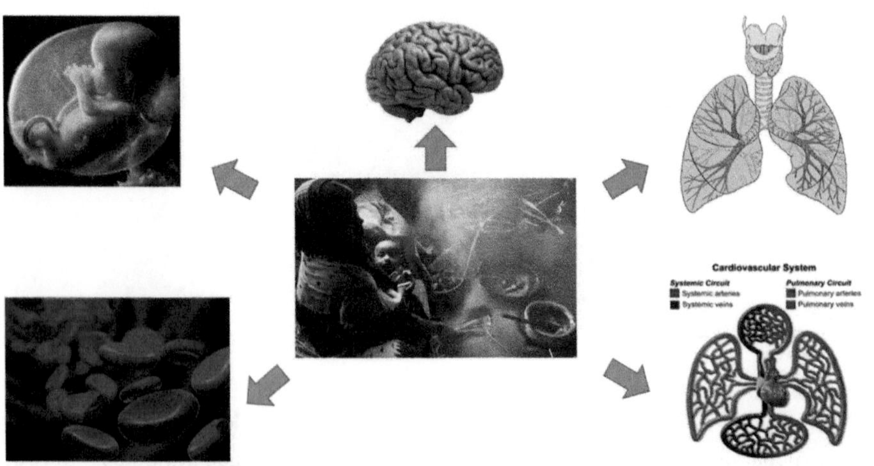

Fig. 6. Schematic representation of the organs systems adversely affected by exposure to biomass emission in HAP.

Table 1
Adverse respiratory health consequences from household air polution exposure related to age at exposure

Exposure Period	Proposed Mechanisms	Intermediator Effect	Health Consequence
Fetal development	Maternal inflammation OS Epigenetic changes Direct particulate damage	Poor placental function Reduced lung growth Delayed immune maturation	Low birthweight/IUGR Low lung function at birth Increased infection risk/pneumonia Lifelong increased risk of COPD, lung cancer
Infancy	Direct particulate damage Systemic inflammation OS DNA damage Epigenetic changes	Anemia Poor lung growth Delayed immune maturation	Respiratory infections/ pneumonia Lifelong increased risk of COPD, lung cancer
Childhood	Direct particulate damage Systemic inflammation OS DNA damage Epigenetic changes	Anemia Reduced lung function Delayed immune maturation	Respiratory infections/ pneumonia Lifelong increased risk of COPD, lung cancer

Abbreviations: COPD, chronic obstructive pulmonary disease; IUGR, intrauterine growth restriction.
Refs.[1,2,8,17–26]

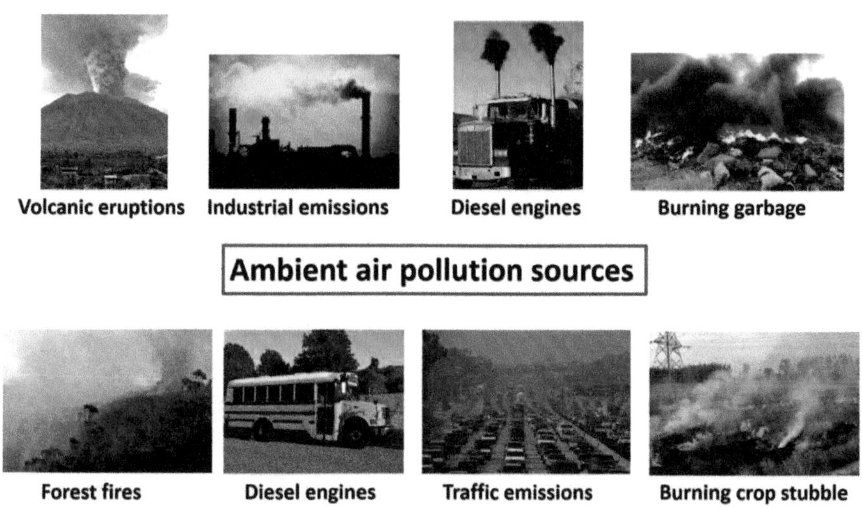

Fig. 7. Sources contributing to ambient air pollution.

Table 2
Air quality standards: guidelines of allowable exposure to criteria air pollutants set by the US Environmental Protection Agency and the World Health Organization

	US Environmental Protection Agency		World Health Organization		
Pollutant	Averaging Time		Averaging Time		Comment
CO	9 ppm 8-h mean (1°)	35 ppm 1-h mean (1°)	Not provided	Not provided	
PM_{10}	150 μg/m^3 24-h mean[a] (1°+ 2°)		20 μg/m^3 annual mean	50 μg/m^3 24-h mean	[a] Averaged over 3 y
$PM_{2.5}$	12 μg/m^3 annual mean[a] (1°) 15 μg/m^3 annual mean[a] (2°)	35 μg/m^3 24-h mean**	10 μg/m^3 annual mean	25 μg/m^3 24-h mean	** 98th percentile, averaged over 3 y
O_3	70 ppb 8-h mean (1°+ 2°)		100 μg/m^3 8-h mean		
NO_2	53 ppb annual mean (1°+ 2°)	100 ppb 1-h mean (1°)**	40 μg/m^3 annual mean	200 μg/m^3 1-h mean	** 98th percentile, averaged over 3 y
SO_2	500 ppb 3-hourly mean (2°)	75 ppb (1°)***	20 μg/m^3 24-h mean	500 μg/m^3 10-min mean	***99th percentile, averaged over 3y

Abbreviations: 1°, primary standards provide public health protection, including protecting the health of "sensitive" populations, such as asthmatics, children, and the elderly; 2°, secondary standards provide public welfare protection, including protection against decreased visibility and damage to animals, crops, vegetation, and buildings; ppb, parts per billion by volume; ppm, parts per million by volume.

[a] WHO guidelines published 2005 with update anticipated in 2020.

Data from Criteria Air Pollutants. EPA. https://www.epa.gov/criteria-air-pollutants. Published March 8, 2018. Accessed March 24, 2020 and Ambient (outdoor) air pollution. World Health Organization. https://www.who.int/news-room/fact-sheets/detail/ambient-(outdoor)-air-quality-and-health. Accessed March 24, 2020.

glutathione-S-transferase enzymes are more susceptible to pollution exposure.[35] These data are consistent with the notion that induction of OS stress is an important mechanism mediating the adverse health effects of IAP.

EXPOSURE TO AIR POLLUTION OUTSIDE THE HOME

Multiple sources contribute to outdoor air pollution. As for HAP and IAP, most ambient air pollution comes from incomplete combustion of fossil fuels. Natural sources, however, also may contribute to ambient air pollution (**Fig. 7**).

By legislation, the US Environmental Protection Agency (EPA) monitors 6 key pollutants in ambient air: lead, PM, CO, NO_2, SO_2, and O_3. These criteria pollutants have national air quality standards set by legislation that define allowable concentrations in ambient air. The WHO and many countries also set allowable exposure levels, with little consistency. **Table 2** shows allowable exposures to criteria pollutants set by the WHO and the EPA.

The global distribution of air pollution is not even, with higher exposures in mega cities in LMICs. **Fig. 8** shows the global distribution of $PM_{2.5}$, with substantially higher levels seen in South Asia and Southeast Asia.

Air pollution exposure has negative impacts on respiratory health. Traffic-related air pollution (TRAP) exposure during childhood is associated with an increased risk of respiratory infections of greater severity[2,36]; lower lung function and reduced lung growth[37,38]; and wheezing illnesses, incident asthma, and asthma exacerbations.[30,39] Accumulating evidence suggests that TRAP exposure induces OS in humans. Children exposed to high levels of TRAP in Mexico City had increased levels of malondialdehyde, an OS-induced product of lipid peroxidation, in exhaled breath condensates.[39] Subjects with null or reduced function mutations in antioxidant defense genes, such as GSTP1, showed increased susceptibility to TRAP exposure,[40] and asthma was more likely in children with TRAP exposure if they showed increased expression of the redox-sensitive transcription factor, NFE2L2 (NRF2) gene.[41]

Acute exposure to TRAP increases respiratory symptoms in children on the day of exposure and with lags of 1 day or 2 days.[42] Increased TRAP levels are associated

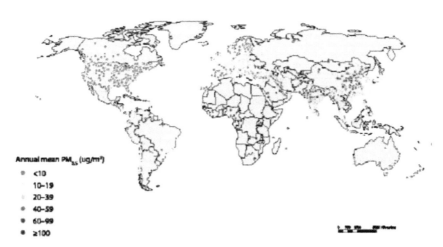

Fig. 8. Global distribution of $PM_{2.5}$ in urban locations. (*From* Inheriting a Sustainable World? Atlas on Children's Health and the Environment. Geneva: World Health Organization; 2017 with permission.)

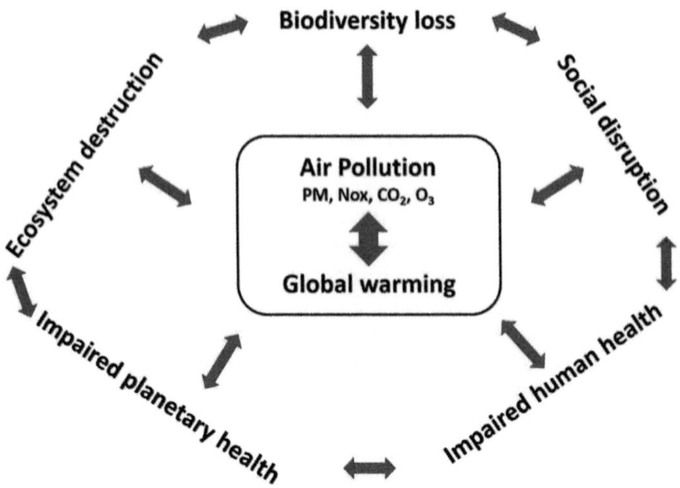

Fig. 9. Schematic representation of the impacts of air pollution and climate change on human and planetary health.

with an increase in school absences for respiratory illnesses, with a peak occurring 5 days after increased O_3 exposure.[43] Sexual dimorphism may occur in TRAP responsiveness, with girls more sensitive in some[44] but not all studies.[45,46] Socioeconomic status also influences the outcomes of TRAP exposure, although not always in a consistent direction.[29,47] Children with asthma generally are more sensitive to TRAP, with increased symptoms, asthma exacerbations, and declines in lung function.[29] Exposure to petrochemical-related VOCs may be dangerous especially for asthmatics.[29]

IMPACT OF CLIMATE CHANGE ON CHILDREN'S RESPIRATORY HEALTH

The link between air pollution and climate change is intricate and obvious. Air pollution increases atmospheric CO_2, which, in turn, induces global warming and climate change[48] (**Fig. 9**). Global warming and climate change increase air pollution, although

Box 2
Extracts from World Health Organization climate change and health

Climate change and health: WHO fact sheet

Climate change adversely affects the social and environmental determinant of disease

Approximately 50,000 excess deaths per year expected (2030–2050) from malnutrition, malaria, diarrhea, and heat stress

Direct costs to health—$2–$4 billion per year by 2030

Countries with weak health infrastructure worse affected

Reducing greenhouse gas emissions can improve health outcomes

From Climate change and health. World Health Organization. https://www.who.int/news-room/fact-sheets/detail/climate-change-and-health. Accessed March 19, 2020.; with permission.

Table 3
Links between climate change and adverse respiratory health outcomes in children

Climate Change Impact	Pathway	Adverse Effect on Children's Respiratory Health
Increased ambient temperature	Urban heat island effects Heat waves Increased temperature variability Altered plant distribution, longer growing seasons and increased pollen production Crop failure and food insecurity	Heat stress Electrolyte disturbance in cystic fibrosis Increased allergic sensitization Increased allergic rhinitis and asthma exacerbations
Decreased air quality	Higher PM Increased surface level O_3 Air stagnation Rising CO_2	Reduced fetal growth and birthweight Lower lung function and lung function growth Altered lung growth and increased bronchial responsiveness Increased incident asthma and asthma exacerbations Increased hospitalization for respiratory illnesses Increased pulmonary infection with serous pathogens in cystic fibrosis
Rising CO_2	Altered plant distribution, longer growing seasons and increased pollen production	Increased allergic rhinitis and asthma exacerbations
Altered rainfall distribution	Altered distribution of disease vectors Crop failure and food insecurity Water insecurity	Altered distribution of vector-borne disease Malnutrition, stunting, and increased susceptibility to respiratory infections
Ocean warming/sea level rise	Severe weather events Drought, floods, cyclones, bushfires Crop failure and food insecurity Water insecurity Population displacement	Increased respiratory infections, asthma exacerbations, emergency department presentations, and hospitalization for respiratory illnesses Increased non–tuberculosis mycobacterium infection Increased chemical exposure Malnutrition, stunting, and increased susceptibility to respiratory infections Adverse mental health outcomes

the precise effect anticipated varies with geographic location.[49] Modeling predicts marked deterioration in air quality over the rest of the twenty-first century, with increases in PM,[49] increases in surface-level O_3,[50] changes in relative humidity,[49] and air stagnation.[51,52]

The WHO predicts an additional 250,000 deaths per year between 2030 and 2050 due to malnutrition, malaria, diarrheal diseases, and heat stress directly attributable to climate change, with direct health costs of between $2 billion to $4 billion per year by 2030 (**Box 2**).

The potential impacts of climate change on respiratory health of children are shown in Table 14.3. Mechanisms include adverse effects on fetal growth and birthweight; increasing lifelong risk of acute and chronic respiratory disease[53–56]; low lung function at birth and decreased lung function growth[19,20]; and increased risk of respiratory infection, including pneumonia, under 5 years of age.[48,57] Climate change–induced increases in surface level O_3[58,59] and in wildfire smoke[60] are predicted to increase health care utilization and hospitalization for asthma and acute respiratory illnesses in children (**Table 3**).

Climate change does represent an opportunity for physicians and gives them a responsibility to act. The American College of Physicians has produced a position paper urging all physician to act[61] and recommends that physicians engage in environmentally sustainable practices that reduce carbon emissions; support efforts to mitigate and adapt to effects of climate change; and educate the public, their colleagues, and lawmakers about the human health risks of climate change, especially respiratory health.

DISCLOSURE

The author has nothing to disclose.

REFERENCES

1. Landrigan PJ, Fuller R, Fisher S, et al. Pollution and children's health. Sci Total Environ 2019;650:2389–94.
2. Goldizen FC, Sly PD, Knibbs LD. Respiratory effects of air pollution on children. Pediatr Pulmonol 2015;51:94–108.
3. Miller MD, Marty MA, Arcus A, et al. Differences Between Children and Adults: Implications for Risk Assessment at California EPA. Int J Toxicol 2002;21:403–18.
4. Ginsberg G, Hattis D, Sonawane B, et al. Evaluation of child/adult pharmacokinetic differences from a database derived from the therapeutic drug literature. Toxicol Sci 2002;66(2):185–200.
5. Aengenheister L, Dugershaw BB, Manser P, et al. Investigating the accumulation and translocation of titanium dioxide nanoparticles with different surface modifications in static and dynamic human placental transfer models. Eur J Pharm Biopharm 2019;142:488–97.
6. Sakamoto M, Chan HM, Domingo JL, et al. Placental transfer and levels of mercury, selenium, vitamin E, and docosahexaenoic acid in maternal and umbilical cord blood. Environ Int 2018;111:309–15.
7. LaKind JS, Berlin CM, Naiman DQ. Infant exposure to chemicals in breast milk in the United States: what we need to learn from a breast milk monitoring program. Environ Health Perspect 2001;109:75–88.
8. Schraufnagel DE, Balmes JR, Cowl CT, et al. Air Pollution and Noncommunicable Diseases: A Review by the Forum of International Respiratory Societies'

Environmental Committee, Part 1: The Damaging Effects of Air Pollution. Chest 2019;155:409–16.
9. Yadav IC, Devi NL. Biomass Burning, Regional Air Quality, and Climate Change. In: Nriagu J, editor. Encyclopedia of environmental health. 2nd edition. Oxford: Elsevier; 2019. p. 386–91.
10. Kulkarni N, Pierse N, Rushton L, et al. Carbon in airway macrophages and lung function in children. New Engl J Med 2006;355:21–30.
11. Dellinger B, Lomnicki S, Khachatryan L, et al. Formation and stabilization of persistent free radicals. Proc Combust Inst 2007;31:521–8.
12. Sly PD, Cormier SA, Lomnicki S, et al. Environmentally Persistent Free Radicals: Linking Air Pollution and Poor Respiratory Health? Am J Respir Crit Care Med 2019;200:1062–3.
13. Gehling W, Dellinger B. Environmentally persistent free radicals and their lifetimes in PM2.5. Environ Sci Technol 2013;47:8172–8.
14. Gehling W, Khachatryan L, Dellinger B. Hydroxyl radical generation from environmentally persistent free radicals (EPFRs) in PM2.5. Environ Sci Technol 2014;48: 4266–72.
15. Moir D, Rickert WS, Levasseur G, et al. A comparison of mainstream and sidestream marijuana and tobacco cigarette smoke produced under two machine smoking conditions. Chem Res Toxicol 2008;21:494–502.
16. Zhang Q, Huang J, Yu G. Polychlorinated dibenzo-p-dioxins and dibenzofurans emissions from open burning of crop residues in China between 1997 and 2004. Environ Pollut 2008;151:39–46.
17. Page CM, Patel A, Hibberd PL. Does smoke from biomass fuel contribute to anemia in pregnant women in Nagpur, India? A cross-sectional study. PloS one 2015; 10:e0127890.
18. Jayaraj NP, Rathi A, Taneja DK. Exposure to Household Air Pollution During Pregnancy and Birthweight. Indian Pediatr 2019;56:875–6.
19. Korten I, Ramsey K, Latzin P. Air pollution during pregnancy and lung development in the child. Paediatric Respir Rev 2017;21:38–46.
20. Latzin P, Roosli M, Huss A, et al. Air pollution during pregnancy and lung function in newborns: a birth cohort study. Eur Respir J 2009;33:594–603.
21. Nandasena S, Wickremasinghe AR, Sathiakumar N. Indoor air pollution and respiratory health of children in the developing world. World J Clin Pediatr 2013; 2:6–15.
22. Qian Z, Zhang B, Liang S, et al. Ambient Air Pollution and Adverse Pregnancy Outcomes in Wuhan, China. Res Rep Health Eff Inst 2016;189:1–65.
23. Rana J, Uddin J, Peltier R, et al. Associations between Indoor Air Pollution and Acute Respiratory Infections among Under-Five Children in Afghanistan: Do SES and Sex Matter? Int J Environ Res Public Health 2019;16:2910.
24. Ranathunga N, Perera P, Nandasena S, et al. Effect of household air pollution due to solid fuel combustion on childhood respiratory diseases in a semi urban population in Sri Lanka. BMC Pediatr 2019;19:306.
25. Sood A, Assad NA, Barnes PJ, et al. ERS/ATS workshop report on respiratory health effects of household air pollution. Eur Respir J 2018;51 [pii:1700698].
26. Yang S-I, Kim H-B, Kim H-C, et al. Particulate matter at third trimester and respiratory infection in infants, modified by GSTM1. Pediatr Pulmonology 2020;55: 245–53.
27. Franklin P, Holt PG, Stick SM, et al. The impact of the indoor environment on the development of allergic sensitization and asthma in children. Australas Epidemiol 2001;8:27–32.

28. Zhang Z, Tan L, Huss A, et al. Household incense burning and children's respiratory health: A cohort study in Hong Kong. Pediatr Pulmonol 2019;54:399–404.
29. Wichmann FA, Müller A, Busi LE, et al. Increased asthma and respiratory symptoms in children exposed to petrochemical pollution. J Allergy Clin Immunol 2009; 123:632–8.
30. Hehua Z, Qing C, Shanyan G, et al. The impact of prenatal exposure to air pollution on childhood wheezing and asthma: A systematic review. Environ Res 2017; 159:519–30.
31. Feleszko W, Ruszczynski M, Jaworska J, et al. Environmental tobacco smoke exposure and risk of allergic sensitisation in children: a systematic review and meta-analysis. Arch Dis Child 2014;99:985–92.
32. Farber HJ, Batsell RR, Silveira EA, et al. The Impact of Tobacco Smoke Exposure on Childhood Asthma in a Medicaid Managed Care Plan. Chest 2016;149(3): 721–8.
33. Makadia LD, Roper PJ, Andrews JO, et al. Tobacco Use and Smoke Exposure in Children: New Trends, Harm, and Strategies to Improve Health Outcomes. Curr Allergy Asthma Rep 2017;17:55.
34. Patelarou E, Tzanakis N, Kelly FJ. Exposure to indoor pollutants and Wheeze and asthma development during early childhood. Int J Environ Res Public Health 2015;12:3993–4017.
35. Dai X, Bowatte G, Lowe AJ, et al. Do Glutathione S-Transferase Genes Modify the Link between Indoor Air Pollution and Asthma, Allergies, and Lung Function? A Systematic Review. Curr Allergy Asthma Rep 2018;18:20.
36. Stern G, Latzin P, Roosli M, et al. A prospective study of the impact of air pollution on respiratory symptoms and infections in infants. Am J Respir Crit Care Med 2013;187(12):1341–8.
37. Boeyen J, Callan AC, Blake D, et al. Investigating the relationship between environmental factors and respiratory health outcomes in school children using the forced oscillation technique. Int J Hyg Environ Health 2017;220:494–502.
38. Schultz ES, Gruzieva O, Bellander T, et al. Traffic-related air pollution and lung function in children at 8 years of age: a birth cohort study. Am J Respir Crit Care Med 2012;186:1286–91.
39. Romieu I, Barraza-Villarreal A, Escamilla-Nunez C, et al. Exhaled breath malondialdehyde as a marker of effect of exposure to air pollution in children with asthma. J Allergy Clin Immunol 2008;121:903–9.e6.
40. MacIntyre EA, Brauer M, Melen E, et al. GSTP1 and TNF Gene variants and associations between air pollution and incident childhood asthma: the traffic, asthma and genetics (TAG) study. Environ Health Perspect 2014;122:418–24.
41. Ungvari I, Hadadi E, Virag V, et al. Relationship between air pollution, NFE2L2 gene polymorphisms and childhood asthma in a Hungarian population. J Community Genet 2012;3:25–33.
42. Spira-Cohen A, Chen LC, Kendall M, et al. Personal exposures to traffic-related air pollution and acute respiratory health among Bronx schoolchildren with asthma. Environ Health Perspect 2011;119:559–65.
43. Gilliland FD, Berhane K, Rappaport EB, et al. The effects of ambient air pollution on school absenteeism due to respiratory illnesses. Epidemiology 2001;12: 43–54.
44. MacIntyre CR, Chughtai AA. Facemasks for the prevention of infection in healthcare and community settings. BMJ 2015;350:h694.
45. Kulkarni N, Cooke MS, Grigg J. Neutrophils in induced sputum from healthy children: role of interleukin-8 and oxidative stress. Respir Med 2007;101:2108–12.

46. Luong LM, Phung D, Sly PD, et al. The association between particulate air pollution and respiratory admissions among young children in Hanoi, Vietnam. Sci Total Environ 2017;578:249–55.
47. Rosenlund M, Forastiere F, Porta D, et al. Traffic-related air pollution in relation to respiratory symptoms, allergic sensitisation and lung function in schoolchildren. Thorax 2009;64:573–80.
48. Mirsaeidi M, Motahari H, Taghizadeh Khamesi M, et al. Climate Change and Respiratory Infections. Ann Am Thorac Soc 2016;13(8):1223–30.
49. Fang Y, Mauzerall DL, Liu J, et al. Impacts of 21st century climate change on global air pollution-related premature mortality. Climatic Change 2013;121: 239–53.
50. Fann N, Nolte CG, Dolwick P, et al. The geographic distribution and economic value of climate change-related ozone health impacts in the United States in 2030. J Air Waste Management Assoc 2015;65:570–80.
51. Horton DE, Skinner CB, Singh D, et al. Occurrence and persistence of future atmospheric stagnation events. Nat Clim Change 2014;4:698–703.
52. Lai LW. Public health risks of prolonged fine particle events associated with stagnation and air quality index based on fine particle matter with a diameter <2.5 mum in the Kaoping region of Taiwan. Int J Biometeorol 2016;60:1907–17.
53. Aguilera I, Garcia-Esteban R, Iniguez C, et al. Prenatal exposure to traffic-related air pollution and ultrasound measures of fetal growth in the INMA Sabadell cohort. Environ Health Perspect 2010;118:705–11.
54. Clemens T, Turner S, Dibben C. Maternal exposure to ambient air pollution and fetal growth in North-East Scotland: A population-based study using routine ultrasound scans. Environ Int 2017;107:216–26.
55. Llop S, Ballester F, Estarlich M, et al. Preterm birth and exposure to air pollutants during pregnancy. Environ Res 2010;110:778–85.
56. Zhao N, Qiu J, Ma S, et al. Effects of prenatal exposure to ambient air pollutant PM10 on ultrasound-measured fetal growth. Int J Epidemiol 2018;47:1072–81.
57. Paynter S, Ware RS, Weinstein P, et al. Childhood pneumonia: a neglected, climate-sensitive disease? Lancet 2010;376:1804–5.
58. Luong LMT, Phung D, Dang TN, et al. Seasonal association between ambient ozone and hospital admission for respiratory diseases in Hanoi, Vietnam. PLoS One 2018;13:e0203751.
59. Sheffield PE, Knowlton K, Carr JL, et al. Modeling of regional climate change effects on ground-level ozone and childhood asthma. Am J Prev Med 2011;41: 251–7.
60. Borchers Arriagada N, Horsley JA, Palmer AJ, et al. Association between fire smoke fine particulate matter and asthma-related outcomes: Systematic review and meta-analysis. Environ Res 2019;179:108777.
61. Crowley RA. Climate Change and Health: A Position Paper of the American College of Physicians. Ann Intern Med 2016;164:608–10.

Inequalities and Inequities in Pediatric Respiratory Diseases

Paulo Camargos, MD, PhD[a], Kimberly Danieli Watts, MD, MS[b,c,*]

KEYWORDS

• Inequality • Inequity • Pediatric respiratory diseases

There is a clear social gradient in intellectual, social, and emotional development. The higher the social position of families, the more do children flourish and the better they score on all development measures. This stratification in early child development arises from inequality in social circumstances.—Sir Michael Marmot. The health gap: the challenge of an unequal world. Lancet, 2015.

INTRODUCTION

The word "inequality" derives from the Latin *inaequalis*, "unequal." At a societal level, equality requires national or global economic integrated governmental policy, such as the implementation of income transfer policies that redistribute wealth through progressive tax and benefit programs. Inequity originates from the Latin *iniquitas* meaning "unfairness, injustice." This is the recognition that systemic policies that are deeply rooted within a country limit the ability of individuals to fully use resources, even if they were equally distributed.

Inequalities in socioeconomic conditions during childhood, such as access to food, housing, health services, education, and essential medicines are accountable for disparities in well-being. This is evident worldwide in the uneven patterns of diseases and health behavior across different socioeconomic groups. Poverty is one of the most critical social determinants of child health, with poverty reduction/cash transfer programs having helped decrease in those younger than 5 years the morbidity and mortality rates from major diseases.[1]

Concerns about social justice have driven movements demanding health equity to improve health conditions and reduce suffering caused by severe inequalities (International Conference on Primary Health Care, Alma Ata 1978). The goal of "Health for All"

[a] Department of Pediatrics, Medical School, Pediatric Pulmonology Unit, University Hospital, Federal University of Minas Gerais, Belo Horizonte, Brazil; [b] Division of Pediatric Pulmonary Medicine, Advocate Children's Hospital, Park Ridge, IL, USA; [c] Rosalind Franklin University of Medicine and Science, North Chicago, IL, USA

* Corresponding author. Advocate Children's Hospital, 1675 Dempster Street, Park Ridge, IL 60068.

E-mail address: kimberly.watts@aah.org

Pediatr Clin N Am 68 (2021) 293–304
https://doi.org/10.1016/j.pcl.2020.09.017 pediatric.theclinics.com

proclaimed that declaration is still far off. There is evidence of a widening gap in health gains between poor and rich countries and between the poor and the rich within countries. A more pragmatic, evidence-based approach toward health equity was more recently agreed on.[2] The International Society for Equity in Health highlights an actionable definition of equity (policy and actions) as "active policy decisions and programmatic actions directed at improving equity in health or in reducing or eliminating inequalities in health."[3]

Socioeconomic status (SES) is a measure of an individual or family social or economic position. It combines several indicators, such as income, education, occupation, and location of residence. Lower SES has been linked to uneven access to health care for many pulmonary diseases such as pneumonia, asthma, cystic fibrosis (CF), chronic obstructive pulmonary disease (COPD), pulmonary hypertension and other chronic respiratory conditions. Current guidelines and management algorithms fail to factor in the effect of SES in the disease process.[4,5]

Respiratory diseases account for significant morbidity and mortality in pediatrics. Health outcomes are unevenly distributed across this population including poor symptom control in asthma and worse survival rates in CF. These outcomes have been associated with both socioeconomic and minority status. It is crucial to understand the origins of these disparities so interventions to improve outcomes and reduce health inequality may be developed.[6]

Seventy percent of the world's population lives in countries where poverty and inequality are rampant. Two hundred sixty-two million school-age children are *not* yet in school, and 10,000 people die each day from lack of access to health services worldwide. The disparity between low and high developed countries is staggering. Around 17% of children born in low human development index countries in 2000 would have died before reaching the age 20, compared with just 1% of children born in high human development countries.[7]

In the United States, there are persistent and widespread inequities in health outcomes based on factors such as race, sex, language, and socioeconomic status. Such inequities have historical roots in structural racism and other forms of systematic discrimination; inequity in health care is a systems-based problem that requires a systems-based approach.[8]

This writing does not mean to be a comprehensive one but rather intends to highlight the negative impact of inequality and inequity on health outcomes in pediatric respiratory diseases and the challenges confronted, explore strategies to mitigate these disparities, and to provide suggested readings to study the subject.

PNEUMONIA/LOWER RESPIRATORY TRACT INFECTIONS

Overview

In 2016, lower respiratory infections (LRIs), mainly due to pneumococcal pneumonia, caused approximately 650,000 deaths in children younger than 5 years worldwide. This mortality rate was unevenly spread across and within countries. Substantial progress has been achieved in reducing the LRIs burden by lessening some primary risk factors, but progress varies by location.[9] The countries with the highest death rate per 100,000 children younger than 5 years were located in sub-Saharan Africa, with rates up to 70 times higher than high-income countries. The fatality ratio is strongly related to sociodemographic index, a composite indicator that includes lagged income *per capita*, average educational attainment in those older than 15 years, and total fertility rate (**Fig. 1**).[9]

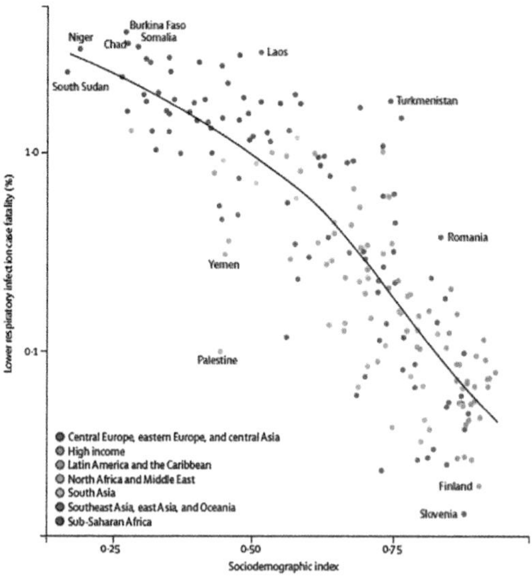

Fig. 1. Fatality ratio and sociodemographic index for children younger than 5 years, 2016. The black line shows lower curve for the relationship between sociodemographic index and lower respiratory infection case fatality ratio. (*From* GBD 2016 Lower Respiratory Infections Collaborators. Estimates of the global, regional, and national morbidity, mortality, and aetiologies of lower respiratory infections in 195 countries, 1990–2016: a systematic analysis for the Global Burden of Disease Study 2016. Lancet Infect Dis 2018;18:1191–210; Reprinted with permission from Elsevier.)

Narrowing the Gap

Childhood malnutrition remains the leading risk factor for mortality due to LRIs in children younger than 5 years of age, which accounted for up to 60% of deaths in 2016. It is estimated that combined interventions to improve nutrition, household and outdoor air pollution, and appropriate antibiotics use could avert one under-5 death due to LRT for every 4000 children treated in countries with the highest LRI burden. Access to timely and appropriate health care is challenging and so the opportunities to reduce mortality due to this preventable cause of death are missing.[9]

Inefficient cooking and heating with solid fuels (wood, coal) in poorly ventilated homes are a major source of exposure to indoor air pollution in developing countries—nearly 3 billion households. This poverty-related global health problem affects about half of the world's children, leading to premature deaths from pneumonia. Impoverished families are more likely to be exposed to smoke from biomass fuels due to cooking in open rather than closed biomass cookstoves.

The relative risk of LRI for children exposed to household solid fuels has been quantified in several studies, both from developing countries and the United States. Strong and consistent association between solid fuel use and an increase in the risk of LRI in exposed children is real. The overall estimate risk of LRI was a pooled *odds ratio* (OR) of 1.8 for children younger than 5 years.[10]

In a randomized controlled trial conducted in Guatemala, 534 households with a pregnant woman or young infants were assigned to either receive a woodstove with chimney (269 cases) or to remain as controls using open woodfires (265 cases). Children younger than 18 months with heavy exposure to woodstove smoke did not have an overall reduction in physician-diagnosed pneumonia. However, there was a 30%

reduction in severe pneumonia, which could have potentially important implications for reducing child mortality. The investigators concluded that more efficient solutions that provide less exposure than woodstoves with chimney might be needed to substantially reduce pneumonia in populations heavily exposed to biomass fuel air pollution.[11]

A recently published report concluded that between 1990 and 2017, reductions in household air pollution could lead to a larger decrease (8.4%) in under-5 LRI mortality than pneumococcal vaccine coverage (6.3%).[12] Effective strategies to reduce the adverse health effects of household air pollution are urgently needed in addition to vaccine availability. Programs to replace indoor biomass burning ovens with ovens using petroleum gas or another cleaner source of energy should be considered.

ASTHMA

Overview

Asthma diagnosis and its management in children varies greatly across the globe. There are consistently high numbers of hospital admissions, avoidable asthma deaths, poor adherence, and high financial burdens. Both diagnosis and management are marred by inequalities with a disproportionate number of children in low-middle income countries without access to or unable to receive appropriate care. Furthermore, overdiagnosis is common in Europe, Australasia, and North America, whereas underdiagnosis is common elsewhere.[13]

In Nigeria, suboptimal asthma control was observed in 19 (17.9%) out of 106 children. Factors such as household smoke exposure, low socioeconomic class, concomitant allergic rhino conjunctivitis, and poor parental asthma knowledge were significantly associated with suboptimal control. Both low socioeconomic class (OR = 6.2) and poor parental asthma knowledge (OR = 7.6) are closely related to low schooling levels.[14]

These kinds of disparities are also present in underserved US populations. For example, asthma prevalence among non-Hispanic black children is approximately 17% and for Puerto Ricans as high as 19.8% %, compared with the national average of 9.6%, and the prevalence among poor children is 13%—more than one and a half times that of children who are not poor.[15,16]

In the United States, Bollinger and colleagues[17] examined the characteristics of underserved minority children with prior intensive care unit (ICU) admissions for asthma. Of those, 93.7% were African American and 92.8% were Medicaid insured. Risk factors for mortality included history of ICU admission, living in extreme poverty (<$10,000/year), having atopy (particularly mouse allergen), using combination controller therapy and overusing albuterol. Controlling for ethnicity, age, and gender, residence in poor and urban areas also exerts influence in increased asthma morbidity. Poverty, poor-quality housing, differences in health care quality, medication compliance, health care access, higher exposure to cockroaches, mice, pollutants, and tobacco smoke, all contribute to increased asthma morbidity in this population.[18]

Lovinsky-Desir and colleagues described the relationship between air pollution exposure and urgent asthma visits by neighborhood asthma prevalence in New York City. Although high asthma prevalence neighborhoods had more air pollution exposure, poverty, stress, and allergen exposure, there was a stronger association between air pollution and urgent asthma visits only in low asthma prevalence neighborhoods. One plausible explanation was that these other factors, namely, poverty, stress, air pollution, are better predictors of asthma health care utilization in poorer communities where overall asthma rates are high.[19]

A cross-sectional survey from 2013 to 2015 revealed that patients in 41 high-income countries have easier access to rescue and controller asthma medications than their counterparts living in nonaffluent societies. Availability and affordability of inhaled albuterol and high-priced inhaled corticosteroids (ICS) reached 91% in high-income countries compared with 54% in low- to middle-income countries surveyed.[20] Considering the number of working days needed to buy medicine is a better measure of comparison than actual prices when looking at drug costs. The affordability of a single beclomethasone 100 μg controller inhaler ranged from around half a day's wages in Afghanistan to almost 14 days in Madagascar. Patients in El Salvador, Ethiopia, Madagascar, and Malawi had to work more than 5 days to buy a single beclomethasone inhaler in a retail pharmacy. A single canister of albuterol costs 4 working days in Burundi, Ethiopia, Indonesia, Madagascar, Mexico, Republic of Guinea, and Mozambique.[21]

Narrowing the Gap

Affordability and availability of antiasthma medicines has unequivocal impact on asthma outcomes. Since 2011, Brazilian has made beclomethasone and albuterol free of charge to patients with asthma. As a result, hospital admission rates due to asthma significantly decreased from 90 to 60/100,000. This suggests that free asthma medication may have a significant public health impact in low- to middle-income countries.[22]

Some studies suggest that on-demand use of ICS for mild asthma might be a reasonable cost-effective alternative with frequent monitoring of asthma control and a switch to daily controller treatment if unsuccessful.[23,24] Valved-holding chambers are also either unavailable or too costly for low-income families around the world. Homemade nonvalved spacers (out of 500 mL soft drink or mineral water bottles and a polystyrene cup) showed comparable bronchodilation to commercial, less affordable spacers or oxygen-driven nebulizers.[25,26]

Brazil tested an asthma management program for low-income settings to reduce health services utilization for acute asthma. A population-based cohort study of 582 children with asthma were enrolled; 470 patients received assistance from a municipal asthma management program and 112 were controls. The study group was provided a written asthma action plan, instruction about the appropriate use of inhaled albuterol, and 317 of the 470 (67.4%) also received beclomethasone. At the end of the study, only 5% of patients in the program versus 34% of controls sought health services because of acute asthma.[27]

In another Brazilian study, an asthma center providing free treatment enrolled 188 patients with severe asthma from low SES, median family income of US$ 2955/y, and a high rate of job loss due to asthma. The total cost of asthma management accounted for 29% of family income. Asthma control scores improved by 50% and quality of life by 74% after proper treatment. When able to return to work, their incomes increased by US$ 711.00/y. Asthma's total cost was reduced by a median of US$ 789.00 per family each year.[28]

Comparable results have been obtained in affluent societies. The Finish established a national drug-reimbursement asthma program. The number of registered patients with persistent asthma increased from 83,000 to 247,583. Despite a threefold increase in the number of patients, the total costs actually decreased by 14%, from €222 million to €191 million. Although the costs for medication and primary care visits went up, the overall annual costs per patient decreased by 72%.[29]

Additional interventions for poor children suffering from asthma in high-income countries have shown promising results including school-based education programs, asthma training for social workers, and environmental control (eliminating exposure to indoor allergens and tobacco smoke), ensuring access to controller medication and evidence-based guidelines.[18]

CYSTIC FIBROSIS

Overview

In 2016, more than half of the US CF population were older than 18 years. The median age and proportion of adults within a given CF population is directly related to their countries' socioeconomic status. Data from 2014 show that Brazil (a low-middle income country) had both lower median age (11.5 vs 20 years) and lower proportion (24.6% vs 50%) of patients older than 18 years in developed countries.[30]

A retrospective analysis of claims from privately insured individual with CF in United States (up to 64 years of age) reported that the average spending nearly doubled from about $67,000 per patient in 2010 to approximately $131,000 per patient in 2016. Spending on outpatient and inpatient care increased by 0.5% and 2.5% per year, respectively, whereas pharmaceutical spending increased by 20.2% per year. The increase in pharmaceutical spending is almost all ascribed to specialty drugs including genetic modulators.[31]

CF medications may be unaffordable for low-middle income countries and also for poor families in developed nations. Unfortunately, not all patients in Latin America, where there is still suboptimal access to various CF interventions, have access to these treatments due to high cost and low rates of reimbursement.[32] A similar scenario occurs for children with CF in the United Kingdom from deprived areas, who are less likely to receive dornase alfa or inhaled antibiotic treatment.[33]

The survival age gap between high-income and low-middle income countries may further increase with the introduction of *CFTR* modulators, a novel class of drugs that directly target the abnormal *CFTR* protein molecular defect. Pharmaceutical spending increased by 33.1% during 2014 to 2016, when a potentiator (ivacaftor) was approved for patients with CF a p.G551D mutation.[34] Since that time additional genetic modulators have been approved with the most recent being triple-drug therapy of elexacaftor and tezacaftor *plus* ivacaftor. Patients aged 12 years or older with at least one copy of the p.F508del mutation are approved at this time for the drug. The cost of this medicine may simply be prohibitive for low-middle countries.

Although CF is usually found in populations of Caucasian descent, particularly those in North America, Europe, and Australasia. CF also occurs in Latin America, Middle Eastern, African, and other populations. Therefore, CF should *not* be excluded in a patient with suggestive clinical findings solely because of that patient's ethnicity. Continued education programs for health professionals would significantly improve the diagnosis and management of CF.

In sharp contrast with affluent societies where newborn screening has dropped the age of diagnosis dramatically and, consequently, improved nutritional status, a population of children with CF attending 2 referral centers in South Africa, some of them originating from Ghana, Malawi, Zimbabwe, and Mozambique, had older age at diagnosis (2–15 months), lower body mass index (BMI) Z-score at diagnosis (minus 3) and lower forced expiratory volume in one second (FEV_1) Z-score at age 10 (minus 3).[35]

Even within high-income countries unequal outcomes may occur. From 1991 to 2010, the overall unadjusted mortality rate for Hispanic patients with CF in the United States was 9.1%, compared with 3.3% among non-Hispanic whites, yielding an unadjusted risk ratio for mortality of 2.7 for Hispanic patients with CF within the United States. After adjusting for several factors, these patients ended up having a 2.8 times higher risk of death.[36]

Rho and colleagues reported in 2018 that Hispanic patients with CF in the United States had an overall lower survival probability (mean age of death of 22.4 ± 9.9 years) compared with non-Hispanic whites (28.1 ± 10.0 years, *P*<.0001). Moreover, Hispanic patients with CF had a 1.27 times higher mortality rate than non-Hispanic whites, after adjusting for several clinical covariates and socioeconomic status. When analyzed by region, Hispanic patients with CF had shorter median survivals in the Midwest, Northeast, and West than non-Hispanic whites, confirming that Hispanic patients with CF have worse overall survival than their non-Hispanic white counterparts.[37]

Patients with CF in the United States of lower socioeconomic status have worse health outcomes. Children from deprived areas weighed less, were shorter, had a lower BMI, were more likely to have chronic *Pseudomonas aeruginosa* infection, and have a lower FEV_1. These inequalities were apparent very early in life and remained thereafter.[33]

Lung transplant could be a life-saving option for many individuals with advanced CF lung disease; however, inequities in the distribution of lung transplant programs globally has led to disparity in lung transplant outcomes. There are only 7 active centers in Brazil. A significant number of patients who are potential candidates for lung transplants die even before making the transplant centers' waiting lists.[38] Conversely, a single transplant center in Italy with 20 years follow-up experience reported one of the highest posttransplant survival rates in the world: 1 year, 93.6%; 5 year, 71.4%; 10 year, 53.6%; 15 year, 36.7%; and 20 year, 31.6%.[39]

Narrowing the Gap

Partnerships between lay organizations, governments, and the pharmaceutical industry are needed to provide sustained, affordable access to treatment of people with CF.[40] Attention to low SES is important so clinicians can help families access programs and grants as well as address adherence issues related to inability to pay for treatments and therapies.[33]

Despite the scarcity of research focusing on literacy and CF, maternal education is a variable included in the US CF Foundation Patient Registry that can be used to assess the role of literacy on CF outcomes, because low health literacy may occur regardless of SES and education level. Conducting interviews in the parents' preferred language and assessing families for literacy and numeracy may reduce literacy-related disparities and improve overall clinical outcomes.[41]

In resource-poor countries, costs of medications fall heavily on the family, and therefore, cost and affordability are major hurdles. The cost of some medicines must come down: medicines can only improve the quality and quantity of life if they are affordable for those who need them.

DISCUSSION

Lack of social protection has implications for any illness. Although waiting for broad and structural public policies directed at reducing inequalities to be implemented by governments, the health sector can offer their own programs and strategies to alleviate that burden and the suffering among children with respiratory diseases.[15]

Inequality levels vary widely between and within countries, even in those nations that share similar levels of development. This highlights the crucial role that national policies and institutions play in affecting inequality, as it directly influences the health status of these societies, especially among children who represent a vulnerable age group.[42]

Medications account for up to 60% of health expenditure in low- to middle-income countries, compared with 18% in 36 high-income countries of the Organization for Economic Co-operation and Development. Many developed countries have public or private programs already in place that subsidize the final cost of medications to consumers. Up to 90% of the population in developing countries purchase medicine through out of pocket payments, making medicines the largest item of family expenditure after food.[43]

Powerful macroeconomic strategies exist to reduce poverty and, consequently, health gaps. It is well known that low levels of child poverty are associated with better early child development, as it is observed in Scandinavian countries, The Netherlands, and Slovenia, use tax and welfare systems toward reducing socioeconomic disparities (**Fig. 2**). Despite their enormous health and socioeconomic differences, the United States, Romania, Bulgaria, and Latvia have roughly, similar levels of child poverty before taxes and transfers; after their implementation in the United States there was no relevant reduction, denoting a still insufficient redistribution of wealth to reduce child poverty in that country.[44]

Nearly 80% of the world's population is exposed to air pollution levels that exceeds WHO regulations. Outdoor air pollution consistently shows an adverse effect on childhood respiratory health, particularly on children with asthma and low SES with an estimated health care cost (34 countries) of approximately US $1.7 trillion in 2010.[45] Implementing strategies to minimize ambient particulate matter pollution (as well as climate change) are urgently needed to protect this vulnerable age group.

To address inequities at a biological and societal levels, research should stratify data based on risk factors that include race, ethnicity, sex, gender, disabilities, and other key social determinants of heatlh.[5,8] The UK Global Health Respiratory Network in 2015 represents a possible change in approaching health disparities. This network combines efforts of world experts in respiratory health from public health and primary and secondary care (pediatrics and adult) to consider respiratory diseases from a wider perspective addressing respiratory health of the poor.[46]

As health professionals, it is critical that we advocate for initiatives that reduce health inequity through societal, private, and governmental sectors. Spearheading research that examines impact of inequality on health outcomes of children and developing comprehensive programs to address these needs are critical to promote change and improve health for children around the world. A profession sworn to heal can no longer passively accept the inequities it has witnessed for decades—or the hand that it has played in them.

The overlapping prejudices embedded in the medical establishment are ultimately harmful not because they hurt feelings but because they alienate patients who need help and lead to bad medicine. These are biases that prevent the profession from taking a more accurate and enlightened view that emphasizes the pervasive environmental and economic roots of patients' health problems.

Covid-19 has highlighted these issues. As this article was being written, the world was struck by the devastating pandemic. Information from countries and cities throughout the world are beginning to report a significant disparity in deaths from this pandemic adversely affecting African Americans, Latinos, and the Navajo Nation and other underserved populations at a staggering rate.[47,48] In the city of Chicago 72% of the cities deaths from Covid-19 were from the African American community that makes up only 30% of the city population. This finding prompted Chicago's Mayor to convene a Racial Equality Rapid Response Team to develop hyperlocal, data-informed strategies to slow the spread of the COVID-19 and improve health outcomes within heavily affected communities. This initiative is to address unmet health

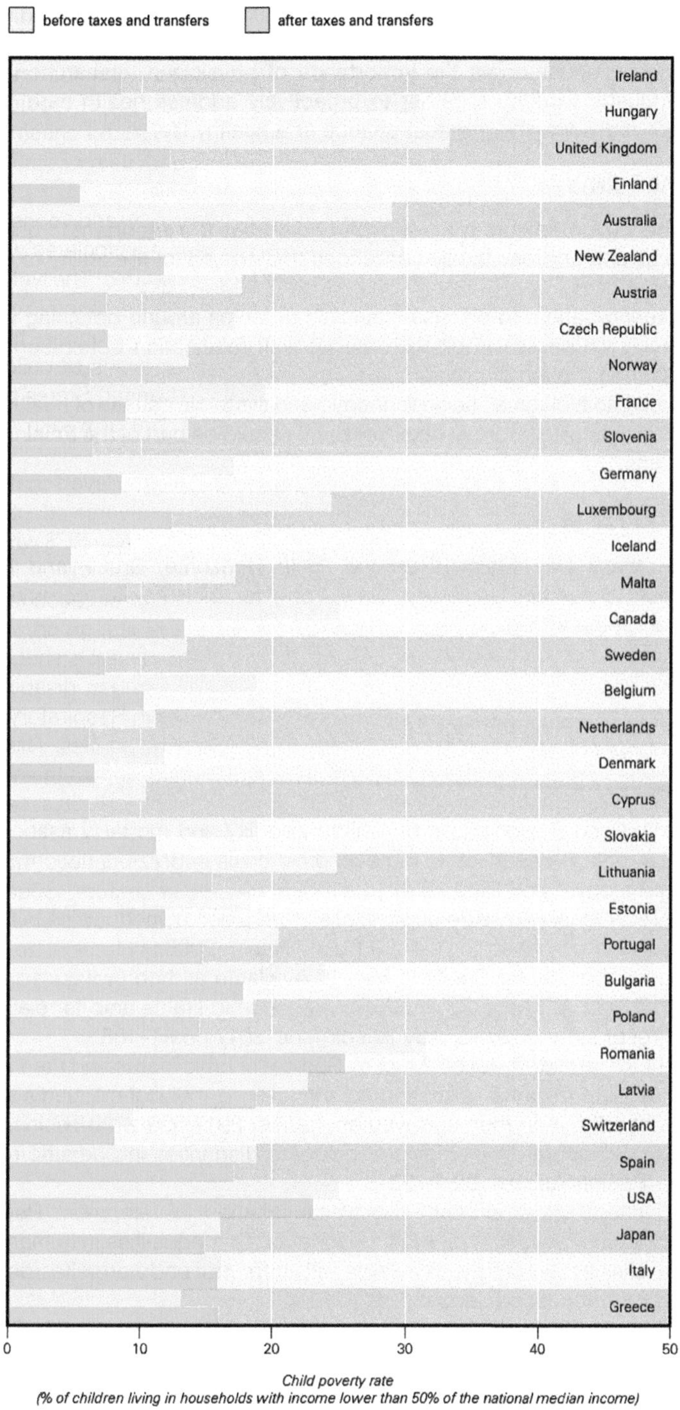

Fig. 2. Relative child poverty rates before taxes and transfers (market income) and after taxes and transfers (disposable income). (Source: UNICEF Innocenti Research Centre. Measuring Child Poverty. Ref.[44])

needs during the pandemic and operationalize a long-term commitment to improving health outcomes in vulnerable communities.[49]

This pandemic underscores the importance of physicians, researchers, government, and industry working together to proactively address health care disparities and give each individual the greatest chance at a healthy life.

CLINICS CARE POINTS

- When caring for patients with respiratory diseases it is important to query issues of access and address family challenges that can affect the ability to receive or implement care.
- Empowering patient to discuss financial hardships around obtaining medicines and having processes in place to assist with medication obtainment will help address the problem of adherence.
- Research into biological, socioeconomic and systemic causes of health care disparities is critical to improve outcomes and should be part of the training of future physicians.

ACKNOWLEDGMENTS

The authors thank Drs. Elaine Drumond, Belo Horizonte, Brazil, and Stephanie Lovinsky-Desir, Columbia University, New York, for their helpful comments to an earlier version of the article.

DISCLOSURE

The authors have nothing to disclose.

REFERENCES

1. Rasella D, Basu S, Hone T, et al. Child morbidity and mortality associated with alternative policy responses to the economic crisis in Brazil: a nationwide microsimulation study. PLoS Med 2018;15:e1002570.
2. Tugwell P, O'Connor A, Andersson N, et al. Reduction of inequalities in health: assessing evidence-based tools. Int J Equity Health 2006;5:11.
3. International Society for Equity in Health. Available at: http://www.iseqh.org.
4. Sahni S, Talwar A, Khanijo S, et al. Socioeconomic status and its relationship to chronic respiratory disease. Adv Respir Med 2017;85:97–108.
5. Stringhini S, Carmeli C, Jokela M, et al. Socioeconomic status and the 25 X 25 risk factors as determinants of premature mortality: a multicohort study and meta-analysis of 1.7 million men and women. Lancet 2017;389:1229–37.
6. Watts KD, Schechter MS. Origins of outcome disparities in pediatric respiratory disease. Pediatr Ann 2010;39:793–8.
7. United Nations Development Programme. Human Development Report 2019 Beyond income, beyond averages, beyond today: inequalities in human development in the 21st century. Available at: http://hdr.undp.org/sites/default/files/hdr2019.pdf. Accessed January 2nd, 2020.
8. Sivashanker K, Gandhi TK. Advancing safety and equity together. N Engl J Med 2020;382:301–3.
9. GBD 2016 Lower Respiratory Infections Collaborators. Estimates of the global, regional, and national morbidity, mortality, and aetiologies of lower respiratory infections in 195 countries, 1990–2016: a systematic analysis for the Global Burden of Disease Study 2016. Lancet Infect Dis 2018;18:1191–210.

10. Balmes JR. Household air pollution from domestic combustion of solid fuels and health. J Allergy Clin Immunol 2019;143:1979–87.
11. Smith KR, McCracken JP, Weber MW, et al. Effect of reduction in household air pollution on childhood pneumonia in Guatemala (RESPIRE): a randomized controlled trial. Lancet 2011;378:1717–26.
12. GBD 2017 Lower Respiratory Infections Collaborators. Quantifying risks and interventions that have affected the burden of lower respiratory infections among children younger than 5 years: an analysis for the Global Burden of Disease Study 2017. Lancet Infect Dis 2020;20:60–79.
13. Lenney W, Adachi Y, Bush A, et al. Asthma: moving toward a global children's charter. Lancet Respir Med 2019;7:299–300.
14. Kuti BP, Omole KO, Kuti DK. Factors associated with childhood asthma control in a resource-poor center. J Fam Med Prim Care 2017;6:222–30.
15. Harris KM. Mapping inequality: Childhood asthma and environmental injustice, a case study of St. Louis, Missouri. Soc Sci Med 2019;230:91–110.
16. Seth D, Saini S, Poowuttikul P. Pediatric inner-city asthma. Pediatr Clin North Am 2019;66:967–79.
17. Bollinger ME, Butz A, Tsoukleris M, et al. Characteristics of inner-city children with life-threatening asthma. Ann Allergy Asthma Immunol 2019;122:381–6.
18. Poowuttikul P, Saini S, Seth D. Inner-city asthma in children. Clin Rev Allergy Immunol 2019;56:248–68.
19. Lovinsky-Desir S, Acosta LM, Rundle AG, et al. Air pollution, urgent asthma medical visits and the modifying effect of neighborhood asthma prevalence. Pediatr Res 2019;85:36–42.
20. Bissell K, Ellwood P, Ellwood E, et al. Essential medicines at the national level: The Global Asthma Network's Essential Asthma Medicines Survey 2014. Int J Environ Res Public Health 2019;16:605.
21. Babar ZU, Lessing C, Mace C, et al. The availability, pricing and affordability of three essential asthma medicines in 52 low- and middle-income countries. Pharmacoeconomics 2013;31:1063–82.
22. Comaru T, Pitrez PM, Friedrich FO, et al. Free asthma medications reduces hospital admissions in Brazil. Respir Med 2016;121:21–5.
23. Martinez FD, Chinchilli VM, Morgan WJ, et al. Use of beclomethasone dipropionate as rescue treatment for children with mild persistent asthma (TREXA): a randomised, double-blind, placebo-controlled trial. Lancet 2011;377:650–7.
24. Camargos P, Affonso A, Calazans G, et al. On-demand intermittent beclomethasone is effective for mild asthma in Brazil. Clin Transl Allergy 2018;8:7.
25. Zar HJ, Brown G, Donson H, et al. Home-made spacers for bronchodilator therapy in children with acute asthma: a randomised trial. Lancet 1999;354:979–82.
26. Duarte M, Camargos P. Efficacy and safety of a home-made non-valved spacer for bronchodilator therapy in acute asthma. Acta Paediatr 2002;91:909–13.
27. Andrade WCC, Camargos P, Lasmar L, et al. A pediatric asthma management program in a low-income setting resulting in reduced use of health service for acute asthma. Allergy 2010;65:1472–7.
28. Franco R, Nascimento HF, Cruz AA, et al. The economic impact of severe asthma to low-income families. Allergy 2009;64:478–83.
29. Haahtela T, Herse F, Karjalainen J, et al. The Finnish experience to save asthma costs by improving care in 1987-2013. J Allergy Clin Immunol 2017;139:408–14.
30. Stephenson AL, Stanojevic S, Sykes J, et al. The changing epidemiology and demography of cystic fibrosis. Presse Med 2017;46:e87–95.

31. Scott D, Grosse SD, Do QN, et al. Healthcare expenditures for privately insured US patients with cystic fibrosis, 2010-2016. Pediatr Pulmonol 2018;53:1611–8.
32. Silva Filho LVRF, Castaños C, Ruíz HH. Cystic fibrosis in Latin America-improving the awareness. J Cyst Fibros 2016;15:791–3.
33. Taylor-Robinson DC, Smyth RL, Diggle PJ, et al. The effect of social deprivation on clinical outcomes and the use of treatments in the UK cystic fibrosis population: a longitudinal study. Lancet Respir Med 2013;1:121–8.
34. Habib AI-R, Kajbafzadeh M, Desai S, et al. A systematic review of the clinical efficacy and safety of CFTR modulators in cystic fibrosis. Sci Rep 2019;9:7234.
35. Owusu SK, Morrow BM, White D, et al. Cystic fibrosis in black African children in South Africa: a case control study. J Cyst Fibros 2019. https://doi.org/10.1016/j.jcf.2019.09.007.
36. Corriveau S, Sykesa J, Stephenson AL. Cystic fibrosis survival: the changing epidemiology. Curr Opin Pulm Med 2018;24:574–8.
37. Rho J, Ahn C, Gao A, et al. Disparities in mortality of Hispanic cystic fibrosis patients in the United States: a national and regional cohort study. Am J Respir Crit Care Med 2018;198:1055–63.
38. Afonso Júnior JE, Werebe E de C, Carraro RM, et al. Lung transplantation. Einstein (São Paulo) 2015;13:297–304.
39. Savi D, Mordenti M, Bonci E, et al. Survival after lung transplant for cystic fibrosis in Italy: a single center experience with 20 years of follow-up. Transplant Proc 2018;50:3732–8.
40. Bell SC, Mall MA, Gutierrez H, et al. The future of cystic fibrosis care: a global perspective. Lancet Respir Med 2019. https://doi.org/10.1016/S2213-2600(19)30337-6.
41. Watts KD. Healthcare inequalities in paediatric respiratory diseases. Paediatr Respir Rev 2012;13:57–62.
42. Alvaredo F, Chancel L, Piketty T, et al. World inequality report 2018. Available at: https://wir2018.wid.world. Accessed December 4, 2019.
43. WHO Policy Perspectives. 2004. Available at: https://apps.who.int/medicinedocs. Accessed December 19th, 2019.
44. UNICEF Innocenti Research Centre. Measuring child poverty: New league tables of child poverty in the world's rich countries. Florence (Italy): Innocenti Research Centre; 2012.
45. Rodriguez-Villamizar LA, Magico A, Osorno-Vargas A, et al. The effects of outdoor air pollution on the respiratory health of Canadian children: a systematic review of epidemiological studies. Can Respir J 2015;22:282–92.
46. Sheikh A, Campbell H, Balharry D, et al. The UK's Global Health Respiratory Network: Improving respiratory health of the world's poorest through research collaborations. J Glob Health 2019;9:020104.
47. Available at: https://www.bbc.com/future/article/20200420-coronavirus-why-some-racial-groups-are-more-vulnerable.
48. Garg S, Kim L, Whitaker M, et al. Hospitalization Rates and Characteristics of Patients Hospitalized with Laboratory-Confirmed Coronavirus Disease 2019 — COVID-NET, 14 States, March 1–30, 2020. MMWR Morb Mortal Wkly Rep 2020;69:458–64.
49. Available at: https://www.chicago.gov/city/en/depts/mayor/press_room/press_releases/2020/april/RERRTUpdate.html.

High-altitude Illnesses and Air Travel

Pediatric Considerations

Nelson Villca, MD[a,*], Adriana Asturizaga, MD[b], Alexandra Heath-Freudenthal, MD, PhD[c]

KEYWORDS

- Barometric pressure (Pb) • Arterial oxygen saturation (Sao_2)
- High-altitude illnesses (HAI) • AMS • HAPE • HACE • Air travel

KEY POINTS

- Physicians caring for pediatric patients with or without underlying conditions should have a basic knowledge of the high-altitude–precipitated physiologic changes.
- Risk factors for high-altitude illness (HAI) are outlined.
- HAI syndromes and their pathophysiology, as well as their prevention and treatment strategies are described.
- Pediatric patients at potential risks of hypoxia while air traveling are considered.

INTRODUCTION

Every year, millions of visitors from low altitudes travel to high-altitude destinations worldwide. Most of these destinations may be reached within a day by modern means of transportation. Many of these mountain travelers are children and adolescents. Rapid ascent to high altitude places the not acclimatized individual at risk of developing high-altitude illness (HAI).

Clinicians working in high-altitude areas should be familiar with the manifestations and management of HAI in the pediatric age group, while all health care workers who advise travelers should have a basic understanding of the best prevention and treatment strategies. Clinicians advising families with children on high-altitude trips should evaluate individual risk factors, provide recommendations to prevent HAI, and determine whether prophylactic medication is appropriate. Common high-elevation destinations include Cusco, Peru (11,000 ft [3300 m]); La Paz, Bolivia (12,000 ft [3640 m]); Everest Base Camp (17,700 ft; 5400 m); and Kilimanjaro, Tanzania

[a] Pediatric Pulmonology, Hospital Materno Infantil, Calle República Dominicana # 100, La Paz – Bolivia; [b] Pediatric Pulmonology, Hospital de la Banca Privada, Av. Héctor Ormachea # 21, La Paz – Bolivia; [c] Pediatric Cardiology, Kardiozentrum, Obrajes, Calle 14 # 669, La Paz, Bolivia
* Corresponding author.
E-mail address: nelues@gmail.com

Pediatr Clin N Am 68 (2021) 305–319
https://doi.org/10.1016/j.pcl.2020.09.015

(19,341 ft; [5895 m]). This article briefly describes the expected physiologic responses and the most relevant HAIs and their prevention and treatment and presents an overview of the most up-to-date recommendations to ensure the safety of children during air travel.

HIGH-ALTITUDE PHYSIOLOGY

The Po_2 is the driving force for the diffusion of oxygen. Oxygen moves from inspired air to the alveolar space via the airways and then diffuses across the alveoli into the blood, where it is carried mainly bound to hemoglobin but also in dissolved form. At the level of the capillaries, oxygen diffuses across vessel walls, through the tissues and into cells, and ultimately into the mitochondria. The partial pressure of oxygen of inspired air (Pio_2) is given by the equation: $Pio_2 = Fio_2 \times (Pb - 47 \text{ mm Hg})$, or $0.21 \times (760-47) = 149$ mm Hg, where *Fio_2* is the fraction of oxygen in inspired air (0.21), *Pb* is the ambient barometric pressure (760 mm Hg), and *47 mm Hg* is the vapor pressure of H_2O at 37°C. Inspired gas is 100% humidified by the time it reaches the alveoli and water vapor pressure is affected by temperature.[1]

As the altitude increases, Pb decreases (**Fig. 1**). Pb and oxygenation decrease in a curvilinear manner with increasing altitude. At any altitude, the proportion of air consisting of oxygen (Fio_2, 21%) remains constant, but with the drop of Pb, the Pio_2 decreases so does the arterial oxygen saturation (Sao_2), resulting in hypoxia. This form of hypoxia is called *hypobaric hypoxia*, and it represents the initial cause of HAI.[1] At sea level, the Pao_2 is approximately 100 mm Hg and the Sao_2 is 95% to 98%.

PHYSIOLOGIC RESPONSES TO HYPOBARIC HYPOXIA

The normal compensatory responses to acute hypobaric hypoxia are termed, *acclimatization*—a series of physiologic changes involving multiple organ systems that occur over varying periods (from minutes to weeks). Acclimatization improves tissue oxygenation by increasing alveolar Po_2 and the efficiency of oxygen diffusion and by enhancing the utilization of oxygen at the cellular level.[1] Acclimatization differs from *adaptation*, which refers to physiologic changes that take place in response to chronic exposure to hypobaric hypoxia over generations and are observed in some populations permanently living at high altitudes.[1]

The human body adjusts well to moderate hypoxia but requires time to do so. The process of acute acclimatization to high elevation takes 3 days to 5 days. Acclimatization prevents HAI, improves sleep, and increases comfort and well-being. Increased ventilation is the first and most important step in acute acclimatization to improve oxygen delivery. Hypoxic stimulation of the peripheral chemoreceptors (carotid bodies) results in increased minute ventilation and is called *hypoxic ventilatory response*. This response increases the alveolar Po_2 and reduces the alveolar Pco_2, resulting in respiratory alkalosis.[1]

As ventilation rises in response to hypoxia, $Paco_2$ falls and pH rises. The central chemoreceptors in the medulla of the brain respond to alkalosis in the cerebrospinal fluid by inhibiting ventilation. Whereas peripheral chemoreceptors are sensitive to changes in pH, central chemoreceptors play the major role in this response. After 2 days to 3 days, the kidneys respond to the respiratory alkalosis with increased excretion of bicarbonate, decreasing the pH toward normal.[2] Increased red blood cell production does not play a role in acute acclimatization, although hematocrit may be increased within 48 hours because of diuresis and decreased plasma volume.[1] An explanation of altitude physiology in more detail may be found in an article by Roach and colleagues.[1]

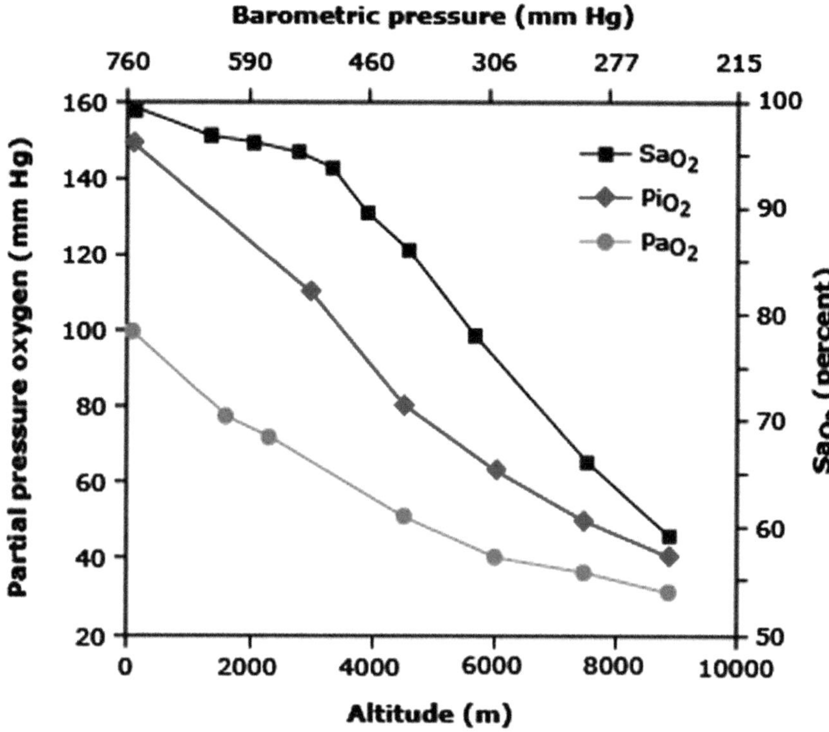

Fig. 1. Oxygenation at different altitudes. Increasing altitude results in a decrease in P_{IO_2}, Pa_{O_2}, and Sa_{O_2}. Note that the difference between P_{IO_2} and Pa_{O_2} narrows at high altitudes because of increased ventilation and that Sa_{O_2} is well maintained while awake until over 3000 m. (*Adapted from* Israëls J, Nagelkerke AF, Markhorst DG, van Heerde M. Fitness to fly in the paediatric population, how to assess and advice. Eur J Pediatr 2018;177(5):633-9; with permission.)

RISK FOR TRAVELERS

Three factors mainly influence the risk of a traveler developing HAI: elevation at destination, rate of ascent, and physical exertion[3,4] (**Box 1**).

Ascent is contraindicated for travelers with sickle cell anemia, severe chronic obstructive pulmonary disease, pulmonary hypertension, heart failure, high-risk pregnancy, cystic fibrosis (forced expiratory volume in the first second of expiration [FEV_1] <30% predicted), unstable angina, recent myocardial infarction (<90 days), arteriovenous malformations, and cerebral space-occupying lesions[4] (**Box 2**).

ACUTE HIGH-ALTITUDE ILLNESS IN CHILDREN AND ADOLESCENTS

Traditionally, 2500 m has been used as the threshold for an increased risk of developing acute HAIs. These are divided into 3 clinical syndromes: acute mountain sickness (AMS), high-altitude cerebral edema (HACE), and high-altitude pulmonary edema (HAPE).[4]

Acute Mountain Sickness

AMS is the most common of the HAIs, with approximately 10% to 25% incidence in nonacclimatized children and adults at elevations between 2000 m (6860 ft) and 3000 m (9840 ft).[5] It is uncommon below 2000 m (6560 ft).

Box 1
Ascent risk associated with underlying medical conditions

- Full-term infants less than 6 weeks old and premature infants less than 46 weeks post–conceptual age.
- Premature infants greater than 36 weeks post–conceptual age with a history of oxygen requirement, BPD, or pulmonary hypertension
- Morbid obesity
- Cystic fibrosis (FEV_1 30%–50% of predicted)
- Poorly controlled chronic conditions (asthma, diabetes, seizure disorder, hypertension, arrhythmia)
- CHDs, such as ASD, VSD, and pulmonary hypertension
- Down syndrome, especially with obstructive sleep apnea
- Sickle cell trait
- Systemic diseases with respiratory compromise (eg, severe scoliosis, neuromuscular disease, obstructive sleep apnea)
- Premature and full-term infants who have experienced respiratory distress in the immediate postnatal period; infants up to 1 year of age with a history of oxygen requirement or pulmonary hypertension

Adapted from Hackett PH and Shlim DR Chapter 3, CDC Yellow Book 2020 Oxford University Press; with permission.

On arrival at high altitude, some individuals may experience a sensation of breathlessness secondary to the hypoxia-induced hyperventilation and palpitations from an increased heart rate. These are normal physiologic responses. Symptoms that represent AMS may develop, however, within 6 hours to 24 hours after a person ascends to 2500 m or higher. Headache is the cardinal symptom,[4] sometimes accompanied by fatigue, loss of appetite, nausea, and occasionally vomiting. Headache onset usually is 2 hours to 12 hours after arrival at a higher elevation and often during or after the first night.[4] In preverbal infants and young children, manifestations of AMS are nonspecific and include loss of appetite, increased fussiness, poor sleep patterns, and decreased playfulness.[6]

Box 2
General measures to prevent high-altitude illness in children

Gradual ascent—avoid abrupt ascent to altitudes above 2800 m (9200 ft).

Acclimatization—take measures to permit the child to become accustomed to higher altitudes:

- When ascending greater than 2500 m (8200 ft), do not spend subsequent nights at elevations more than 500 m higher than the previous night.
- Rest day (no ascent and no vigorous activity) for every 1000 m (3280 ft) increase in altitude
- When possible, spend at least 5 days at an intermediate altitude (typically 3000–4000 m) before proceeding to higher elevations.

If a child has an acute upper or lower respiratory infection or otitis media, extra caution should be exercised during rapid ascent above 2500 m (8200 ft)

Data from Garlick V, O'Connor A, Shubkin CD. High-altitude illness in the pediatri population: A review of the literature on prevention and treatment. Curr Opin Pediatr. 2017;29(4):503-509.

Diagnosis of AMS is a clinical one that relies on commonly observed manifestations. No radiographic or laboratory testing ordinarily is required, unless the diagnosis of AMS is unclear. For most children and adults, the symptoms usually resolve within 1 day to 2 days.[7,8]

Treatment is based on symptom severity.[4,7] Mild AMS may be treated with acetaminophen or ibuprofen for headache and dimenhydrinate for vomiting. Moderate AMS may require supplemental oxygen and acetazolamide. Supplemental oxygen is more effective than acetazolamide at rapidly relieving the symptoms of moderate to severe AMS. If symptoms persist or are getting worse while the traveler is resting at the same elevation, or in spite of medication, the traveler must descend.[4,5] For prevention and pharmacologic prophylaxis, acetazolamide speeds acclimatization and effectively treats AMS but is better for prophylaxis than treatment.[7,8]

If acetazolamide is used, duration of treatment depends on the ascent profile. Individuals ascending to a fixed sleeping altitude may start acetazolamide the day before ascent and continue treatment for 48 hours. If further ascent is planned, acetazolamide may be continued until maximum elevation is attained.[8] The pediatric dose of acetazolamide for prevention of AMS is 2.5 mg/kg per dose twice a day (maximum single dose 125 mg)[9] (**Box 3**).

AMS has a spectrum of manifestations that in the most serious scenarios rarely may develop as HAPE or HACE.

High-altitude Pulmonary Edema

HAPE is a form of noncardiogenic pulmonary edema. This condition rarely may develop in some apparently healthy children and active young adults after a rapid ascent to altitudes above 2500 m (8200 ft),[6] although altitude alone should not be used to rule out a diagnosis. This occurs most commonly after sustained hypobaric hypoxia of 24 hours or longer. The overall incidence of HAPE is approximately 1 in 10,000 visitors, and many of these are children.[10] Some individuals tolerate high altitude at first but become ill if they attempt to climb to higher altitudes.

Infants and young children may manifest only pallor and depressed consciousness or other nonspecific symptoms, such as increased fussiness, crying, decreased appetite, decreased playfulness, and disrupted sleep.[11] In older children and adolescents, initial symptoms are increased breathlessness with exertio, and eventually breathlessness at rest, associated with weakness and productive cough of pinky frothy sputum.[12,13]

Physical examination reveals tachypnea, low oxygen saturation as measured by pulse oximetry (Spo_2), tachycardia, and diffuse crackles on lung auscultation. Chest radiographs show patchy infiltrates consistent with noncardiogenic pulmonary edema (**Fig. 2**). HAPE may be misdiagnosed as pneumonia in children residing at high altitude due to the overlap in radiographic findings and physical examination.

An estimated 20% of the general population responds to a hypoxic stimulus with a pronounced increase in the pulmonary vascular resistance (PVR); this phenomenon is known as *hypoxic pulmonary vasoconstriction.* Individuals with these reactions are referred to as *hyperreactors*. Current thinking regarding the pathophysiology of HAPE centers around the increased pulmonary arterial pressure with altitude and hypoxemia and that, in hyperreactors, this response is exaggerated. This reaction may result in severe pulmonary arterial hypertension at rest or with exercise. An increase in pulmonary vasoreactivity has been documented in children and adults diagnosed with HAPE. It may lead to increased pulmonary edema secondary to augmented alveolar-capillary permeability and elevated hydrostatic pressures.[13,14]

Box 3
Recommendations for children with preexisting illnesses

Infants and children with certain underlying diseases are at particular risk for serious complications, including exacerbation of their preexistent condition or life-threatening illnesses:

- Sickle cell disease—these patients should ascend cautiously if at all, because sickle cell crisis may occur at altitudes as low as 1500 m [4920 ft].
- Asthma—these patients may find that their symptoms improve because of a relative lack of allergens at high altitudes. They seem to have no higher risk of HAI than patients without asthma. These patients don't need to avoid high altitudes.
- Other chronic lung disease—children with cystic fibrosis or BPD are at increased risk of significant hypoxemia and should undergo oxygen saturation monitoring during altitude travel.
- Cardiac diseases with increased pulmonary artery blood flow—patients with cardiac lesions involving an increase in pulmonary blood flow, such as ASD, VSD, and PDA, with or without pulmonary hypertension, are at risk of developing HAPE. Patent foramen ovale is not considered a contraindication to high-altitude exposure.
- Children with trisomy 21 have increased pulmonary vascular reactivity and a higher risk of pulmonary hypertension than healthy children, in addition to their increased risk of congenital cardiac defects. They also are more likely to have obstructive sleep apnea and hypoventilation. These factors place them at a higher risk of HAPE, even at low altitudes. Thus, travel to high altitude with these patients should be handled cautiously or avoided, if possible.
- Infants with a history of oxygen therapy or pulmonary hypertension—infants less than 6 weeks of age and those less than 1 year of age with a history of oxygen requirement or pulmonary hypertension have several physiologic limitations that place them at risk for hypoxemia, pulmonary hypertension, and, even right heart failure when rapidly exposed to high altitude. They should get the consent of the specialist before traveling to HA.

Data from Hackett, P and Gallaher SA. High altitude disease: Unique pediatric considerations UpToDate June 2020.

HAPE may be fatal with delayed diagnosis and treatment.[12] Treatment of HAPE in lowland children and adolescents who ascend to high altitude is directed to the prompt administration of supplemental oxygen and reduction of pulmonary artery pressure.[12,13] Most symptoms are amenable to treatment: headaches with nonsteroidal analgesics (eg, ibuprofen) and shortness of breath with bed rest in the Fowler position (patient's head of bed placed at a 45º angle), limiting cold exposure,

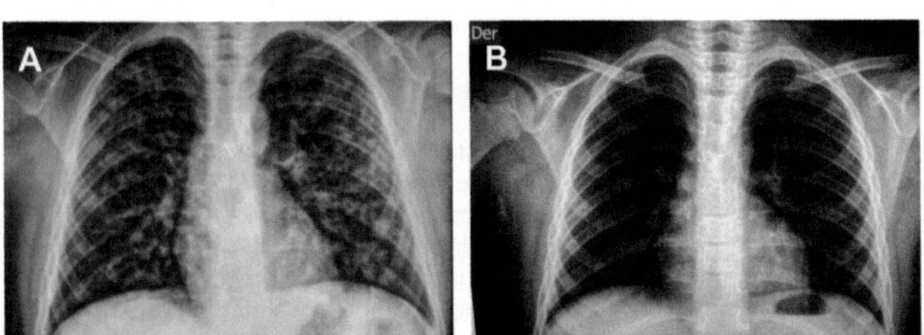

Fig. 2. (*A*) Chest radiograph from a 6 years-old child with HAPE showing characteristic patchy alveolar infiltrates. (*B*) Normal chest radiograph after 24 h. (*Courtesy of* G. Zubieta-Calleja, MD, FPVRI, La Paz, Bolivia.)

administering oxygen via nasal cannula or partial rebreathing mask, evacuation to a lower altitude, and simulating descent using hyperbaric therapy.[12–14]

Of these treatments, descent (simulated or actual) rarely is needed but may resolve the symptoms rapidly, usually within 24 hours to 48 hours, and supplemental oxygen often is effective and appears superior to any pharmacologic therapy. Gamow bag has been reported to be a useful treatment device.[13,14] A Gamow bag is a portable hyperbaric bag used for the treatment of HAIs. By increasing air pressure around the patient, the chamber simulates descent of as much as 7000 ft, thus relieving symptoms.[12,13]

Most children with mild HAPE are treated as outpatients with supplemental oxygen and remain at the same altitude with their families.[13] HAPE resolution in children is rapid, often in 1 day to 3 days. Acetazolamide is not recommended as prophylactic or active treatment of HAPE.

Children may develop HAPE when traveling from low altitude to high altitude for vacation (classic HAPE) or when returning to high-altitude homes from low altitude (re-entry HAPE); or, developing HAPE even with a respiratory illness at high altitude without any change in elevation (high-altitude resident pulmonary edema).[13]

A small proportion of young children with HAPE may have an underlying predisposing condition. Thus, an echocardiogram is warranted to exclude underlying cardiopulmonary abnormalities, including structural heart disease and pulmonary arterial hypertension, because they may surface when exposed to hypoxic conditions, even in apparently healthy individuals without previous unusual clinical history.[13,14]

High-altitude Cerebral Edema

HACE may occur as a complication of AMS and/or HAPE, but it is rare. Symptoms include ataxia, confusion, and altered mental status.[15–17] HACE also may occur in the presence of HAPE.[15–17]

Diagnosis is clinical. With the exception of brain magnetic resonance imaging, laboratory testing is useful only to exclude other diagnoses. Unlike AMS, HACE requires immediate intervention. Descent is the definitive treatment. Dexamethasone is a critical rescue medication. It should be administered immediately upon the suspicion of HACE at an initial dose of 1-2 mg/kg intramuscularly (IM), or intravenously (IV) once, then 0,25 mg/kg/dosis PO every 6 hours. Sufficient oxygen should be given to maintain Spo_2 greater than 90%. Hyperbaric therapy with a portable, manually inflated hyperbaric chamber (Gamow bag) may be lifesaving. All treatments play important roles in facilitating descent or delaying progression of the illness until evacuation may be executed.[15–17]

MEDICATIONS

Acetazolamide prevents AMS when taken before ascent; it also may help speed recovery if taken after symptoms have developed.[4] The drug works by acidifying the blood and reducing the respiratory alkalosis associated with high altitudes, thus improving respiration and arterial oxygenation and speeding acclimatization. An effective dose that minimizes the common side effects of increased urination and paresthesia of the fingers and toes is 125 mg every 12 hours, beginning the day before ascent and continuing the first 2 days at elevation or longer if ascent continues. Allergic reactions to acetazolamide are uncommon. The recommended pediatric dose is 5 mg/kg/d in divided doses, up to 125 mg twice a day and 250 mg twice a day for those children older than 12 years of age (**Table 1**).

HIGH ALTITUDE AND CONGENITAL HEART DISEASE

At high altitudes, a delayed postnatal adaptation due to a slow decrease in neonatal PVR and a genetic predisposition to vascular hyperreactivity may result in an elevated

Table 1
Medications to prevent and treat high-altitude illness

Medication	Use	Route	Dose
Acetazolamide	AMS, HACE prevention	Oral	125 mg twice a day; 250 mg twice a day if >100 kg Pediatrics: 2.5 mg/kg every 12 h
	AMS treatment[a]	Oral	250 mg twice a day Pediatrics: 2.5 mg/kg every 12 h
Dexamethasone	AMS, HACE prevention	Oral	2 mg every 6 h or 4 mg every 12 h Pediatrics: should not be used for prophylaxis
	AMS, HACE treatment	Oral, intravenous, intramuscular	AMS: 4 mg every 6 h HACE: 8 mg once, then 4 mg every 6 h Pediatrics: 0.15 mg/kg/dose every 6 h up to 4 mg

[a] Acetazolamide also may be used at this dose as an adjunct to dexamethasone in HACE treatment, but dexamethasone remains the primary treatment of that disorder.

pulmonary artery pressure and supplemental oxygen dependency in the first weeks of life. A child with ventricular septal defect atrial septal defect or patent ductus arteriosus may not necessarily have the typical symptoms associated with increased pulmonary blood flow, such as sweating, tachypnea, and delayed growth. Therefore, large defects may be missed in this group of patients.[18]

Screening newborn children for critical congenital heart disease (CHD) focuses using differential pulse oximetry as well as clinical parameters. It is worthy to considerate, the oxygen saturation parameters decrease with high altitude, for example, an SPO2 of 90% is perfectly normal at 11.000 feet or 3600m above sea level. As discussed previously, altitude hypoxemia induces pulmonary hypertension, which commonly found in left-to-right shunt forms of CHD. The pulmonary pressure decreases immediately after surgical correction. The authors currently screen newborns at high altitude for all forms of CHD using echocardiography. Heart malformations affect 1% of all newborns worldwide; however, congenital heart disease incidence increases with altitude and is twice as frequent at 3600 m.[18] CHD distribution varies at high altitude in all patients groups including in children with Trisomy 21.

PREGNANCY

Pregnant women should discuss traveling to high altitude with their physician. Travel by pregnant women from low altitude to high altitude or vice versa may induce premature labor due to changing Pbs on the amniotic sac. Morphologic changes in the placenta occur in response to lowered maternal arterial oxygen concentration. The incidence of preeclampsia is significantly higher at high altitude.[19] Although the birthweight is higher in native mothers, a progressive decrease in birthweight of newcomers with rising altitude has been reported. Maternal smoking may worsen this tendency.[20]

AIR TRAVEL—PEDIATRIC PATIENTS

Pediatric health care providers frequently are faced with the question of whether it is safe to allow their patients to travel by air. Approximately 10% of emergencies involve children. The 3 most common medical emergencies are respiratory, neurologic, and infectious disease.[21] As discussed previously, the main effect of increasing altitude is a decrease in Pb. At sea level, the Pb is 760 mm Hg. Commercial airlines cruise at approximately (11,582 m [38,000 ft]), equivalent to a Pb of approximately 190 mm Hg (25% of Pb at sea level). In a pressurized cabin, the minimal Pb is 564 mm Hg (75% of Pb at sea level); with this reduction in Pb, the Po_2 decreases from 160 mm Hg to 119 mm Hg. To compensate for the decrease in Po_2, the body adapts by increasing minute ventilation and cardiac output (tachycardia), which produces a decrease in alveolar Pco_2 and an increase in alveolar Po_2.[2] Another significant effect of the decrease in Pb is the expansion of air volume. This phenomenon affects all air trapped in an enclosed, gas-filled space in the human body, during ascent and descent. In addition to the drop in Pb, medical problems during flight may be precipitated by other conditions: low cabin humidity, air recirculation with increased risk of transmitting infectious diseases, and prolonged immobility.

The medical history, the timing of the most recent exacerbation of preexisting condition, previous flight experience, and the estimated flight duration are essential to probe. Long flights, more than 6 hours, increase the risk of hypoxia.[22] The current respiratory condition should be evaluated. Pulse oximetry at rest and activity may show hypoxemia but a normal result cannot exclude on-board hypoxemia.

A possible method to estimate the effect of a decrease in Po_2 is the hypoxia challenge testing (HCT), also known as high-altitude simulating test (HAST). An individual is placed in a whole-body plethysmograph and given a mixture of 15% oxygen in nitrogen for 30 minutes.[23] Supplemental oxygen during flight should be recommended if Spo_2 falls to less than 85% or less than 90%, depending on age (<1 or $\geq$1 year of age, respectively).[24]

PEDIATRIC PATIENTS AT RISK FOR THE EFFECTS OF HYPOXIA

Although the paucity of studies done in this population makes specific recommendations difficult, a recently published comprehensive review by Israëls and colleagues[25] provides an excellent overview of the available data. The pediatric patients most at risk for the effects of hypoxia are premature newborns and children with chronic or acute lung disease, anemia, cardiopulmonary conditions, and neuromuscular disorders (see **Table 2**).

For healthy term infants, it is recommended to delay air travel for 1 week after birth. Premature infants without chronic lung disease are considered appropriate to fly over 3 months of adjusted gestational age.[25] Due to an increased risk of apnea, however, these infants should be advised to abstain from flying during a lower respiratory tract infection or significant upper respiratory tract infection, until 6 months of adjusted gestational age, and to have oxygen available if they present signs of respiratory distress. Premature neonates with bronchopulmonary dysplasia (BPD) should be evaluated by HCT due to a high risk of desaturation during flight.[25]

For children greater than 5 years of age with chronic pulmonary disease (eg, cystic fibrosis) and FEV_1 less than 50% of predicted or severe respiratory disease, HCT is advised in order to decide on supplemental oxygen while flying.[25] Patients currently receiving supplemental oxygen should have the flow rate doubled and abstain from flying, if the flow rate at sea level greater than 4 L/min. If children received long-term oxygen therapy up to 6 months previously, a hypoxia test should be obtained and in-flight oxygen should be available.[25]

For pediatric patients with certain neuromuscular conditions receiving intermittent ventilator support, HCT should be performed and in-flight oxygen should be

Table 2
Risk factors for in-flight medical emergencies and advice on assessment in specific pediatric patients

Patient Group	In-flight Risk Factor	Risk of	Assessment	Advice
Anemia	Low Po_2	Syncope, decreased O_2 delivery	Hemoglobin	If hemoglobin <8.5 g/dL: transfusion or abstain from flying.
Asthma	Limited medical care	Exacerbation	—	Emergency medicine in cabin
BPD	Low Po_2	Hypoxia	If <1 y of age: HCT	Spo_2 during HCT <85%: recommend on-board oxygen. Spo_2 during HCT <90%: consider on-board oxygen. Currently receiving oxygen: double flow rate. Current flow >4 L/min: refrain from flying
Chronic pulmonary disease on long-term O_2 support (in previous 6 mo)	Low Po_2	Hypoxia	If no current oxygen support: HCT	Spo_2 during HCT <90%: recommend on-board O_2 Currently receiving flow: as for BPD
Chest wall deformity	Low Po_2	Hypoxia with insufficient compensation	Nightly ventilator support: HCT	Desaturation during HCT: on-board O_2
CHD	Low Po_2	Hypoxia	Respiratory and circulatory status	Cyanotic heart disease: flying seems safe. If NYHA class IV, abstain from flying or, if essential, on-board O_2
Cystic fibrosis	Low Po_2	Hypoxia	If FEV_1 <50%: HCT	Spo_2 during HCT <90%: recommend on-board O_2.
	Low humidity	Exacerbation	—	Consider extra dose of nebulized medication.
Seizure disorder	Limited medical care	Convulsion	—	Emergency medication in cabin

Immunodeficiency	Recirculation of air	Respiratory infection	—	Hand hygiene and, if possible, seating ≥2 rows from passengers with respiratory infection
Neonate, term	Low Po_2	Apnea	—	Abstain from flying if <1 week old.
Neonate, preterm, no chronic lung disease	Low Po_2	Apnea, hypoxia	Check for signs of respiratory infection.	Abstain from flying until 3 mo of corrected age. Lower respiratory tract infection: abstain from flying if <6 mo of corrected age.
Neonate, preterm, chronic lung disease	Low Po_2	Hypoxia	Respiratory status	Currently receiving O_2: double flow rate. Current flow >4 L/min: abstain from flying.
Neuromuscular disease	Low Po_2	Hypoxia with insufficient compensation	Nightly ventilator support: HCT	Spo_2 during HCT <90%: recommend on-board O_2.
Otitis media	Pressure	Barotitis, pain	Otoscopy	Nasal decongestants, analgesics
Pneumonia	Low Po_2	Hypoxia	Respiratory status, Spo_2	Abstain from flying until afebrile, clinically stable, and Spo_2 ≥94% at sea level.
Pneumothorax	Pressure	Tension pneumothorax	Chest radiograph	Abstain from flying until 7 d after resolution (14 d in case of trauma).
Pulmonary hypertension	Low Po_2	Increase in pulmonary hypertension		Insufficient data Consider on-board oxygen.
Upper airway infection (recent)	Pressure	Barotitis	Otoscopy	Nasal decongestant Chewing or sucking during ascent and descent
Sickle cell disease	Low Po_2, humidity	Venoocclusive crisis		Adequate fluid intake, prevent cooling down.
Thrombophilia (high-risk)	Immobility	DVT	—	Compression stockings

(*continued on next page*)

Table 2
(*continued*)

Patient Group	In-flight Risk Factor	Risk of	Assessment	Advice
Trapped air, intrathoracic (eg, cystic lung disease)	Pressure	Pneumothorax	If possible, determine size	Insufficient data for advice; discuss with specialist.
Trapped air, intracranial (eg, pneumocephalus)	Pressure	Intracranial herniation	If possible, determine amount of trapped air.	Insufficient data for advice; discuss with specialist.
Trapped air, in mechanical device (balloon, drain)	Pressure	Trauma	—	(Partially) deflate before ascent.

Adapted from Israëls J, Nagelkerke AF, Markhorst DG, van Heerde M. Fitness to fly in the paediatric population, how to assess and advice. Eur J Pediatr. 2018;177(5):633-639; with permission.

available.[25] For patients with acute upper or lower respiratory tract infection or other infections, the advice is to abstain from flying until afebrile and clinically stable and oxygen saturation is greater than 94% at sea level.[25] For children with known anemia, recent hemoglobin should be greater than or equal to 8.5 g/dL during flight. It is recommended to cancel the flight or give a transfusion.[25]

The main risks of hypoxia on underlying cardiopulmonary conditions are a further fall of Spo_2 in cyanotic heart disease and a pulmonary hypertensive crisis. These patients should be evaluated by their specialist to decide if on-board oxygen is required. Patients with symptoms of heart failure at rest (New York Heart Association [NYHA] class IV) are advised to abstain from flying. If, nevertheless, flying seems to be inevitable, on-board oxygen is advised.[25]

Children with severe restrictive lung disease (chest wall deformities or neuromuscular disease) might not be able to increase minute ventilation to compensate for the drop in Po_2. These patients should undergo an HCT to assess the need for on-board O_2.[26]

The most common complication of changes in air pressure is pain and inflammation of the tympanic membrane, called *barotitis*. To prevent barotitis, children are advised to chew, drink, or suck during ascent and descent. Current otitis media may lead to intense pain during flight. Nasal decongestants and adequate analgesics are advised while on board.[27]

Pneumothorax in a child is a contraindication for air travel due to the risk of developing a tension pneumothorax. After a pneumothorax, it is important to ensure resolution before air travel and to delay travel for 7 days after a spontaneous event and for 14 days after a traumatic pneumothorax.[24]

The pediatric patients most at risk for the effects of low cabin humidity are those with cystic fibrosis and sickle cell disease. In children with cystic fibrosis, the thick mucus in the airways may become even more dehydrated due to low humidity, which in turn might exacerbate the pulmonary disease.[28] In patients with sickle cell disease, the low air humidity with increased insensible losses, low fluid intake, cold, and decrease in Po_2 all starer risk factors for a venoocclusive crisis. These patients should be advised to prevent cooling down and ensure adequate fluid intake.[29]

Children who are immunodeficient or immunosuppressed are at risk for the effects of recirculation of air in a constricted space. Moreover, children with respiratory infections might spread the organism to other passengers. Most aircrafts incorporate special filters to remove viruses that travel in large droplets and all bacteria and fungi[30] and tat circulate the air from top to bottom, which decreases the flow from passenger to passenger. The risk of acquiring an airborne illness is highest when sitting in the 2 rows nearest to an index case on flights over 8 hours.[30]

This is a risk for deep venous thrombosis (DVT). This risk is lesser in children, however, than in adults. For patients with a highest risk of DVT (history of DVT or active malignancy), a preflight prophylactic dose of low-molecular-weight heparin may be considered, especially for flights longer than 8 hours.[24]

MEDICAL EMERGENCIES DURING FLIGHT

Children with chronic disease should carry emergency medication with them. Asthma exacerbations are a common medical problem during flight, which emphasizes the need to carry bronchodilators in the cabin with an appropriate route of administration and oral steroids. For patients with seizure disorder, the risk is increased due to the combination of hypoxia, jet lag, and fatigue. It is advised they carry an anticonvulsant of rapid action.[30]

CLINICS CARE POINTS

- Newborn present longer postnatal adaptation and may need supplementary oxygen to complete the process.
- Spirometry values are higher than at sea level (SL) and asthma attacks are less common.
- Low arterial partial pressure of oxygen and pulse oximetry, as well as higher pulmonary artery pressures determines a unique distribution and natural history of CHD. Patients with left to right shunt frequently show a late onset of irreversible pulmonary hypertension.
- AMS) and HAPE) may be easily treated. Descent is and rarely need, except on mountain climbing. These complications may be triggered by respiratory infections and latent pulmonary hypertension.
- Children with pre-existing conditions involving low oxygen saturation should get advice by specialists before flying.

ACKNOWLEDGMENT

The authors are deeply grateful to Dr Nelson L. Turcios for his outstanding assistance with his careful reading and editing of earlier versions of the article.

DISCLOSURE

The authors have nothing to disclose.

REFERENCES

1. Roach RC, Lawley JS, Hackett PH. High-altitude physiology. In: Auerbach PS, editor. Wilderness medicine. 7th edition. PA: Elsevier; 2017.
2. West JB, Schoene RB, Luks AM, Milledge JS. High altitude medicine and physiology. 5th edition. Boca Raton (FL): CRC Press; 2013.
3. Gallagher SA, Hackett PH, Rosen JM. High altitude: physiology, risk factors, and general prevention. UpToDate; 2020. Available at: https://www.uptodate.com/contents/high-altitude-illness-physiology-risk-factors-and-general-prevention/print.
4. Hackett PH, Shlim DR. Chapter 3, CDC yellow book. Oxford (England): Oxford University Press; 2020.
5. Bloch J, Duplain H, Rimoldi SF, et al. Prevalence and time course of acute mountain sickness in older children and adolescents after rapid ascent to 3450 meters. Pediatrics 2009;123:1.
6. Yaron M, Niermeyer S, Lindgren KN, Honigman B. Evaluation of diagnostic criteria and incidence of acute mountain sickness in preverbal children. Wilderness Environ Med 2002;13:21.
7. Garlick V, O'Connor A, Shubkin CD. High-altitude illness in the pediatric population: a review of the literature on prevention and treatment. Curr Opin Pediatr 2017;29(4):503–9.
8. Davis C, Hackett P. Advances in the prevention and treatment of high altitude illness. Emerg Med Clin North Am 2017;35(2):241–60.
9. Hackett P, Gallaher SA. High altitude disease: unique pediatric considerations. UpToDate; 2020. Available at: https://www.uptodate.com/contents/high-altitude-disease-unique-pediatric-considerations/contributors.
10. Giesenhagen AM, Ivy DD, Brinton JT, et al. High altitude pulmonary edema in children: a single referral center evaluation. J Pediatr 2019;210:106.

11. Duster MC. Derlet MN High-altitude illness in children. Pediatr Ann 2009; 38(4):218.
12. Hackett PH, Luks AM, Lawley JS, Roach RC. High-altitude medicine and pathophysiology. In: Auerbach PS, Cushing TA, Harris SN, editors. Auerbach's wilderness medicine. 7th edition. Philadelphia: Elsevier; 2017. p. 8.
13. Liptzin DR, Abman SH, Giesenhagen A, et al. An approach to children with pulmonary edema at high altitude. High Alt Med Biol 2018;19(1):91–8. https://doi.org/10.1089/ham.2017.0096.
14. Stream JO, Grissom CK. Update on high-altitude pulmonary edema: pathogenesis, prevention, and treatment. Wilderness Environ Med 2008;19(4):293–303. https://doi.org/10.1580/07-WEME-REV-173.1.
15. Gallagher SA, Hackett PH. Acute mountain sickness and high altitude cerebral edema. UpToDate; 2018. Available at: https://www.uptodate.com/contents/acute-mountain-sickness-and-high-altitude-cerebral-edema.
16. Simancas-Racines D, Arevalo-Rodriguez I, Osorio D, et al. Interventions for treating acute high altitude illness. Cochrane Database Syst Rev 2018;2018(6). https://doi.org/10.1002/14651858.CD009567.pub2.
17. Jensen JD, Vincent AL. High altitude cerebral edema (HACE). In: StatPearls [Internet]. Treasure Island (FL): StatPearls Publishing; 2020. Available at: https://www.ncbi.nlm.nih.gov/books/NBK430916/.
18. Heath A, Freudenthal F, Taboada C, et al. Textbook of pulmonary vascular disease. Chapter 85. In: Pulmonary hypertension and congenital heart defects at high altitude. New York: SPRINGER SCIENCE+BUSINESS MEDIA; 2011. p. 10013.
19. Julian CG, Moore LG. Human genetic adaptation to high altitude: evidence from the Andes. Genes (Basel) 2019;10(2). https://doi.org/10.3390/genes10020150.
20. Jean D, Moore LG. Travel to high altitude during pregnancy: frequently asked questions and recommendations for clinicians. High Alt Med Biol 2012;13(2):73–81.
21. Qureshi A, Porter KM. Emergencies in the air. Emerg Med J 2005;22:658–9.
22. Lee AP, Yamamoto LG, Relles NL. Commercial airline travel decreases oxygen saturation in children. Pediatr Emerg Care 2002;18(2):78–80.
23. Vetter-Laracy S, Osona B, Peña-Zarza JA, et al. Hypoxia challenge testing in neonates for fitness to fly. Pediatrics 2016;137(3):e20152915.
24. Ahmedzai S, Balfour-Lynn IM, Bewick T, et al. On behalf of the British Thoracic Society Standards of Care Committee. Managing passengers with stable respiratory disease planning air travel: British Thoracic Society recommendations. Thorax 2011;66(suppl 1):i1-30.
25. Israëls J, Nagelkerke AF, Markhorst DG, van Heerde M. Fitness to fly in the paediatric population, how to assess and advice. Eur J Pediatr 2018;177(5):633–9. https://doi.org/10.1007/s00431-018-3119-9.
26. Mestry N, Thirumaran M, Tuggey JM, et al. Hypoxic challenge flight assessments in patients with severe chest wall deformity or neuromuscular disease at risk for nocturnal hypoventilation. Thorax 2009;64(6):532–4. https://doi.org/10.1136/thx.2008.099143.
27. Wright T. Middle-ear pain and trauma during air travel. BMJ Clin Evid 2015;2015: 0501.
28. Withers A, Wilson AC, Hall GL. Air travel and the risks of hypoxia in children. Paediatr Respir Rev 2011;12(4):271–6. https://doi.org/10.1016/j.prrv.2011.02.002.
29. Willen SM, Thornburg CD, Lantos PM. Travelers with sickle cell disease. J Travel Med 2014;21(5):332–9. https://doi.org/10.1111/jtm.12142.
30. Lang M. Air travel and children's health issues. Pediatr Child Health 2007;12(1): 45–50.

Risk Factors for Severity in Children with Coronavirus Disease 2019

A Comprehensive Literature Review

Sophia Tsabouri, MD, PhD*,[1], Alexandros Makis, MD, PhD[1], Chrysoula Kosmeri, MD, PhD, Ekaterini Siomou, MD, PhD

KEYWORDS

• Children • Coronavirus • COVID-19 • Risk factor • Severity

KEY POINTS

- The ongoing coronavirus disease 2019 (COVID-19) pandemic has affected hundreds of thousands of people.
- Children have so far accounted for 1.7% to 2% of diagnosed cases of COVID-19.
- Children often have milder disease than adults, and child deaths have been rare.
- Risk factors for severe disease from COVID-19 in children are reported to be young age and underlying comorbidities, although this is not confirmed in all studies.
- It is unclear whether male gender and certain laboratory and imaging findings can also be considered as risk factors, because of insufficient data.

INTRODUCTION

Until recently, 6 different coronaviruses (CoVs) had been identified in humans (human CoVs [HCoVs]): HCoV-OC43, HCoV-229E, HCoV-NL63, HCoV-HKU1, severe acute respiratory syndrome (SARS)-CoVs, and MERS-CoVs. Endemic HCoV-OC43 and HCoV-229E were described in the 1960s, and HCoV-NL63 and HCoV-HKU1 in 2004 and 2005, respectively.[1,2] The first serious CoV disease outbreak occurred in China in 2002, when the novel SARS-CoV emerged, which was thought to have been transmitted from civet cats or bats to humans.[3,4] The second novel CoV emerged in Saudi Arabia in 2012, the Middle East respiratory syndrome

Funding: None.
Conflicts of interest: The authors have no conflicts to disclose.
Department of Paediatrics, Child Health Department, School of Medicine, University of Ioannina, Stavros Niarchos Avenue 45500, Ioannina, Greece
[1] Equal contributors.
* Corresponding author.
E-mail addresses: stsabouri@gmail.com; tsabouri@uoi.gr

Pediatr Clin N Am 68 (2021) 321–338
https://doi.org/10.1016/j.pcl.2020.07.014

(MERS)–CoV,[5] which is transmitted from dromedary camels to humans.[6] Collectively, these 2 CoV diseases did not affect children widely, because of the short-term nature of the epidemic of SARS and the rigid transmission route of MERS.

Since December 2019, SARS-CoV-2 has been recognized as the causal factor of severe pneumonia and potential damage to vital organs in humans. The first cases of SARS-CoV-2 originated in Wuhan in the Hubei province of China, and subsequently spread to other countries throughout the world.[7] In February 2020, the World Health Organization (WHO) designated the disease CoV disease 2019 (COVID-19).

A substantial number of studies have already been published on adults with COVID-19, but reports on children with COVID-19 are scarce. This article analyzes the current knowledge on the risk factors for the progression and severity of COVID-19 in infants and children. The possible mechanisms of aberrant clinical features of COVID-19 in children are also presented. To the best of our knowledge, this is the first review addressing the risk factors associated with the progression and severity of COVID-19 in children.

METHODS

Original research studies published in English between February 26, 2020 and June 10, 2020 were identified using PubMed and Scopus. The search used combinations of the key words "COVID-19," "SARS-CoV2," "mechanism," :risk factor," "severity," and "child." In addition, the reference lists of the retrieved articles were checked for other relevant articles. The initial search yielded 293 articles, of which, after screening of their titles, 72 studies were considered relevant to the aim of this review. Studies on adults and neonates were not included, and 7 studies were excluded because they were in Chinese. Pediatric case reports of COVID-19 were included only if they provided information about risk factors for severe disease. Thus, 23 studies were eventually selected, as shown in **Fig. 1**, and are discussed here. The factors that may introduce bias into the findings of this article are restriction to articles in English, together with database and citation bias.

Most of the studies originated in China, the United States, Italy, Spain, and South Korea, despite the large number of patients diagnosed with COVID-19 throughout the world. Some published studies relating to COVID-19 in children do not provide detailed information on the mechanisms, triggering factors, or clinical features, which led to the deterioration of the status of the patients. In addition, the current studies do not provide a uniform definition of severe or critical disease. The information from all the studies related to the risk factors for severe COVID-19 in infants and children is summarized in **Table 1**.

EPIDEMIOLOGY OF CORONAVIRUS DISEASE 2019

COVID-19 worldwide is less common in children than in adults. A review of 72,314 cases by the Chinese Center for Disease Control and Prevention showed that less than 1% of the cases were in children younger than 10 years and 1% of the cases were in children aged 10 to 19 years.[8] In the United States, among 149,082 reported cases of COVID-19, 1.7% were in children aged less than 18 years.[9] From the currently available data, it seems that children tend to have asymptomatic or mild disease more commonly than adults,[8,10] but severe cases and even deaths have been reported worldwide in patients younger than 18 years. In a cohort study of 32,583 confirmed cases of COVID-19 from Wuhan, China, 4.1% of severe and critical cases were in patients aged less than 20 years.[11]

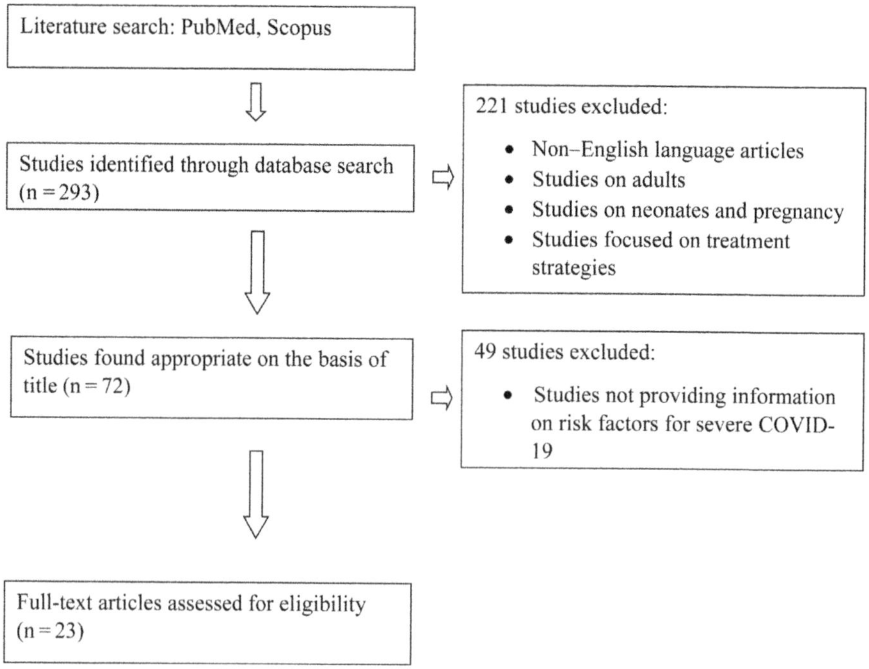

Fig. 1. The literature search on risk factors for severe COVID-19 in childhood (February 26 to June 10, 2020).

According to a large retrospective study conducted in China, 4 HCoVs, HCoV-OC43, HCoV-229E, HCoV-NL63, and HCoV-HKU1, were more common in children, because their prevalence was 4.3%, and the highest prevalence was among infants aged 7 to 12 months.[12] Infection by these 4 strains usually causes acute respiratory disease, with severe manifestations in some children.[13] Regarding SARS-CoV, only 6 case series have been reported, including a total of 135 pediatric cases, from Canada, Hong Kong, Taiwan, and Singapore.[14] A milder form of the disease was observed in children compared with adults, and no child death was recorded.[15] In the MERS-CoV epidemic, pediatric cases were even fewer, because only 2 small case series of children were reported, both originating from Saudi Arabia, 1 of 31 children with a mean age of 10 years[16] and 1 of 7 children with a mean age of 8 years.[17] In both studies, 42% of the infected children were asymptomatic,[16,17] and in 1, 2 of the 7 had severe disease,[17] whereas in the other, 2 of the 31 children died (6%).[16]

RISK FACTORS FOR SEVERITY IN CORONAVIRUS DISEASE 2019 AND OTHER CORONAVIRUS INFECTIONS

The Impact of Age

Severe acute respiratory syndrome–coronavirus-2

In a series of 2135 children with suspected and confirmed COVID-19 from China, severe disease was defined as the occurrence of dyspnea, central cyanosis, and oxygen saturation of less than 92%. Critical disease was defined as progression to acute respiratory distress syndrome, shock, encephalopathy, myocardial injury, coagulation dysfunction, and acute kidney injury.[10] Severe and critical cases were reported in 10.6% of the children aged less than 1 year, 7.3% of those aged 1 to 5 years, 4.1%

Table 1
Studies on severity and risk factors of coronavirus disease 2019 in children (February 26 to June 10, 2020)

First Author	Region	Study Period	Number of Children	Mean Age (% of Young Children)	Underlying Diseases Present (Diseases)	Severity	Risk Factors
Bialek et al[9]	United States (33% from New York City, 23% from the rest of New York State, 15% from New Jersey, 29% from other jurisdictions)	February 12 to April 2, 2020	2572	11 (<1 y, 15%)	23% (chronic lung disease, cardiovascular disease, immuno-suppression)	5.7%–20% hospitalized, 0.58%–2% admitted to ICU, aged <1 y: 15%–62% hospitalized, 3 deaths	Children aged <1 y, underlying condition
Dong et al,[10] 2020	Chinese CDC, cases from Hubei province and Anhui, Henan, Hunan, Jiangxi, Shanxi, and Chongqing	January 16 to February 8, 2020	2135 suspected and confirmed cases	7 (<1 y, 17.6%)	Not available	90% had asymptomatic to moderate disease Severe or critical disease in 10.6% <1 y, 7.3% 1–5 y, 4.1% 6–10 y, 3% >16 y; 1 14-year-old boy died	Young age
Lu et al,[30] 2020	Wuhan Children's Hospital, China	January 28 to February 26, 2020	171	6.7 (<1 y, 18%)	3 patients (hydronephrosis, leukemia, intussusception)	3 patients with invasive mechanical ventilation (all with underlying condition), 1 death	Underlying condition
DeBiasi et al,[22] 2020	Children's National Hospital Washington	March 15 to April 30, 2020	177	9.6	39% (asthma, neurologic condition, DM, obesity, cardiac problem, hematological disease, oncological condition)	9 critically ill patients	Adolescents and young adults

Parri & Leng,[32] 2020	Italy, 17 pediatric emergency departments, the CONFIDENCE study	March 3 to March 27, 2020	100	3.3 (40% <1 y, 14% <5 y)	27%, cystic fibrosis; neurologic, hematological, cardiac, immunologic, oncological conditions; metabolic disease; prematurity syndrome	1% had severe disease, 1% were in critical condition	Underlying medical condition, young age
Chao et al,[44] 2020	Single tertiary children's hospital, New York City	March 15 to April 13, 2020	67	13.1	Obesity and asthma	33 admitted to ICU	Higher levels of CRP, procalcitonin, and proBNP and platelet count
Whittaker et al,[24] 2020	8 hospitals in United Kingdom	March 23 to May 16, 2020	58	9	3 had asthma, 1 neurodisability, 1 epilepsy, 1 sickle cell disease, 1 alopecia	All had multisystem inflammatory syndrome, 50% developed shock, and 14% coronary artery aneurysm	Increased CRP and ferritin levels, older age, black or Asian race
Shekerdemian et al,[29] 2020	46 North American ICUs	March 14 to April 3, 2020	48	13	83%	All admitted to ICU, 23% had multiorgan failure, 2% needed extracorporeal membrane oxygenation, 4% died	Underlying comorbidities
Tagarro et al,[35] 2020	30 hospitals in Madrid, Spain	March 2 to March 16, 2020	41	1	27% had underlying disease	60% hospitalized, 9.7% admitted to ICU, 9.7% needed respiratory support (1 had underlying condition)	Perhaps young age, underlying condition

(*continued on next page*)

Table 1
(*continued*)

First Author	Region	Study Period	Number of Children	Mean Age (% of Young Children)	Underlying Diseases Present (Diseases)	Severity	Risk Factors
Qiu et al,[43] 2020	3 hospitals, Zhejiang, China	January 17 to March 1, 2020	36	8.3 (<5 y, 28%)	Not available	All patients had mild or moderate type	Radiographic presentation, decreased lymphocyte counts, increased body temperature, high levels of procalcitonin, D-dimers, and creatine kinase-MB
Belhadjer et al,[49] 2020	14 ICUs in France and Switzerland	March 22 to April 30, 2020	35	10	28% had comorbidities (asthma, overweight)	Multisystem inflammatory syndrome–acute cardiac failure	Cytokine storm and macrophage activation
Bandi et al,[23] 2020	University COVID-19 clinic, Chicago, IL	12 March to 20 April, 2020	25	9.7 y	Not available (1 sickle cell acute pain crisis)	20% hospitalized, 12% admitted to ICU, 1 intubated	Older age African American race
Zheng et al,[33] 2020	10 hospitals, Hubei, China	February 1 to February 10, 2020	25	3 (<3 y 40%)	8% (congenital heart disease, malnutrition, suspected hereditary metabolic diseases)	Most patients had mild disease Two had critical disease (both with underlying disorder)	Underlying disorders

Cheung et al,[51] 2020	Columbia University Irving Medical Center/ New York-Presbyterian Morgan Stanley Children's Hospital in New York City	April 18 to May 5, 2020	17	8	3 mild asthma	Multisystem inflammatory syndrome	Inflammatory markers, troponin T, and NT-proBNP levels
Verdoni et al,[48] 2020	Bergamo province, Italy	February 18 to April 20, 2020	10	7.5	None	Multisystem inflammatory syndrome	Older age, features of macrophage activation
Riphagen et al,[47] 2020	ICU, United Kingdom	Mid-April, 2020	8	9	None	Multisystem inflammatory syndrome	Afro-Caribbean descent Male gender
Sun et al,[34] 2020	ICU of Wuhan Children's Hospital, China	January 24 to February 24, 2020	8	7 (3 children $\leq$1 y)	1 acute lymphoblastic leukemia	All admitted to ICU	Increased levels of CRP, LDH, procalcitonin, abnormal liver function, cytokine storm, abnormalities on chest CT
Liu & Zhang,[19] 2020	3 branches of Tongji Hospital, Wuhan, China)	January 7 to January 15, 2020	6	3 (4 children $\leq$3 y)	None	All 4 patients $\leq$3 y had pneumonia, 1 admitted to ICU	Uoung age
Cui et al,[18] 2020	Hubei Province, China	January 28, 2020	1	55 d	None	Pneumonia, myocardial injury, acute liver injury	Young age
Shi et al,[42] 2020	Hubei Province, China	February 3, 2020	1	2 mo	None	Severe pneumonia, need for noninvasive ventilation	Young age, coinfection with RSV

Abbreviations: CDC, Center for Disease Control and Prevention; CRP, C-reactive protein; CT, computed tomography; DM, diabetes mellitus; ICU, intensive care unit; LDH, lactate dehydrogenase; MB, myocardial band; NT-proBNP, N-terminal pro–b-type natriuretic peptide; proBNP, pro–b-type natriuretic peptide; RSV, respiratory syncytial virus.

of those aged 6 to 10 years, and 3% of the children aged greater than 16 years. One 14-year-old boy died, but no further information was provided about this patient, and the study gave no data on underlying comorbidity or other possible risk factors. It is of note that, of the 2135 children, only 728 had laboratory confirmation, and the severe symptoms in the suspected cases may have been be caused by pathogens other than SARS-CoV-2. Two case reports from the same country, China, referred to children with severe disease, a 55-day-old female infant and a 3-year-old girl with no apparent risk factor apart from the young age.[18,19]

Cases have been reported of infants in China and in Vietnam that, despite their young age, had mild disease, including 10 diagnosed with COVID-19 who were otherwise healthy, with mild or no symptoms.[20,21] In a study of 177 children from the Children's National Hospital in Washington, DC, the adolescents and young adults were more commonly critically ill than the younger children.[22] Another study from the United States reported that the mean age of COVID-19–positive children was significantly higher than those testing negative (9.72 vs 4.85 years). In that study, the ethnicity was examined, and African American children had a significantly higher rate of positive tests for COVID-19: 6.8% versus 1.7% of white children.[23] In a study in the United Kingdom, among 58 children, race (black or Asian) was described as a risk factor for COVID-19.[24]

Other coronaviruses

In the United States, in the case of other CoVs, specifically 229E, HKU1, NL63, and OC43, age less than 2 years has been reported as a risk factor for severe disease, defined as the need for respiratory support.[25] In contrast, in a series of 44 children in China with SARS-CoV, an age of greater than 12 years was associated with severe illness, requiring methylprednisolone therapy and oxygen supplementation.[15]

In adults, older age has been reported to be an independent risk factor for severity and mortality, not only in SARS-CoV-2 but also in the previous epidemics of SARS and MERS.[26,27]

The Impact of Male Gender

Male gender is a risk factor for severe CoV disease in adults.[28] A predominance of men was reported in all age subgroups among 2490 pediatric cases of COVID-19 in a series in the United States, but no details were given about the impact of gender on the severity of the disease.[9] Among 2143 Chinese children with COVID-19 in the study of Dong and colleagues,[10] no significant difference was reported in the number of cases between boys and girls, and no detailed information was given on the gender of the severe and critical cases. In a cross-sectional study of 48 children with COVID-19 admitted to US and Canadian intensive care units (ICUs), 52% were boys.[29] Severe disease has been reported in girls and the current data suggest that, in children, male gender is not an independent risk factor of severe COVID-19.

Underlying Medical Comorbidity

Severe acute respiratory syndrome–coronavirus-2

In a series of 171 children with COVID-19 from the city in China, Wuhan, where SARS-CoV-2 was first described, 3 patients required ICU support and invasive mechanical ventilation, all of whom had underlying comorbidities. One was a 10-month-old male infant with intussusception who developed multiorgan failure and died 4 weeks after admission.[30] The second child had leukemia, in the maintenance chemotherapy phase, and the third, aged 13 months, had bilateral hydronephrosis and calculus of the left kidney.[30,31] It was not reported whether any of the 168 children who did not need ICU admission had an underlying condition.

In the recently published The Coronavirus Infection in Pediatric Emergency Departments (CONFIDENCE) study from Italy, which included 100 children, 27% had an underlying medical condition. Of the 9 children needing respiratory support, 5 were aged less than 1 year and 6 had an underlying condition. The severe (1) and critical (1) cases were both in children with underlying medical conditions.[32]

Among 25 pediatric cases of COVID-19 from Hubei province in China, two 1-year-old boys needed invasive mechanical ventilation, both of whom had congenital heart disease. One of them also had malnutrition and a suspected hereditary metabolic disease, and the other had coinfection with *Enterobacter aerogenes*.[33]

The first report from the United States concerning children with COVID-19 is of 2572 pediatric cases. Among the children for whom hospitalization status was known, 20% were hospitalized. Because of lack of information on specific disease features, hospitalization was considered to be an indicator of serious illness, and it was most often reported in children younger than 1 year. An underlying medical condition was noted in 77% of hospitalized children, in contrast with 12% of those not hospitalized. The most common comorbidities were chronic lung disease (including asthma), cardiovascular disease, and immune suppression. Three deaths were reported, but their association with COVID-19 is still under investigation.[9] In another US study, among 48 children admitted to an ICU, 83% had a significant preexisting comorbidity.[29] Severe and critical cases have also been reported in children with no underlying comorbidity. Sun and colleagues[34] reported 8 severe and critical cases of children in a hospital in Wuhan, 7 of whom were previously completely healthy. In this study, severe cases were defined as the coexistence of tachypnea, oxygen saturation less than 93%, and arterial partial pressure of oxygen less than or equal to 300 mm Hg, whereas critical cases were defined as the presence of septic shock or the need for mechanical ventilation or ICU admission. The age range of the patients in the 8 severe cases was from 2 months to 15 years, 6 were boys, and only 1 of them had an underlying medical condition (acute lymphocytic leukemia).[34]

Information from a registry of 310 hospitals in Madrid, Spain, showed that, of 41 children with COVID-19, 60% were hospitalized, 4 children were admitted to an ICU, and 4 needed respiratory support. Of these children, 1 had a previous condition (recurrent wheezing) and no patient died.[35] In a recent report from Paris, France, of 27 children with severe COVID-19, 70% had an underlying medical condition. Of the 5 children who died, 3 had no underlying comorbidity, suggesting that comorbidities may be a risk factor for severe disease and fatality but that other mechanisms may also be implicated in the severity of the disease.[36]

It seems, therefore, that although underlying medical comorbidity may be a risk factor for severe disease in childhood, it is not the only risk factor for progression of the disease and development of complications. It would be of interest to gather further information on the children with underlying medical problems and assess the percentages with severe or mild disease, and their other risk factors. To date, there is lack of such data in the literature, although, in adults, specific comorbidities are well documented as risk factors not only for admission to the ICU but also for mortality.[37]

Other coronaviruses

Severe pediatric disease from other CoVs reported in the United States, specifically 229E, HKU1, NL63, and OC43, defined as need for respiratory support or pediatric ICU admission, has been associated with underlying comorbidity, and, in particular, cardiovascular, chronic respiratory, and genetic/congenital conditions.[25] Ogimi and colleagues[38] in the United States showed that both an immunocompromised state and underlying pulmonary disorder were associated with lower respiratory tract disease or severe lower respiratory tract disease from HCoV. No significant difference was found regarding the severity of illness among hospitalized children with different HCoV types.[25]

The 2 deaths reported in children with MERS-CoV in Saudi Arabia were in a 2-year-old child with cystic fibrosis[39] and a 9-month-old infant with infantile nephrotic syndrome,[40] whereas a 14-year-old girl with Down syndrome needed hospital admission but eventually recovered.[39]

Coinfection with Another Pathogen

Severe acute respiratory syndrome–coronavirus-2

Coinfection with other pathogens may be a risk factor for severe disease. One child in Wuhan with a history of congenital heart disease and severe illness was found to have coinfection with *E aerogenes*.[33] In a study of 20 pediatric cases from the same region, 40% had an underlying coinfection, but there was no report on their severity.[41] A severe case of COVID-19 has been reported in a Chinese 2-month-old infant who had coinfection with respiratory syncytial virus (RSV).[42]

Other coronaviruses

The presence of copathogens with more than 1 HCoV strain (229E, HKU1, NL63, and OC43) or other respiratory pathogens is a risk factor for febrile illness. Patients infected with a single strain of HCoV were more likely to present pulmonary rales than those infected by more than 1 HCoV strain or other respiratory pathogens.[12] The presence of RSV has been associated with lower respiratory tract disease or severe lower respiratory tract disease from HCoV.[38]

Laboratory Findings

This article reports only the available laboratory information on the severe cases compared with mild cases, according to the current literature; several publications did not provide relevant data.

Severe acute respiratory syndrome–coronavirus-2

Based on currently available data, it is not possible to document a pattern of laboratory values in pediatric COVID-19 according to the severity of the disease. In the study of Qiu and colleagues[43] from China, no laboratory data were reported for severe cases, but only for 36 children with moderate and mild disease. Moderate cases (19 patients) compared with mild cases (17 patients) were associated with increased body temperature, a decrease in lymphocyte counts, higher levels of procalcitonin and creatine kinase-MB (myocardial band), and increased D-dimer levels.[43] Laboratory data from 8 severe pediatric cases in the same country showed normal or increased leukocyte count, and high levels of C-reactive protein (CRP), procalcitonin, and lactate dehydrogenase, whereas half had abnormal liver function tests.[34] In a study of 67 children in the United States, admission to an ICU was associated with higher levels of CRP, procalcitonin, and pro–B-type natriuretic peptide and an increased platelet count.[44]

Henry and colleagues[45] reviewed 2020 case reports and case series providing laboratory data on pediatric cases of COVID-19. In that review, 69.6% of the children had a normal leukocyte count and the investigators commented that the absence of lymphopenia in children may in part be explained by the milder disease. Another assumption was that increased procalcitonin level could be caused by a bacterial coinfection as a complication of COVID-19.[45] Procalcitonin level was increased in 80% of Chinese pediatric patients in the study of Xia and Shao,[41] and, in that series, 40% of the children had a coinfection.

Other coronaviruses

Neutrophilia was a predictor of severe illness among 44 children with SARS.[15] Lymphopenia was detected in 10 children with SARS, of whom 4 needed oxygen therapy and 2 needed assisted ventilation.[46]

RISK FACTORS FOR PEDIATRIC MULTISYSTEM INFLAMMATORY SYNDROME ASSOCIATED WITH SEVERE ACUTE RESPIRATORY SYNDROME–CORONAVIRUS-2

A syndrome of fever and multisystem inflammatory syndrome (MIS) has recently been described in children with COVID-19. Some of these children presented with shock and multiorgan failure and others had characteristics of Kawasaki disease or a combination of Kawasaki-like disease and shock, named the Kawasaki disease shock syndrome.[47,48] These children presented with acute cardiac decompensation,[49] and some developed coronary artery aneurysms.[24] Among 44 children hospitalized in the United States with MIS, 84.1% had gastrointestinal symptoms as the presenting clinical complaint.[50]

Most studies to date have reported that MIS presents in children at an older age, with a median age of 8 to 10 years.[24,49,51] In a retrospective study of 35 children with MIS, admitted to ICUs in France and Switzerland, comorbidities were present in 28% of the children, including asthma and being overweight,[49] but most of the children in other studies reported from Europe, specifically Italy and the United Kingdom, were previously healthy.[24,48] In a study of 8 children from the United Kingdom with MIS, 6 were Afro-Caribbean and 5 were male.[47] It has been suggested that black and Asian races may be predisposed to this clinical complication.[24] These limited data indicate a possible gender and race predilection for MIS.

The laboratory findings in children with MIS were characterized by a marked increase in levels of inflammatory markers such as CRP and ferritin,[24] and a cytokine storm, with specific increase in the level of interleukin (IL)-6 and macrophage activation.[49,51] The patients often had a significant increase in B-type natriuretic peptide and troponin T.[48] MIS is considered to be a result of a continuous immune response rather than injury from an acute SARS-CoV-2 infection. The disease presented 2 to 3 weeks after the peak of the infection and most children had negative COVID-19 polymerase chain reaction but positive viral serology.[52]

WHAT MECHANISMS PLAY A ROLE IN THE ATYPICAL PICTURE OF CORONAVIRUS DISEASE 2019 IN CHILDREN?

The SARS-CoV-2 is a β CoV of group 2B, with more than 70% similarities in genetic sequence to SARS-nCoV.[53] The established scientific evidence on SARS-novel coronavirus has enabled elucidation of the host defense mechanisms against SARS-CoV-2 and helped to explain the lower susceptibility of children to the virus and the variability between children. The reasons for the different pattern of COVID-19 in children are still unclear, but several hypotheses have been put forward.

Environment-Epigenetics

The effect of the environment must be considered a factor with significant impact on infection with COVID-19. Children have healthier airway tracts, because of having less exposure to cigarette smoke, air pollution, chemicals, and industrial pollutants than adults. In adults, these environmental factors, and especially smoking, have a negative epigenetic impact on epithelial and immune cells, leading to increased vulnerability to all respiratory viruses, including SARS-CoV-2.[54,55] CoVs are known to alter the epigenetic cellular mechanisms of the host associated with viral entry, replication, and innate immune control.[56]

Most children hospitalized with COVID-19, especially those in the ICU, were less than 3 years of age.[33,35] This finding may be explained by the immaturity of the immune system in this age period, the low likelihood of wearing face masks in this age group, and the subsequent high viral load.[57]

Another reason for the different clinical picture of COVID-19 in children is that they have fewer underlying disorders that may predispose to severe COVID-19 than adults.[58] The severity of COVID-19 is higher in children with preexisting conditions, such as asthma, malignancies, cardiovascular disorders, and immunosuppression.[33,35] In certain chronic diseases, including systemic lupus erythematosus (SLE), epigenetic dysregulation might enable viral entry, replication, and a disproportionate immune response to SARS-CoV-2.[59]

Entry of the Virus into the Cells

Angiotensin-converting enzyme 2 (ACE2) is a zinc-containing metalloenzyme located on the surface of endothelial and other cells that counters the activity of the related angiotensin-converting enzyme (ACE) by reducing the amount of angiotensin-II.[60] ACE2 serves as the entry point into cells for NL63 and SARS-CoV, and recent studies indicate that ACE2 is also likely to be the receptor for SARS-CoV-2 and the key region responsible for the interaction.[61,62]

Differences in the distribution, maturation, and functioning of ACE2 in the developing phase of childhood is a possible reason for milder SARS-CoV-2 infection. Newborn infants and children have higher ACE activities, with serum levels showing an increase until puberty and progressive reduction after maturity.[63] In contrast, ACE2 expression in rat lung has been found to decrease dramatically with age.[64] Studies have provided evidence that ACE2 also protects against the severe acute lung injury that can be activated by sepsis, SARS, and avian influenza A H5N1 virus infection.[65] It may be that children are protected against SARS-CoV-2 because ACE2 is less mature at younger ages.

Epigenetic alteration of ACE2, which is further exacerbated by virus infections, is another potential mechanism in the severity of COVID-19 in patients with chronic diseases such as SLE.[59]

Another aspect in the variability of severity is the genetic variation of ACE among different populations. The polymorphism D/I in ACE1, an enzyme with amino acid identity and function similar to ACE2, could explain the varying rate of COVID-19 infection between European countries, and, specifically, the prevalence of COVID-19 infections has been shown to be correlated with the ACE D allele frequency.[66]

Immune Antiviral Response

Frequent exposure of children to viral infections boosts the immune system and possibly enhances the response to SARS-CoV-2, and the presence of other concurrent viruses in the airway mucosa may limit the replication and the viral load of SARS-CoV2.[67] It has been shown that the number of viral copies is correlated with the severity of COVID-19.[68]

The immune system undergoes significant changes from birth to adulthood, especially in lymphocyte biology,[69] and the interaction of lymphocytes with SARS-CoV-2 may be different in children from that in adults. It is of note that, when documented, lymphocytopenia is frequent in adults with COVID-19 (83%)[70] but not in children

(3%).[30,45] However, in the 2003 SARS epidemic, lymphocytopenia was reported in 77% of infected children.[15] The changing level of T lymphocytes with age may also be a reason for the mild disease phenotype in childhood.[71]

Interferon-mediated response to HCoVs is essential for the disease course. Virus-induced suppression of interferon-induced pathways leads to viral replication and disease progression, along with the production of other proinflammatory cytokines, such as IL-2, IL-6, and tumor necrosis factor, in the lower respiratory tract and other tissues.[72] In some cases, the increase of cytokine levels is uncontrolled, leading to the detrimental cytokine syndrome, with a poor outcome.[73] The percentage of children with COVID-19 with increased levels of inflammatory markers is reported to be low, and this could be a cofactor for nonsevere disease.[45] In contrast, an unusual immune response accompanied by cytokine storm and macrophage activation is thought to result in MIS, which has been linked to COVID-19 in children.[24]

Another immunologic aspect that could be related to the mild disease in children is trained innate immunity, because of the routine use of various vaccines, including bacillus Calmette-Guérin(BCG). BCG vaccination induces epigenetic changes in monocytes, and increased cytokine production in response to several different pathogens.[74] In mice, BCG also enhances nonspecific defense against influenza virus infection.[75]

Several studies have identified links between inadequate vitamin D concentrations and the development of upper and lower respiratory tract infections in infants and young children. Although the mechanism of the vitamin D effect on immunity is complex, currently available data support the hypothesis that cathelicidins and defensins can reduce viral replication rates and the levels of proinflammatory cytokines.[76] Studies in small children with influenza have shown that high doses of vitamin D resulted in fast relief from symptoms, a rapid decrease in viral load, and early disease recovery. In addition, high daily doses of vitamin D have been shown to be effective in the prevention of seasonal influenza.[77]

SUMMARY

Although children are less susceptible to COVID-19, and the clinical picture in childhood is often distinct from that in adults, in both age groups chronic underlying medical problems can predispose to severe disease. In contrast with adults, in whom older age is an independent risk factor for severity and mortality, very young age is considered a risk factor for severity in children, although this has recently been questioned, and MIS occurs in older children.

Although a distinct pattern of laboratory findings has not emerged as being associated with severity of the disease in pediatric cases of COVID-19, lymphopenia seems to be a risk factor for severe disease in children. Increased levels of the inflammatory markers procalcitonin and CRP could be caused by a bacterial coinfection as a complication of COVID-19. The recently described pediatric MIS seems to be the result of continuous immune response rather than an injury from an acute SARS-CoV-2 infection, but further studies are needed to reach definitive conclusions.

Several other aspects could be implicated in the severity of COVID-19 in children, such as coinfection with RSV, responsiveness of the immune system, vaccination history, levels of vitamin D, and genetic polymorphisms, but the present paucity of data limits the ability to draw such conclusions.

It is important to further study the potential risk factors for severe disease in children and to clarify the underlying mechanisms in order to improve the management of children with COVID-19 and to help in the development of new forms of treatment.

CONTRIBUTORS

S. Tsabouri and A. Makis designed the study, and S. Tsabouri, A. Makis, and C. Kosmeri did the literature search. A. Makis, C. Kosmeri, and E. Siomou were responsible for the data collection. S. Tsabouri and C. Kosmeri collected and analyzed the data. S. Tsabouri, A. Makis, C. Kosmeri, and E. Siomou analyzed data and wrote the article.

REFERENCES

1. McIntosh K, Dees JH, Becker WB, et al. Recovery in tracheal organ cultures of novel viruses from patients with respiratory disease. Proc Natl Acad Sci U S A 1967;57(4):933–40.
2. Woo PC, Lau SK, Chu CM, et al. Characterization and complete genome sequence of a novel coronavirus, coronavirus HKU1, from patients with pneumonia. J Virol 2005;79(2):884–95.
3. Drosten C, Gunther S, Preiser W, et al. Identification of a novel coronavirus in patients with severe acute respiratory syndrome. N Engl J Med 2003;348(20): 1967–76.
4. Luk HKH, Li X, Fung J, et al. Molecular epidemiology, evolution and phylogeny of SARS coronavirus. Infect Genet Evol 2019;71:21–30.
5. Cauchemez S, Fraser C, Van Kerkhove MD, et al. Middle East respiratory syndrome coronavirus: quantification of the extent of the epidemic, surveillance biases, and transmissibility. Lancet Infect Dis 2014;14(1):50–6.
6. de Groot RJ, Baker SC, Baric RS, et al. Middle East respiratory syndrome coronavirus (MERS-CoV): announcement of the Coronavirus Study Group. J Virol 2013;87(14):7790–2.
7. Paules CI, Marston HD, Fauci AS. Coronavirus infections-more than just the common cold. JAMA 2020. https://doi.org/10.1001/jama.2020.0757.
8. Wu Z, McGoogan JM. Characteristics of and Important Lessons From the Coronavirus Disease 2019 (COVID-19) outbreak in china: summary of a report of 72314 cases from the chinese center for disease control and prevention. JAMA 2020. https://doi.org/10.1001/jama.2020.2648.
9. CDC COVID-19 Response Team. Coronavirus Disease 2019 in Children - United States, February 12-April 2, 2020. MMWR Morb Mortal Wkly Rep 2020;69(14): 422–6.
10. Dong Y, Mo X, Hu Y, et al. Epidemiology of COVID-19 Among Children in China. Pediatrics 2020;145(6):e20200702.
11. Pan A, Liu L, Wang C, et al. Association of public health interventions with the epidemiology of the COVID-19 Outbreak in Wuhan, China. JAMA 2020; 323(19):1–9.
12. Zeng ZQ, Chen DH, Tan WP, et al. Epidemiology and clinical characteristics of human coronaviruses OC43, 229E, NL63, and HKU1: a study of hospitalized children with acute respiratory tract infection in Guangzhou, China. Eur J Clin Microbiol Infect Dis 2018;37(2):363–9.
13. Corman VM, Muth D, Niemeyer D, et al. Hosts and sources of endemic human coronaviruses. Adv Virus Res 2018;100:163–88.
14. Stockman LJ, Massoudi MS, Helfand R, et al. Severe acute respiratory syndrome in children. Pediatr Infect Dis J 2007;26(1):68–74.
15. Leung CW, Kwan YW, Ko PW, et al. Severe acute respiratory syndrome among children. Pediatrics 2004;113(6):e535–43.

16. Al-Tawfiq JA, Kattan RF, Memish ZA. Middle East respiratory syndrome coronavirus disease is rare in children: an update from Saudi Arabia. World J Clin Pediatr 2016;5(4):391–6.
17. Alfaraj SH, Al-Tawfiq JA, Altuwaijri TA, et al. Middle East respiratory syndrome coronavirus in pediatrics: a report of seven cases from Saudi Arabia. Front Med 2019;13(1):126–30.
18. Cui Y, Tian M, Huang D, et al. A 55-Day-Old Female Infant infected with COVID 19: presenting with pneumonia, liver injury, and heart damage. J Infect Dis 2020;221(11):1775–81.
19. Liu W, Zhang Q. Detection of Covid-19 in Children in Early January 2020 in Wuhan, China. N Engl J Med 2020;382(14):1370–1.
20. Le HT, Nguyen LV, Tran DM, et al. The first infant case of COVID-19 acquired from a secondary transmission in Vietnam. Lancet Child Adolesc Health 2020;4(5):405–6.
21. Wei M, Yuan J, Liu Y, et al. Novel coronavirus infection in hospitalized infants under 1 year of age in China. JAMA 2020;323(13):1313–4.
22. DeBiasi RL, Song X, Delaney M, et al. Severe COVID-19 in children and young adults in the Washington, DC Metropolitan Region. J Pediatr 2020;223:199–203.e1.
23. Bandi S, Nevid MZ, Mahdavinia M. African American children are at higher risk for COVID-19 infection. Pediatr Allergy Immunol 2020. https://doi.org/10.1111/pai.13298.
24. Whittaker E, Bamford A, Kenny J, et al. Clinical characteristics of 58 children with a pediatric inflammatory multisystem syndrome temporally associated with SARS-CoV-2. JAMA 2020. https://doi.org/10.1001/jama.2020.10369.
25. Varghese L, Zachariah P, Vargas C, et al. Epidemiology and clinical features of human coronaviruses in the pediatric population. J Pediatric Infect Dis Soc 2018;7(2):151–8.
26. Choi KW, Chau TN, Tsang O, et al. Outcomes and prognostic factors in 267 patients with severe acute respiratory syndrome in Hong Kong. Ann Intern Med 2003;139(9):715–23.
27. Hong KH, Choi JP, Hong SH, et al. Predictors of mortality in Middle East respiratory syndrome (MERS). Thorax 2018;73(3):286–9.
28. Onder G, Rezza G, Brusaferro S. Case-fatality rate and characteristics of patients dying in relation to COVID-19 in Italy. JAMA 2020. https://doi.org/10.1001/jama.2020.4683.
29. Shekerdemian LS, Mahmood NR, Wolfe KK, et al. Characteristics and Outcomes of Children With Coronavirus Disease 2019 (COVID-19) Infection Admitted to US and Canadian Pediatric Intensive Care Units. JAMA Pediatr 2020. https://doi.org/10.1001/jamapediatrics.2020.1948.
30. Lu X, Zhang L, Du H, et al. SARS-CoV-2 Infection in Children. N Engl J Med 2020;382(17):1663–5.
31. Yang P, Liu P, Li D, et al. Corona Virus Disease 2019, a growing threat to children? J Infect 2020;80(6):671–93.
32. Parri N, Lenge M. Children with Covid-19 in Pediatric Emergency Departments in Italy. N Engl J Med 2020;383(2):187.
33. Zheng F, Liao C, Fan QH, et al. Clinical Characteristics of Children with Coronavirus Disease 2019 in Hubei, China. Curr Med Sci 2020;40(2):275–80.
34. Sun D, Li H, Lu XX, et al. Clinical features of severe pediatric patients with coronavirus disease 2019 in Wuhan: a single center's observational study. World J Pediatr 2020;16(3):251–9.

35. Tagarro A, Epalza C, Santos M, et al. Screening and severity of coronavirus disease 2019 (COVID-19) in Children in Madrid, Spain. JAMA Pediatr 2020. https://doi.org/10.1001/jamapediatrics.2020.1346.
36. Oualha M, Bendavid M, Berteloot L, et al. Severe and fatal forms of COVID-19 in children. Arch Pediatr 2020;27(5):235–8.
37. Zhou F, Yu T, Du R, et al. Clinical course and risk factors for mortality of adult inpatients with COVID-19 in Wuhan, China: a retrospective cohort study. Lancet 2020;395(10229):1054–62.
38. Ogimi C, Englund JA, Bradford MC, et al. Characteristics and outcomes of coronavirus infection in children: the role of viral factors and an immunocompromised state. J Pediatric Infect Dis Soc 2019;8(1):21–8.
39. Memish ZA, Al-Tawfiq JA, Assiri A, et al. Middle East respiratory syndrome coronavirus disease in children. Pediatr Infect Dis J 2014;33(9):904–6.
40. Thabet F, Chehab M, Bafaqih H, et al. Middle East respiratory syndrome coronavirus in children. Saudi Med J 2015;36(4):484–6.
41. Xia W, Shao J. Clinical and CT features in pediatric patients with COVID-19 infection: Different points from adults. Pediatr Pulmonol 2020;55(5):1169–74.
42. Shi B, Xia Z, Xiao S, et al. Severe Pneumonia Due to SARS-CoV-2 and respiratory syncytial virus infection: a case report. Clin Pediatr (Phila) 2020;59(8):823–6.
43. Qiu H, Wu J, Hong L, et al. Clinical and epidemiological features of 36 children with coronavirus disease 2019 (COVID-19) in Zhejiang, China: an observational cohort study. Lancet Infect Dis 2020;20(6):689–96.
44. Chao JY, Derespina KR, Herold BC, et al. Clinical characteristics and outcomes of hospitalized and critically ill children and adolescents with coronavirus disease 2019 (COVID-19) at a Tertiary Care Medical Center in New York City. J Pediatr 2020;223:14–9.e2.
45. Henry BM, Lippi G, Plebani M. Laboratory abnormalities in children with novel coronavirus disease 2019. Clin Chem Lab Med 2020;58(7):1135–8.
46. Hon KL, Leung CW, Cheng WT, et al. Clinical presentations and outcome of severe acute respiratory syndrome in children. Lancet 2003;361(9370):1701–3.
47. Riphagen S, Gomez X, Gonzalez-Martinez C, et al. Hyperinflammatory shock in children during COVID-19 pandemic. Lancet 2020;395(10237):1607–8.
48. Verdoni L, Mazza A, Gervasoni A, et al. An outbreak of severe Kawasaki-like disease at the Italian epicentre of the SARS-CoV-2 epidemic: an observational cohort study. Lancet 2020;395(10239):1771–8.
49. Belhadjer Z, Méot M, Bajolle F, et al. Acute heart failure in multisystem inflammatory syndrome in children (MIS-C) in the context of global SARS-CoV-2 pandemic. Circulation 2020. https://doi.org/10.1161/CIRCULATIONAHA.120.048360.
50. Miller J, Cantor A, Zachariah P, et al. Gastrointestinal symptoms as a major presentation component of a novel multisystem inflammatory syndrome in children (MIS-C) that is related to COVID-19: a single center experience of 44 cases. Gastroenterology 2020. https://doi.org/10.1053/j.gastro.2020.05.079.
51. Cheung EW, Zachariah P, Gorelik M, et al. Multisystem Inflammatory Syndrome Related to COVID-19 in previously healthy children and adolescents in New York City. JAMA 2020. https://doi.org/10.1001/jama.2020.10374.
52. Panupattanapong S, Brooks EB. New spectrum of COVID-19 manifestations in children: Kawasaki-like syndrome and hyperinflammatory response. Cleve Clin J Med 2020. https://doi.org/10.3949/ccjm.87a.ccc039.
53. Hui DS, Azhar EI, Madani TA, et al. The continuing 2019-nCoV epidemic threat of novel coronaviruses to global health - The latest 2019 novel coronavirus outbreak in Wuhan, China. Int J Infect Dis 2020;91:264–6.

54. Buro-Auriemma LJ, Salit J, Hackett NR, et al. Cigarette smoking induces small airway epithelial epigenetic changes with corresponding modulation of gene expression. Hum Mol Genet 2013;22(23):4726–38.
55. Cai H. Sex difference and smoking predisposition in patients with COVID-19. Lancet Respir Med 2020;8(4):e20.
56. Schäfer A, Baric RS. Epigenetic landscape during coronavirus infection. Pathogens 2017;6(1):8.
57. Kam KQ, Yung CF, Cui L, et al. A Well Infant with Coronavirus Disease 2019 (COVID-19) with High Viral Load. Clin Infect Dis 2020;71(15):847–9.
58. Jordan RE, Adab P, Cheng KK. Covid-19: risk factors for severe disease and death. BMJ 2020;368:m1198.
59. Sawalha AH, Zhao M, Coit P, et al. Epigenetic dysregulation of ACE2 and interferon-regulated genes might suggest increased COVID-19 susceptibility and severity in lupus patients. Clin Immunol 2020;215:108410.
60. Hamming I, Timens W, Bulthuis ML, et al. Tissue distribution of ACE2 protein, the functional receptor for SARS coronavirus. A first step in understanding SARS pathogenesis. J Pathol 2004;203(2):631–7.
61. Wang Q, Zhang Y, Wu L, et al. Structural and Functional Basis of SARS-CoV-2 Entry by Using Human ACE2. Cell 2020;181(4):894–904.e9.
62. Xu X, Chen P, Wang J, et al. Evolution of the novel coronavirus from the ongoing Wuhan outbreak and modeling of its spike protein for risk of human transmission. Sci China Life Sci 2020;63(3):457–60.
63. Bénéteau-Burnat B, Baudin B, Morgant G, et al. Serum angiotensin-converting enzyme in healthy and sarcoidotic children: comparison with the reference interval for adults. Clin Chem 1990;36(2):344–6.
64. Xie X, Chen J, Wang X, et al. Age- and gender-related difference of ACE2 expression in rat lung. Life Sci 2006;78(19):2166–71.
65. Gu H, Xie Z, Li T, et al. Angiotensin-converting enzyme 2 inhibits lung injury induced by respiratory syncytial virus. Sci Rep 2016;6:19840.
66. Delanghe JR, Speeckaert MM, De Buyzere ML. The host's angiotensin-converting enzyme polymorphism may explain epidemiological findings in COVID-19 infections. Clin Chim Acta 2020;505:192–3.
67. Nickbakhsh S, Mair C, Matthews L. Virus-virus interactions impact the population dynamics of influenza and the common cold. Proc Natl Acad Sci U S A 2019; 116(52):27142–50.
68. Liu Y, Yan LM, Wan L, et al. Viral dynamics in mild and severe cases of COVID-19. Lancet Infect Dis 2020;20(6):656–7.
69. Simon AK, Hollander GA, McMichael A. Evolution of the immune system in humans from infancy to old age. Proc Biol Sci 2015;282(1821):20143085.
70. Guan WJ, Ni ZY, Hu Y, et al. Clinical characteristics of coronavirus disease 2019 in China. N Engl J Med 2020;382(18):1708–20.
71. Kotylo PK, Fineberg NS, Freeman KS, et al. Reference ranges for lymphocyte subsets in pediatric patients. Am J Clin Pathol 1993;100(2):111–5.
72. He L, Ding Y, Zhang Q, et al. Expression of elevated levels of pro-inflammatory cytokines in SARS-CoV-infected ACE2+ cells in SARS patients: relation to the acute lung injury and pathogenesis of SARS. J Pathol 2006;210(3):288–97.
73. Vaninov N. In the eye of the COVID-19 cytokine storm. Nat Rev Immunol 2020; 20(5):277.
74. Kleinnijenhuis J, Quintin J, Preijers F, et al. Long-lasting effects of BCG vaccination on both heterologous Th1/Th17 responses and innate trained immunity. J Innate Immun 2014;6(2):152–8.

75. Netea MG, Schlitzer A, Placek K, et al. Innate and adaptive immune memory: an evolutionary continuum in the host's response to pathogens. Cell Host Microbe 2019;25(1):13–26.
76. Zisi D, Challa A, Makis A. The association between vitamin D status and infectious diseases of the respiratory system in infancy and childhood. Hormones (Athens) 2019;18(4):353–63.
77. Zhou J, Du J, Huang L, et al. Preventive effects of vitamin d on seasonal influenza A in infants: a multicenter, randomized, open, controlled clinical trial. Pediatr Infect Dis J 2018;37(8):749–54.

Printed and bound by CPI Group (UK) Ltd, Croydon, CR0 4YY
03/10/2024
01040480-0010